Frequency-Specific Microcurrent in Pain Management

Please note the previous printing included a DVD with the book.
The content is now only available online via: http://booksite.elsevier.com/9780443069765.

For Elsevier:

Publisher: Alison Taylor
Development Editor: Sheila Black
Project Manager: Beula Christopher
Design: Stewart Larking
Illustration Manager: Merlyn Harvey
Illustrator: Graeme Chambers

Frequency-Specific Microcurrent in Pain Management

Carolyn R. McMakin MA DC

Clinical Director
Fibromyalgia and Myofascial Pain Clinic
Portland, Oregon
President
Frequency Specific Seminars
Vancouver, Washington, USA

Foreword by

Leon Chaitow ND DO
Registered Osteopath and Naturopath
Honorary Fellow and Former Senior Lecturer
School of Life Sciences, University of Westminster
London, UK
Fellow, British Naturopathic Association

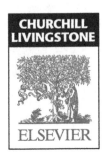

Edinburgh London New York Oxford Philadelphia St Louis Sydney Toronto 2011

CHURCHILL
LIVINGSTONE
ELSEVIER

ISBN 978-0-443-06976-5

British Library Cataloguing in Publication Data
A catalogue record for this book is available from the British Library

Library of Congress Cataloging in Publication Data
A catalog record for this book is available from the Library of Congress

NOTICE
Knowledge and best practice in this field are constantly changing. As new research and experience broaden our understanding, changes in research methods, professional practices, or medical treatment may become necessary.

Practitioners and researchers must always rely on their own experience and knowledge in evaluating and using any information, methods, compounds, or experiments described herein. In using such information or methods they should be mindful of their own safety and the safety of others, including parties for whom they have a professional responsibility.

To the fullest extent of the law, neither the Publisher nor the authors, contributors, or editors, assume any liability for any injury and/or damage to persons or property as a matter of products liability, negligence or otherwise, or from any use or operation of any methods, products, instructions, or ideas contained in the material herein.

The frequencies and protocols discussed in this book have not been evaluated for safety or efficacy by the US Food and Drug Administration or any other governmental health service. Without dissection and biopsy and further research there is no way to know with certainty what the frequencies presented in this text book are actually doing to the specific conditions and tissues.

In thousands of treatments the tissue "acts as if" the frequencies are correct and responds as if the frequencies are doing exactly what they are alleged to do but the author, the publisher and FSM can make no claims about being able to change specific conditions or tissues until further research has been done. The descriptions of the conditions being treated and the tissues being affected are a model for what we think is happening. The descriptions of clinical effects seen during treatment are presented in good faith.

That caution being given the frequencies presented in the technique chapters that follow will be discussed as if the descriptions are correct. The frequencies, concepts and protocols that follow have not been shown to treat and can make no claims about addressing any specific organ or treating any disease state. The principles of biologic resonance as they apply to human health and the body are experimental and should be added as adjuncts to traditional methods of diagnosis and treatment.

Practitioners should proceed accordingly and evaluate each patient in accordance with the standards of care for their discipline depending on the patient's presenting symptoms and condition.

ELSEVIER your source for books, journals and multimedia in the health sciences

www.elsevierhealth.com

Working together to grow libraries in developing countries

www.elsevier.com | www.bookaid.org | www.sabre.org

ELSEVIER BOOK AID International Sabre Foundation

The Publisher's policy is to use paper manufactured from sustainable forests

Printed in China

This book is dedicated to the courageous pain patients who say yes to yet one more day every day, who struggle with physical, emotional, mental and financial challenges the rest of us can only imagine, who are faced with misunderstanding, skepticism and prejudice in medicine and society that can sear the soul and drive hope to the most distant edge of consciousness. It is dedicated to those patients who went to the distant edge and found enough hope to say yes one more time to yet another doctor, risked yet one more disappointment and took the chance of being helped by a new therapy. It is dedicated to those who have been helped by FSM and who have had the courage to redefine their lives and find the answer to the question, "Who am I if I am not in pain?"

And it is dedicated to those who have not been helped. When we didn't know enough, or guess right or try the right thing or when it just wasn't time or when it just wasn't possible. This book is the promise I made that we would keep looking for a solution for you, that we would find the right frequency combination, the right application, the right diagnosis and the clear understanding that it takes to bring hope a little closer.

It is dedicated to those who couldn't make the leap just yet but who thought about it, to those who left pain free for the first time in years and for some reason never came back for the second or third treatment that might have allowed them to remain pain free. It is dedicated to the right amount of courage on the right day and at the right time for them to step onto wings of hope just one more time and have the right amount of grace to be healed.

It is dedicated to Harry VanGelder where the concept and the frequencies began.

Contents

In the late 1990s I began to receive feedback from patients with chronic pain conditions – such as fibromyalgia syndrome (FMS), and myofascial pain syndrome (MPS) – that they had received or were receiving profound relief of their pain and other symptoms from a "new" form of electrotherapy – frequency-specific microcurrent (FSM).

Skepticism is a well developed attribute in my make-up, particularly where intransigent conditions such as fibromyalgia are concerned, and specifically where "novel" treatment methods are involved. An opportunity arose around that time to visit a clinic in Portland, Oregon, where FSM was being used extensively as part of the treatment of patients with a variety of chronic pain conditions. Watching people being treated and having the chance to speak with them and the practitioners involved severely dented the skepticism and I resolved to explore the topic further.

This I did via correspondence with the lead author of this book (who was at that time owner of the clinic in question), as well as doing a great deal of reading on the subject, including of early 20th century texts on microcurrent and a variety of related topics, because the use of this modality is by no means new, as is explained in Chapter 1.

Coincidentally, soon after, I also had the chance to receive FSM treatment for two minor but chronic symptoms. I had strained my left elbow some years previously, which left me with intermittent aching and periodic acute flare-ups, particularly after the tissues of the joint had been overloaded during application of osteopathic soft tissue techniques. Over the years the elbow had been stubbornly unresponsive to conventional treatments (physical therapy, medication), as well as to osteopathic, naturopathic, acupuncture and chiropractic attention. I happened to mention my elbow problem to Carolyn McMakin when we were both attending a conference in Tampa.

Dr McMakin provided a single FSM treatment while I sat near the back of the lecture theatre, as she (with her portable FSM unit) was seated in the row behind. A damp towel, in which a graphite glove linked to the unit was wrapped, was placed around the aching elbow. Dr McMakin's hand was in the other glove (also connected to the unit), and this palpated, or rested close to, the base of my neck. Over the next 15 minutes or so, as I continued to pay attention to the presenter on stage, I felt absolutely no sensation from the FSM application, but recall Dr McMakin's gloved hand periodically palpating the tissues of my lower neck/upper thoracic spine, as she occasionally altered the settings on her machine.

By the end of the treatment the nagging ache in the joint had eased considerably, and over the subsequent few days all symptoms vanished and they have not returned. A subsequent opportunity occurred, a year or so later, to receive attention via FSM for recurrent neurological symptoms in my lower legs, which had defied diagnosis and treatment from multiple sources (mainstream and complementary). Once again the results were excellent.

These experiences, along with reading on the subject, as well as continued anecdotal, and early research evidence, contributed to the removal of my initial skepticism.

I now regularly recommend patients with chronic pain to seek out FSM treatment from well qualified and trained healthcare professionals, and I am happy to promote the concepts wherever possible.

As of now, the precise mechanisms involved in the beneficial results are only partially understood, although research strongly suggests that at least one of the main effects of the minute current is to stimulate cellular production of ATP (adenosine triphosphate), the form of energy used by cells. The additional access to ATP by damaged or dysfunctional tissues may, it seems, stimulate the local healing processes, encouraging tissue regeneration, reducing excessive inflammation and pain, and so enhancing repair.

Since the current involved in FSM is so minute (in the region of a millionth of an amp), it mimics the electrical processes that occur naturally in nerves, and is in no way injurious. Safety and efficacy are arguably the two most potent attributes of any form of treatment, and studies to date – as outlined in this book – offer support for these two claims.

Is FSM treatment always successful? Clearly not, but it is often successful where other forms of treatment fail, in the face of some of the most intransient chronic pain situations imaginable – and, importantly, it does no harm.

Is pain the only focus of FSM? By no means, since enhanced self-healing potential can involve a wide array of conditions, from inflammatory bowel disease to fractures, as well as various degenerative diseases. In Chapter 1 some of these are mentioned, and in later chapters they are explored more fully.

Is FSM a "cure-all"? No, but if research continues to confirm both the safety and the efficacy of its use, then FSM might be seen to be potentially useful – and sometimes curative – in a huge number of conditions.

It may be helpful to reflect that most disease, dysfunction and pain emerge from a background of failed adaptation. Therefore the potential to enhance the ability of tissues and organs to repair themselves, and so be better able to handle adaptive loads more efficiently, can be seen to offer virtually universal applicability. This would not, however, alter the obligation, in healthcare settings, to also aim to remove or reduce the current adaptive load (i.e. biochemical, biomechanical and/or psychosocial stressors) wherever possible.

Carolyn McMakin is a pioneer and her book is a statement of where she is on that journey. There remains a great deal still to do to verify, refine, explore, explain and define the most useful ways of employing FSM, and this text is a big step forward in that direction.

Leon Chaitow, ND, DO
London, 2010

The first time I felt one particular frequency melt a hard tight muscle into something resembling smooshy pudding, my ideas about how therapy can affect biological tissue changed forever. My ideas about biological tissue itself changed forever. The changes didn't take hours or months, but seconds. My concept of how energy and matter can interact changed over time. Over the next few years with the help of referring physicians, patients, colleagues and students, FSM developed into a system that could be taught. Once it was determined that it could be taught and the results became predictable, the system became more and more refined and people began asking for a text book.

The practice of FSM developed clinically. It was not a matter of looking at the research, because there wasn't any. It was not even a matter of looking at a list of frequencies and picking correct combinations the first time out. FSM developed and is still developing by a series of educated guesses and through trial and error. The physiology of injured and dysfunctional tissue becomes more relevant when the specific pathology and the specific tissue dictate the treatment. The frequency combinations and treatment protocols were tried based largely on educated intuition. If there was a dramatic beneficial effect that was reproducible, then a literature search was done to confirm that the treatment made sense. In the text book the material is organized the other way around. The literature describing the known pathologies of various conditions is placed first in the chapter, making it appear as if it guided the treatment process. It is only fair to admit up front that this is an illusion. It was convenient, but not inevitable that the pathologies described by the literature ended up matching the pathologies thought to be removed by the frequencies.

This trial-and-error, learn-as-you-go process, led to some regrettable errors. There were patients treated for diabetic peripheral neuropathies during one year who had no benefit from treatment because the nerve was used as the target tissue. Once an overdue reading of a neurology textbook revealed that the problem was in the blood vessels and the target tissue was changed, results improved and

patients recovered. Fibromyalgia patients had their pain return within days until it was discovered that treating with frequencies to remove the scar tissue in the cord would increase range of motion and make pain relief more lasting. My apologies to the patients who arrived during this steep learning curve.

It became clear over time that the clinical effects were predictable, teachable and reproducible. But the model for the mechanism of how the results were being produced was pretty sketchy until Dr. James Oschman shared his knowledge and experience. Jim first watched FSM work when a mutual friend was treated for myofascial pain in a small meeting room in Washington DC in 2000. He sent the articles that eventually became the groundbreaking book, Energy Medicine: The Scientific Basis (Elsevier 2000) and the model began to take shape in 1999. He helped refine the model when he spoke at the first FSM International Symposium in 2003 and has continued to refine it at each of the three FSM symposia since then. His friendship and generous advice have been invaluable and the proposed mechanisms for how FSM produces its effects would not be as well understood without his expertise.

Dr. Leon Chaitow was a speaker at the Anglo European Chiropractic College conference on spine trauma where the outcomes of FSM treatment in fibromyalgia associated with cervical trauma were first presented. His stature, bushy eyebrows and reputation were so intimidating that I avoided meeting him. A mutual friend finally introduced us by email and suggested I write a chapter for his Fibromyalgia book. I met him at Focus on Pain and treated his shoulder and he became self-described FSM advocate. He introduced me to his editor and the idea for this textbook was born. It would never have been conceived or completed without his mentorship and support.

The editorial team at Elsevier has been patient with this first-time author and busy traveler and it is much appreciated.

Special thanks go to George Douglas, my mentor, partner and friend for 18 years whose help made FSM and, at times, even my life possible. It is dedicated to my children Wendy and Adam for their support and understanding for the hours and weeks

FSM took away from our lives so that we could give the gift of hope to patients and their doctors. Dr. Jeffrey Bland and Dr. Kristi Hughes brought FSM to their audiences and changed our lives completely. My dear Dr. David Simons shared his love, support, inspiration and experience and helped move FSM forward in ways too numerous to mention.

I thank everyone who worked at the clinics and made all that we learned possible and the seminar staff who make the seminars possible so we can figure out how to teach it.

And finally my special thanks go to the FSM practitioners – our colleagues – the dedicated, talented medical physicians, chiropractors, naturopaths, physical, occupational and neuromuscular therapists and acupuncturists who have taken the course and changed their paradigm forever of what is possible, and who bring FSM, hope and healing to patients every day.

This text book is a snapshot in time of what has been found to be effective in various conditions. All of the warnings and precautions we know about are included. I have made most of the mistakes mentioned. Take them seriously. When you become aware of what you can do with the correct frequencies, it is awe-inspiring and humbling. FSM continues to evolve and each practitioner who treats a patient contributes to a larger body of clinical outcomes and helps refine the treatments. Eventually basic science research will elucidate the mechanisms and controlled trials will help convince the skeptics. In the meanwhile, those who use FSM will help to change patients' lives and in so doing change their own. I hope you enjoy the process.

Carolyn R. McMakin, MA, DC
Vancouver, Washington, 2010

Microcurrent Device Safety Statement

All microcurrent devices are classified for regulatory convenience by governmental health agencies in the category of TENS devices. The current used in microcurrent devices is 1000 times less than that of a TENS device and the two devices are not in any way similar in function, design or clinical effect.

The manufacturers and distributors of these devices cannot and do not make any claims for their use beyond those approved by the FDA for TENS devices.

The information in this text book refers to frequency effects delivered by any two-channel micro-amperage current device. No manufacturer or distributor of any microcurrent device has sponsored or participated in the creation of this text book. This text is meant for educational purposes only and does not reflect the opinion or view held by any manufacturer or distributor of any microcurrent device, including those mentioned in this text.

TENS devices require a prescription and licensing that includes the right to use electrical stimulation devices on patients.

The protocols included in this text are intended to be used by trained healthcare professionals.

TENS devices all carry the following warnings or contraindications:

1. Do not run current through a pregnant uterus.

   The precaution in pregnancy is stronger for FSM than for TENS. Once a woman is known to be pregnant FSM should not be used to treat any condition expect perhaps herpes. The changes in endorphins, cytokines and prostaglandins seen with the use of certain frequencies may have unknown and unanticipated effects on the developing fetal nervous system and on the prostaglandin levels required to maintain a pregnancy. Before a woman is known to be pregnant the fetal nervous system is not developed enough that the frequency effects would affect it.
   This precaution is theoretical and there have been no cases ever reported of FSM causing any difficulty with fetal development or pregnancy.
2. Do not run current through the brain.
3. Do not use current on people with demand-type pacemakers unless the practitioner or patient has received approval from the pacemaker manufacturer's technical support department. In clinical use patients have been treated above the clavicle and below the waist with no ill effects.
4. Do not run current through the eye.
5. Do not use over carotid sinus especially in patients with a known sensitivity to carotid sinus reflex.

Patients with any other implanted electronic device should not be subjected to stimulation unless specialist medical opinion has first been obtained.

Warnings

Safety of TENS devices in pregnancy has not been established.

TENS is not effective for pain of central origin.

TENS devices have no curative value.

TENS provides symptomatic treatment and as such suppresses sensation of pain which may be protective.

Considerations

Patients with implanted metal pins, metal plates, pumps, artificial joints, and stents have been treated with no problems reported. Microamperage current is physiologic. If it is unproblematic for the metal to be in the normal body current, then it is equally unproblematic for it to be in microcurrent.

The history of frequency-specific microcurrent

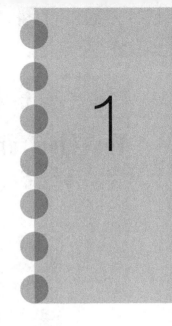

1

"It's easy to walk on water once you know where the rocks are."

Anonymous

The history of electromagnetic therapies

Starting in the late 1800s there was a tremendous upwelling of interest in electromagnetism and electrical effects. In the early 1900s, medical physicians and osteopaths were interested in using electromagnetic therapies and frequencies as a way of treating patients. The devices and techniques were used by thousands of doctors but were not accepted by the medical establishment. Albert Abrams, MD used electromagnetic therapies in his San Francisco clinic from 1914 until his death in 1937. He founded the Electromedical Society and the journal Electromedical Digest as a way for practitioners to communicate and share their research and treatment findings (ERA 1980). In 1934 the American Medical Association, in its efforts to standardize medical education and treatments, decreed that drugs and surgery were the accepted tools of medicine and anyone using electromagnetic therapies would lose their license to practice which at that time was granted by the AMA. The research and clinical use of electromagnetic therapies in medicine came to a halt and by the early 1950s the necessary devices were rendered illegal in the United States by the FDA, after which, electromedical practice gradually died out although

the early devices remained in use in private medical and osteopathic practices around the US, Canada and England.

Where the frequencies came from

In the late 1940s, after his service in World War II, Harry Van Gelder, an osteopath and naturopath trained in England and Australia bought a small private osteopathic practice in Vancouver BC that came with one of these early electromedical machines and a list of frequencies. He taught himself to use the machine and apply the frequencies, and achieved a degree of notoriety as a successful healer. Using the machine, the frequencies, osteopathic manipulation, homeopathy and nutrition he treated patients from all over Canada and the US for ailments ranging from back pain to cancer and his fame grew along with his success. In 1955 he moved his practice and his family back to Australia, returning in 1972, to practice in Ojai, California. Using the same tools and achieving the same level of success, his notoriety grew and patients once again found him from all over the US and Canada.

In 1980 a chiropractic student named George Douglas heard about Dr. Van Gelder's practice in Ojai and spent three months working with him to learn his methods. Dr. Douglas came home with the list of frequencies and put them in a drawer as a memento. After graduating from Western States Chiropractic College in Portland Oregon in 1983, he began teaching in the student health center where

DOI: 10.1016/B978-0-443-06976-5.00001-0

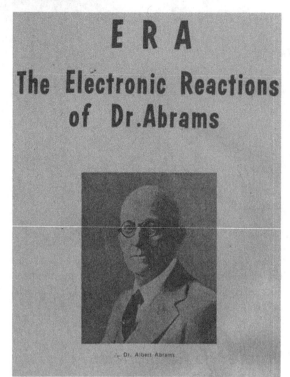

Figure 1.1 • Albert Abram's, a medical physician practicing in San Francisco from 1910 until 1937, founded the Electromedical Society and Electromedical Digest. The "Electronic Reactions of Abrams" pamphlet was published in the 1960s by the now defunct Borderland Research.

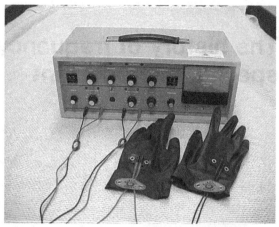

Figure 1.2 • The original Precision Microcurrent could deliver frequencies accurate only to two digits. If the switch was set to 19 the .1, 1, and 10 multiplier could form 1.9, 19, and 190 but not 191, which was needed for tendons or 195 which was used for the bursa. The two-digit specific unit gave way to the three-digit unit in 1999.

I met him in 1991 when I was a third year chiropractic student. In 1992 Dr. Douglas purchased a Precision Microcurrent instrument because it had two channels, as did Dr. Van Gelder's antiquated machine, and he had the idea that it might be useful as a way of delivering the frequencies.

First uses of microcurrent and the frequencies

Microcurrent was introduced in the United States as a physical therapy modality in the late 1970s by a chiropractor and acupuncturist Dr. Thomas Wing. Dr. Wing used four low frequencies such as .3Hz, .6Hz, 10Hz, and 30Hz delivered with single channel microcurrent unit using cotton tipped probes and eventually a double channel microcurrent called the "Myomatic I" (I = interferential). Because of its ability to increase ATP production (Cheng 1982) microcurrent was being used by Dr. Wing and others to increase the rate of healing in injured athletes, to control pain, to increase the rate of fracture repair and wound healing and to treat myofascial pain.

Microcurrent delivers subsensory current in millionths of an ampere compared to the milliamps current, one thousand times stronger, used in other widely used electrotherapies such as interferential and TENS which makes muscles contract and can be felt as a buzzing or pulsing. One micro amp (μA) is the same 1/1000 of a milliamp (mA). The current cannot be felt and is the same level of current that the body itself produces in every cell and tissue.

Microcurrent and the frequencies were used on family and friends for two years starting in 1993 when I graduated from Chiropractic College producing some positive response and no negative effects from use of the frequencies or the current. I bought a small chiropractic practice in 1994 and introduced microcurrent into my practice in 1995 as a way of treating fibromyalgia and myofascial pain patients. We used standard adhesive electrode pads to connect the machine to the patient and set the microcurrent machine for various frequencies and observed the responses. Not all of the frequencies produced beneficial results but none of them produced any adverse effects so we felt comfortable exploring further to see what was possible.

Open-minded friends interested in the treatment concept volunteered to be treated. A family friend came over one afternoon and after hearing about our new discovery asked us to try treating his back. Twenty years previously he had fallen off of a ladder and landed flat on his back creating a massive bruise the length of his trunk. His back was still sore and tender to touch 20 years after the injury and he wanted to see if it could be changed. The muscles in his back felt stiff, hardened and almost crunchy as the adhesive electrode pads were applied on the four corners of his torso and microcurrent and the frequencies on Van Gelder's list for reducing fibrosis, "deep old bruise" and mineral deposits were used on the injured tissue. Much to our surprise, the pain disappeared and the tissue became soft, non-tender and pliable in 30 minutes giving a glimmer of what was to come.

Clinical practice using frequencies

By 1996, I had a typical suburban chiropractic practice focused on musculoskeletal pain and injury. The joint manipulation, adjusting, massage and manual trigger point therapy taught in Chiropractic College were the tools available to treat patients. I was a new practitioner in a small practice, seeing about 35 patients a week, and wanting to expand my patient services, I bought a microcurrent device used by estheticians intended to provide facial anti-aging skin treatments. This skin care microcurrent used a pair of graphite conducting gloves to carry the current to the patient's skin. Before and after photographs showed dramatic improvement in lines, wrinkles and jowls, and it was likely that patients would pay cash for such treatments and increase the practice revenue. I never suspected where it would end up.

In January 1996, one of the afternoon patients was a crane operator who had been injured in an auto accident four months before. His job required that he look down from his control station at the top of the crane and turn his head as he moved train cars and ship containers around a large freight yard. The auto accident had injured the muscles in his neck and created myofascial trigger points that made him dizzy when he activated these muscles. He had a sturdy thick neck, and three months of manual trigger point therapy had produced only minimal improvement in symptoms. His neck muscles felt firm, hardened and almost crunchy. In fact, they felt exactly like my friend

Chuck's chronically painful, long-ago injured back muscles had felt the week before.

The similarity between the feeling of the neck muscles and Chuck's back muscles made me think of using the frequencies and microcurrent. The graphite gloves were attached to the skin care microcurrent unit across the hall and fit perfectly when moved to the leads on the two-channel Precision Microcurrent machine in the patient's treatment room. I wondered out loud if the frequencies would have the same effect on this patient's neck muscles as they had on Chuck's back muscles. The patient asked whether it would hurt, and when told that it wouldn't, he encouraged me to give it a try.

The frequencies we used to treat our friends and family were written on the back of a business card stored in the top of the machine. The frequencies were set on the machine, it was turned on, the gloves were moistened to allow proper conduction of the imperceptible current and the gloves were placed on the patient's neck. The treatment had the immediate and totally unexpected effect of making the muscles go completely soft or "smooshy". It was as if the tissue changed state from a solid to a gel. The taut bands disappeared instantly, as did the patient's pain, and the treatment was complete in 30 minutes. In five years of training and practice doing manual massage and trigger point therapy no tissue had ever changed the way this tissue did. Surprise and disbelief were replaced by curiosity when the effects proved to be permanent and the symptoms resolved completely in one additional treatment.

The next patient who came in with pain from myofascial trigger points had the same positive response to the same frequencies. The muscle went smoosh, the taut bands disappeared, the pain went away and the changes became permanent in a very few treatments. Within the week every patient who came in was being treated for their muscle pain with microcurrent and frequencies. In every case muscles went smoosh, taut bands disappeared, pain went away and the changes were sometimes permanent and sometimes not. Local doctors began referring their fibromyalgia and myofascial pain patients to the clinic after hearing me speak at a continuing education course on fibromyalgia offered at Portland State University in 1995. The small chiropractic clinic became the Fibromyalgia and Myofascial Pain Clinic of Portland, developing a reputation and a client base of difficult to treat chronic pain patients. Soon, every patient who came into the clinic with pain was being treated with the graphite gloves and the

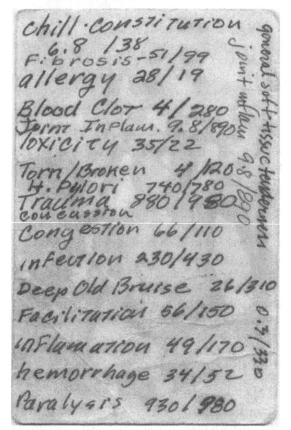

Figure 1.3 • The original frequency list was written on the back of a business card for reference.

frequencies and the positive responses grew more consistent. By March, dozens of patients had responded well and there was some real excitement about our results. Then quite suddenly, two people changed the practice forever.

FSM clinical practice expands

Dr. Paul Puziss, an open minded orthopedic surgeon specializing in arthroscopic shoulder surgery, worked well with chiropractic physicians and had an appreciation for the effects of myofascial trigger points as pain generators. Dr. Puziss operated on a clinic patient and, following the six-week surgical recovery, Dr. Puziss sent him back for what he thought would be months of standard manual trigger point therapy. Dr. Puziss saw the patient for his follow-up after only two microcurrent treatments and called the clinic immediately asking, "What did you do? I have never seen anyone recover motion so quickly after a surgery!" He listened to the explanation of the new treatment method and responded by sending every failed shoulder pain patient in his practice to the clinic in the spring of 1996. Shoulder patients, as it turns out, have very particular patterns of muscle, nerve and joint dysfunction and learning the techniques to treat them successfully took the better part of a year. The lessons learned from these early patients formed the basis of what has been taught in FSM seminars ever since.

In March 1996, a colleague at a local continuing education seminar asked politely, "How are things going?" She listened to the stories of our incredible success using microcurrent to treat myofascial trigger points, and within weeks she started referring patients. Over the next six months she referred dozens of her most difficult, impossible-to-treat, post-injury, chronic pain patients and their response to frequencies and current taught us how to use FSM.

In 60 days, the small chiropractic practice became a chronic pain clinic, doubled in size from 45 patients a week to 90 patients a week, and maintained this pace for the next four years. The lessons learned about treating chronic pain patients during that period are the foundation of what is taught today as Frequency-specific Microcurrent.

Developing the protocols

The results produced in treating simple myofascial trigger points were nothing short of miraculous and the patients for whom it was not effective eventually became the exception not the rule. Patients who had been helped told friends and family and the practice continued to grow. Assistants were needed to keep the office working efficiently. In June of 1996, Kristi Hawkes, a student at the National College of Naturopathic Medicine (NCNM) in Portland, began working ten hours a week in the clinic, helping with FSM treatments as a student "preceptor". We wanted to demonstrate to ourselves that our positive results were not due to the placebo effect from the patient's or the doctor's positive expectation. We set up an ongoing experiment where Kristi operated the machine and the patients were treated with the machine facing away from me. For a few months, nothing was said in the treatment room that would give the patient encouragement and in some cases somewhat discouraging comments were made to see if expectation made a difference. Some treatments were started with the machine turned off to see if there was a noticeable difference in tissue response. Each time the machine was off the usual softening of the muscles did not occur and it was noticed immediately. The pain reduction and tissue softening response only happened when the machine was on and never happened if the machine was off. It became apparent that it was not any positive expectation or magic hands that produced the changes in tissue. It had to be the treatment itself, and we closed that experiment.

The technique needed to be fine tuned and standardized. There were frequencies to remove pathologies such as inflammation, fibrosis, chronic inflammation, toxicity and scar tissue and frequencies for tissues such as muscle, fascia and nerve. The machine had two channels that could deliver frequencies. Channel A fired 2 milliseconds before channel B fired. Which frequency went on which channel? Did it matter? In what order did we need to run them to achieve optimal results? What conditions would respond and what conditions would not? In June of 1996 none of these questions had answers. The clinic spent three months trying different combinations of tissue and condition frequencies on A and B channels in different patients on different days until we found that we achieved the best responses with the condition on channel A and the tissue on channel B.

The results became more consistent but patients still needed ten or fifteen treatments before the improvements became permanent. How could we get faster, more long lasting results? One of the interns went to the rare book room at the National College of Naturopathic Medicine (NCNM) and looked up frequencies in Electromedical Digest. This journal was published from 1920 to 1951 and had articles by physicians who treated patients with electromagnetic therapies. One of the interns, Ryan Wilson, found a list of frequencies used by Albert Abrams in his San Francisco clinic in the back of a 1927 issue of the magazine.

Albert Abrams was a controversial figure in his day but attracted the attention and support of the famous muckraking writer Upton Sinclair. Sinclair went to San Francisco in 1922 intending to write about Abrams and expose him as a fraud and a quack. What he saw in Abram's clinic caused him to write an article for Pearson's magazine titled "House of Wonders". He saw Abrams diagnose and successfully treat pain and lethal conditions of the day such as tuberculosis, cancer, pneumonia, and influenza. Abrams

founded the Electromedical Society and Electromedical Digest and funded them until his death in 1937. When we added Abrams' frequencies for tissue fibrosis at the beginning of the myofascial trigger point treatments, our outcomes improved and patients began to recover more quickly.

Why use graphite gloves?

Wanting to find out if the way the current was applied made a difference, we tried adhesive electrode pads such as those used on TENS devices and we tried the graphite conducting gloves that came with the facial microcurrent machine to connect the leads from the machine to the patient. The two red, or positive current, leads were plugged into the jacks on the back of one of the graphite gloves and the two black, or negative current, leads were plugged into the jacks on the back of the other graphite glove. The practitioner wore latex gloves inside the graphite gloves to prevent the current from going through the doctor instead of the patient.

The graphite gloves consistently produced a better response than the adhesive electrode pads for reasons that are still not clear. There is a theory but there is not an easy way to test it so it will remain a theory. The graphite gloves are effectively cylinders of conductive material that allow the electrons in the current to flow around them before going into the patient. Physics tells us that moving electrons create a magnetic field that is perpendicular to their path. When the current flows through the gloves the electron path is circular and the magnetic field created has to be passing through the patient. Adhesive electrodes create a point of current entry on a flat surface and do not create a circular path. It seems likely that the magnetic field from the circular path creates the enhanced effect seen with the graphite gloves but not everyone agrees with this theory.

The first FSM course

By October of 1996, it was apparent that this treatment technique was extremely promising. But was it real? Could the results be reproduced or was there some complex placebo effect operating in our clinic that had not been discovered? In a fee-for-service clinic you cannot ethically conduct the double-blind placebo-controlled studies that are the medical gold standard for proving efficacy of a treatment. Patients and insurance companies pay for treatment, not research, and there wasn't enough clinical data to attempt university collaboration or grant funding for a controlled research trial even if we had known how to apply for one.

The most obvious way to tell if the treatment was reproducible was to teach it and see if people new to the technique could achieve the same results. There were some hurdles before we could teach the technique and make equipment available. The graphite gloves were only available to the purchasers of the $7000 facial toning machine sold by Bio-Therapeutics. David Suzuki, president of Bio-Therapeutics and Microcurrent Technologies finally relented in the face of impassioned pleading and agreed to sell the graphite gloves to practitioners who took the FSM course.

A logo and a name for this new technique had to be created so the flyers to advertise the course would look professional. On a Friday night in November, Ryan Wilson and Kristi Hawks joined me for a brainstorming session at a local pub at the end of a long and busy week. With the noisy Friday night happy hour crowd chattering in the background, Frequency-specific Microcurrent emerged from the long list of crossed off names on the pad as the simplest and most descriptive. As the three of us talked, Ryan doodled on napkins with a felt tipped pen. Variations on a theme were tried and discarded until the current form of the Frequency-specific Microcurrent logo took shape and was voted in. A grateful patient who owned a sign shop took the napkin and turned it into a graphics file and "FSM" had a name and a face.

The first FSM seminar was scheduled in mid-January 1997 at NCNM, the Portland Naturopathic College. We sent out flyers to licensed chiropractors, naturopaths and naturopathic students in Oregon. Twenty-five students attended the first one-day course. The syllabus totaled 17 typed pages. Part of that syllabus presented the early microcurrent applications promoted by Dr. Thomas Wing when he introduced microcurrent to the US in the 1970s. The most commonly used frequencies were .3Hz, for increasing healing, .6Hz for stimulation of acupuncture points, 30Hz for pain control, and 300Hz for reducing edema and stimulating lymphatic flow. Dr. Wing's protocols were all included in the first syllabus.

The flyers, syllabus and frequency summary sheet were created on the clinic computer at night after patients had gone home and the flyers were folded, sealed and stamped at home on the kitchen table. The copy shop printed the ten page syllabus the day before the seminar and the summary sheet was two short columns on one side a sheet of paper. The first class was taught on a chalk board and included demonstrations, a practice session and a very nervous instructor. Dr. Douglas purchased a fruit platter at a local grocery store for the snack breaks, and brought an electric tea kettle, paper cups and tea bags from home for warm drinks. We made it up as we went along and somehow got through the day. A few attendees caught the bug and contacted the local distributor for Precision Microcurrent to purchase a machine and began using the technique. By June of 1997 the answer to our question appeared in the form of practitioners reporting successful, reproducible results. The frequency-specific response was real.

Teaching the seminars

FSM was first taught to discover whether it was reproducible. The classes continued because it would have been immoral to stop teaching them. So many pain patients were helped with FSM in the clinic that it seemed important to train other practitioners so they could pass along this relief to many more pain patients. The seminars became easier and attracted more students when we gained approval for continuing education credit in Oregon for chiropractors and naturopaths later in 1997.

The two-day seminars were presented as a low key home grown event four times a year in Portland at

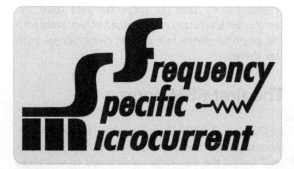

Figure 1.4 • The FSM logo was devised in felt pen on the back of a napkin in a local pub on a Friday night in November of 1996. A patient with a graphics business turned it into the FSM logo used today.

the National College of Naturopathic Medicine until 2000. NCNM resides in a grand 1900s vintage brick building tucked away on a side street in central Portland. Sometimes the boiler didn't work in the winter and we wore coats and gloves in the frigid lecture room, sometimes the guard would forget to open the building on Saturday morning and the group would stand in the rain for 30 minutes awaiting his arrival. But the room rental price was right, the staff was friendly and supportive and the school setting was familiar and comforting. The syllabus grew to 40 typed pages, the summary sheet increased to two columns of frequencies and protocols on both sides of a sheet of paper; Dr. Wing's material was deleted and only FSM treatment protocols were presented.

The practice became overwhelmingly busy with more and more difficult patients referred from chiropractic, medical and naturopathic physicians all over Oregon. Every patient we helped seemed to know six people like themselves and they sent their friends and family in droves. It was the perfect learning environment and a wonderful, if hectic, place to practice and gather experience. Interns, assistants and associates came and went. In 1997, Kristi Hawks, now Dr. Kristi Hughes, moved back home to Minnesota to set up practice and eventually became a captivating teacher and lecturer and one of the busiest most knowledgeable naturopathic physicians in the country.

The first collected case report presentation

In February 1997, a Chiropractor who belonged to the American Back Society (ABS) heard me talking about FSM at a medical meeting and suggested that our results would be perfect for a workshop presentation at the ABS national meeting in San Francisco in December 1997. FSM outcomes in the treatment of myofascial trigger points were collected for the year and the following is an excerpt from the resulting paper.

Results in clinical practice – 1996

250 new patients were treated in 1996 and the results in 137 cases of "simple" chronic myofascial pain in various body regions uncomplicated by disc injury, neuropathy, or severe arthridities, most due to prior trauma or chronic overuse were examined. Symptom duration ranged from 8 months to 22 years. The majority of patients had been treated by one or more prior therapies including prescription drugs, physical therapy, surgery, chiropractic, acupuncture, trigger point therapy and massage. Of those 137 patients, 128 completed treatment. Pain was reduced in 126 of those 128 from an average 5–8/10 to a 0–2/10. Two patients had pain reduced from the 5–8/10 range to 3–4/10 range. Treatment duration varied between 6 and 60 visits depending on the severity, complexity and chronicity of the case. Patients were told to return if the pain reoccurred or motion became limited. Only six patients have returned for occasional follow-up treatments. The results seem to be long lasting and possibly permanent. No follow-up questionnaires were sent so the exact long-term results cannot be documented.

Results in clinical practice – 1997

Further refinements in treatment techniques and frequencies resulted in improved patient response and reduced the number of treatments required. Data was retrieved from the charts of 100 new patients seen between January and June of 1997 and the results are quite encouraging. There were 50 patients with head, neck or face pain resulting from chronic myofascial complaints. There were five acute cervical and 21 with chronic low back complaints. The rest were shoulder, other extremity or thoracic pain. Most of the patients were referred to the clinic by a medical physician, chiropractor, naturopathic physician or another patient. We defined chronic as pain lasting longer than 90 days after the precipitating trauma.

The outcomes were described as simple averages. The average chronicity was 4.7 years in head, neck and face pain and after 11.2 treatments over a 7.9 weeks treatment period the average pain levels decreased from a 6.8/10 to 1.5/10. There was no control group but the patients in some sense served as their own control since 88% (44/50) had failed with some other therapy. Seventy-five percent of patients (33/44) had failed with medical care, 54% (24/44) had failed with chiropractic, 38% (17/44) had failed with physical therapy, 11% (5/44) with naturopathic care, and 6% (3/44) with acupuncture. Many patients had used two or more of these therapies with minimal to no permanent relief.

The outcomes were better in low back pain than in neck pain group even though the low back pain was

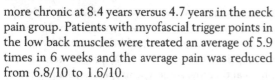

more chronic at 8.4 years versus 4.7 years in the neck pain group. Patients with myofascial trigger points in the low back muscles were treated an average of 5.9 times in 6 weeks and the average pain was reduced from 6.8/10 to 1.6/10.

In general, patients were treated twice a week with FSM, manipulation and massage. As they improved, their treatments were reduced to once a week, then once every two weeks. Half the neck pain patients took 10 or more treatments to obtain maximum improvement. It took two years to learn that cervical patient recovery took 11 treatments in 8 weeks compared to the low back patient's 6 treatments in 6 weeks because their myofascial pain was complicated by or perpetuated by nerve irritation, disc and facet joint injuries and ligamentous laxity from trauma or degeneration. The low back patients all had simple myofascial pain due to trigger points with no complicating factors.

This was the next lesson in the specificity of response. Trigger points perpetuated by nerves, discs, facets and ligaments do not respond to the treatments for trigger points directed solely at the muscle. When the treatment protocols for nerves, discs, facets and ligaments were developed two years later and used with an accurate assessment and diagnosis, patient recovery became more efficient and consistent.

At the American Back Society national meeting in December 1997, 450 people attended a plenary lecture in the morning by an orthopedic surgeon who stated that myofascial pain from trigger points must be the result of emotional conversion since these patients never improved. The speaker was polite and curious and asked for a copy of the paper when he was told that myofascial pain and trigger points were treated easily and effectively with this new method. In general, FSM and the clinical outcomes were well received by clinicians and skeptically assessed by researchers and this first exposure to the world of medical meetings turned out to be a good education.

FSM goes public

Shortly after the American Back Society meeting, there was a call for papers in the area of head, neck and face pain from a peer reviewed journal called "Topics in Clinical Chiropractic" (TICC) which accepted case reports. I decided to write up the cervical cases that had been presented at the American Back Society meeting and submit them to this journal. The paper was accepted and in August 1998 FSM had its first publication (McMakin 1998).

In July of 1998, I was correcting the galley proofs of the TICC paper while sitting in the back row listening to a lecture by Jeff Bland, PhD. Dr. Bland gave seminars all over the US presenting the biochemical and physiologic mediators of health and illness and a new concept he called "Functional Medicine". He was one of my favorite speakers and his annual hour-long lectures were a must. When he saw the galley proofs of the article he asked for a reprint when it was published.

When he received the reprint Jeff called and asked if I would agree to be interviewed as a "Clinician of the Month" for his tape series called "Functional Medicine Update" that went out to over 5000 subscribers in the US and around the world. The interview was taped in February of 1999 and distributed in April 1999. Jeff Bland and that interview started a process that would change FSM forever.

There were 400 calls to the clinic requesting information and the FSM seminar, now two days long but still written on a chalk board, began attracting medical physicians and chiropractors from all over the United States. Shirley Hartman MD, a general practitioner and acupuncturist, flew from Florida to Portland to take the seminar and was the first one ever or since to have all of the frequencies memorized by Sunday afternoon. She loved the seminar but spent $85 in cab fare being lost and trying to find NCNM in its obscure location in downtown Portland. After that, the seminars moved to a small hotel near the airport for the next five years. Dana Pletcher a chiropractor from Chicago and Catherine Willner, MD a neurologist from Durango, Colorado heard the functional medicine update interview and took the seminar in the early years. Dr. Pletcher sponsored the FSM seminar in Chicago and Dr. Hartman brought FSM to Jacksonville Florida for the next four years. Dr. Willner ended up pioneering FSM treatments for the nervous system, lectures on FSM and the nervous system at the FSM Advanced course and has become an ardent supporter and friend.

New discoveries – treating nerve pain

In 1996 and 1997 the treatments for myofascial pain and trigger points were developed. In 1998 we discovered nerve pain could be treated. A patient came in with arm pain that was clearly from nerve irritation instead of trigger points and said, "For goodness sake, think of something and try something, anything to get rid of this." It was a matter of thinking it through. There was a frequency to remove inflammation and a frequency from Van Gelder's list of tissues for the nerve. It seemed reasonable that nerve pain would come from inflammation in the nerve. Using the basic technique of removing "pathology" from a tissue, we used 40Hz on channel A to remove inflammation and 390Hz on channel B to direct the effect to the nerve as a tissue. In 1998 the Precision Microcurrent could only deliver frequencies accurate to two places. It had two digits and a three place multiplier of .1, 1 and 10. So if the two digit switch was set at 39 and the multiplier was set at 10 the frequency delivered was 390Hz. The frequency for the nerve from Van Gelder's list was 396Hz – 390Hz was as close as we could get and it seemed to work fairly well.

The DC current is delivered as a ramped square wave pulse that can be alternating or polarized positive or negative. In his book, The Body Electric, Robert Becker (1985) described the human body as having a natural polarity more positive at the top and negative at the feet, more positive in the middle and negative at the ends of the hands and feet. In physical therapy classes at the Chiropractic College, they taught us that positive polarized current sedates nerves and causes vasoconstriction. It seemed reasonable to sedate painful nerves and to follow the normal polarization of the body by using a positive polarized current.

The glove with the two positive red colored leads was placed at the neck and the glove with the negative black colored leads was placed at the hand for nerve pain in the arm, with the current polarized positive. The patient's pain dropped from 7 out of 10 to a zero in 30 minutes and the patient went home pain free and acting as if she was a little "stoned". Unlike treatments for muscles, treating the nerve created an induced euphoria that became as predictable as it was profound. The response to the first nerve pain treatment was even more amazing and unexpected than the response to the first myofascial treatment since nerve pain is otherwise very difficult or impossible to treat.

But there were no laurels to rest on; nerve pain did not stay gone like myofascial trigger points. It came back, especially if the patient lifted anything or spent time with the neck or the low back flexed forward. Once the pain could be eliminated, the bar was raised to see if the relief could be made permanent. This meant that the team had to learn how to rehabilitate the discs in the neck and low back that were causing the nerve inflammation.

There were frequencies for the discs so we began treating the discs with FSM and found that disc pain and nerve pain resolved more quickly when both tissues were treated. Often, patients with disc and nerve pain in the neck or low back also had local low back or neck pain that was coming from the posterior joints in the spine called facet joints. The facet joint symptoms improved only when the frequencies to remove inflammation and scar tissue from the joint tissues were used in treatments. The patients were wonderful teachers. One day when his facet joints were being treated a patient said, "It feels as if the pain is in the bone!" When the frequencies to reduce inflammation in the bone and its outer covering, the periosteum, were added to the treatment his back pain went away. This discovery began the next steep learning curve.

Improving clinical skills

Because the treatments were so specific, the diagnosis had to be correct for the treatment to be effective. We discovered over time that if the treatment was effective the diagnosis was correct. If the treatment was ineffective the diagnosis was refined and a new treatment was designed based on the new assessment. Sometimes an effective treatment for one problem led to the resolution of that problem only to reveal a different underlying problem that had been hidden by the first.

For example, a patient injured three years previously in an auto accident would present with neck and midscapular, shoulder and arm pain. When treatment resolved the myofascial trigger points and softened the tight painful neck muscles, neck range of motion increased and arm pain improved but then the local neck pain and midscapular pain became much worse. After numerous repetitions of this pattern, we eventually discovered that an x-ray taken from the side with the neck flexed forward and then extended back revealed the problem. The flexion–extension x-ray showed that the ligaments holding the vertebra together had been stretched and injured in the accident. The lax ligaments at C5–6 which had been splinted by the tight muscles were now unsupported because the muscles were relaxed and the upper of the two vertebra was sliding forward on the lower one each time the patient

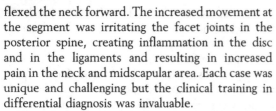

flexed the neck forward. The increased movement at the segment was irritating the facet joints in the posterior spine, creating inflammation in the disc and in the ligaments and resulting in increased pain in the neck and midscapular area. Each case was unique and challenging but the clinical training in differential diagnosis was invaluable.

The clinic developed a reputation for treating chronic pain of all types and treated more and more difficult, chronic and complicated pain patients every year from 1998 until the clinic closed in 2007. Most but not all patients recovered as we searched to find the combination of approaches that make the difference between success and failure.

Discovering the treatment team

We found that a team approach to treatment was the key. Successful disc rehabilitation in the neck, thoracic spine and low back depended on reduction of inflammation, reduction of nerve pain and enhanced tissue repair from FSM. But exercise rehabilitation to strengthen and stabilize the spine was crucial to create lasting results – the problem was finding a physical therapist that understood complicated patients and would not make them worse with heavy weights or inappropriate therapies. A chance conversation in a beachside pizza parlor led to the discovery of the second member of the team. The Ola Grimsby Institute (OGI) trained physical therapists specializing in spinal stabilization at New Heights Physical Therapy clinic and created appropriate exercises with light weights on pulleys individualized for each patient to strengthen the muscles, improve circulation at the spine, and correct poor biomechanics and posture.

The third member of the team appeared when we found Dr. Roy Slack, a physiatrist or physical medicine physician, who specialized in spinal injections. He was well trained, compassionate and exquisitely skilled. He used light anesthesia and was sensitive to the patient's comfort during the procedure. There were times when an injection of steroids and Marcaine into a facet joint or the epidural space near an injured disc was the only way to make a dramatic reduction in inflammation and allow the patient to tolerate exercises at the PT clinic and benefit from the FSM therapies for nerve and muscle at our clinic. The team was in place and results continued to improve.

None of this should suggest that every patient recovered completely. Quite the contrary, as the patients and their problems became more and more complex the percentage permanently "cured" seemed to decline. The physical, emotional and financial hurdles to be overcome were often insurmountable and many patients left treatment still in pain. But most patients left with some improvement and all had a better understanding of their condition.

Discovering the treatment for fibromyalgia from spine trauma

In 1999, Advanced Pain Management Group (APMG), Portland's only multidisciplinary medical pain management clinic, decided to include a chiropractor and FSM. At APMG between March and December of 1999 the patients who required prescribed narcotics, injections, spinal morphine pumps or spinal electrical stimulators and who had pain problems that were orders of magnitude more difficult to treat than patients seen by the average chiropractor provided the beginning of the next leap on the learning curve.

In April 1999, an APMG patient presented with severe full body pain following a series of physical traumas in the preceding seven years. She had pain in the neck, arms, and hands, mid back, low back, legs and feet that she rated as a 7–8/10. She did not tolerate narcotics for various reasons and was sent for FSM as a last resort.

All of the muscles in her neck and upper back were taut and exquisitely tender to touch – even light touch would make her flinch and break into a sweat. It could not be the muscles, discs or facet joints. After treating those conditions for three years it was obvious that they were not capable of creating such intense widespread pain and muscle tension. The only tissue that could possibly cause such widespread neck to foot pain was the spinal cord and it seemed likely that the pathology creating the spinal cord irritation would be inflammation. Since we had a frequency from Van Gelder's list for the spinal cord (10Hz) and a frequency to reduce inflammation (40Hz) there was a way to test the hypothesis with a treatment. Robert Becker's description of the body's polarity dictated that the positive leads be placed at her neck, the negative leads at her feet and the current be polarized positive.

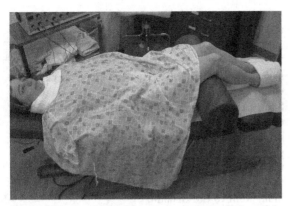

Figure 1.5 • The first patients treated with the fibromyalgia protocol had one graphite glove wrapped in a wet towel around the neck and another towel wrapped in a wet glove around the feet. Clinic associate, Sonja Pettersen, ND helped with the seminars and modeled for this photograph.

The response was immediate and surprising. The patient began to relax and the neck and back muscles gradually softened. The pain began to recede first in the feet and legs and then the back and neck and finally the arms were pain free. In 30 minutes the induced euphoria response we had come to expect with nerve pain treatment was more profound than any ever seen. The patient stopped talking, closed her eyes and began to breathe more slowly and deeply. She could be roused but would not talk willingly. At the end of 90 minutes she was completely pain free. What had happened, how it worked and how long it would last were all mysteries. As it turned out, her pain stayed down from a 7/10 to a 3–5/10 for three days after each treatment and then gradually returned. The patient lived three hours drive from the clinic and came in to be treated three times. She had to borrow money to pay for the gasoline to get to Portland from the coast for the third treatment. It was her final treatment and we both knew the relief was not likely to last. She brushed off my apology and said she was content because her pain would be down for her daughter's birthday party the next day.

Over the next few months there were ten patients with similar pain patterns and similar history of trauma who had the same response to the same treatment. The pain would be gone in 60 to 90 minutes, the patient would get so stoned that she could not talk and the pain would come back within one to two days. Dr. Eric Long, well known for his skill in doing nerve conduction studies, differential diagnosis and treatment of chronic pain, referred a patient because he heard that "something different" was

being done for pain patients. Her case was particularly challenging and her stoicism and courage in the face of intractable pain was inspiring. She was treated with the new protocol and at the end of an hour she was pain free, peaceful and looked years younger. She was grateful for the temporary relief and was told that we were working on finding a way to create more permanent improvement.

We had no idea how the spinal cord influenced full body pain and no idea how we were influencing it with frequencies and current. More important, after the experience with medical skeptics at the American Back Society meeting, it was clear that no one would believe the results unless we had objective data to prove that something measurable was changing. Dr. Long was glad that his patient had been helped but said that nerve conduction testing was much too imprecise to document such changes and he had absolutely no idea of how to document what had happened. The excitement about the successful treatment was matched only by the frustration of having no idea what exactly was happening, how it worked or how to make it permanent.

By the end of 1999, 25 patients with this pain pattern and history had been treated. The diagnosis was "fibromyalgia" associated with some sort of physical trauma affecting the spine. Patients were told that the trauma had injured a disc in the neck and created inflammation in the spinal cord and that the inflammation was amplifying the impulses coming up pain pathways in the spinal cord from the arms and legs. The pain level was usually high, rated by the patient as being between a 5 and 9/10 even if the patient was on narcotics. The patients, mostly female, had a history of auto accidents or falls, surgeries that involved intubation for general anesthesia or lifting injuries. The pain diagrams began to look familiar. There were always x's or circles at the front and back of the neck, points of the shoulders, arms, elbows, hands, midscapular area, back, low back, legs and feet. A patient whose fibromyalgia did not begin with some sort of trauma never complained of pain in the hands or feet.

The physical examination findings were always similar. The knee reflexes were always hyperactive, indicating a significant degree of irritation in the spinal cord. (Normal knee or patellar tendon reflexes are normal because descending inhibitory impulses from the brain come down to the L3 nerve root in the spine in time to dampen the reflex arc. If the conduction of descending inhibitory nerve impulses in the spinal cord is reduced due to inflammation in the spinal cord the reflex has enough time to become hyperactive but

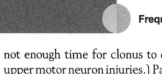

not enough time for clonus to develop as happens in upper motor neuron injuries.) Patients whose fibromyalgia did not begin with some trauma had normal or even reduced patellar reflexes. There was always hypersensitivity at specific nerve roots, usually in nerves coming from the neck. Only patients whose fibromyalgia started with trauma had these findings and only these patients responded to the 40Hz and 10Hz frequencies applied with polarized positive current from neck to feet treatment protocol. The key to successful treatment was once again accurate diagnosis.

Understanding the CTF treatment – developing the model

In June of 1999, I met an old friend at a medical meeting in Canada who had moved from Portland to England to teach at Anglo European Chiropractic College (AECC) in Bournemouth. He was very pleased to hear about the positive results with this very difficult group of pain patients and asked that the outcomes and model be presented in March 2000 at the joint spring conference of Anglo European Chiropractic College and the British Chiropractic Association whose topic was "Cervical Trauma and Chronic Pain". The paper, due in January, had to answer the questions: How would a disc injury create amplification of the pain impulses going up the spinal cord from the hands and feet? What happened to discs when they were injured but not herniated? What effect do injured discs have on the nerve and the spinal cord? Why do they have hyperactive reflexes? Why doesn't it heal?

In December, a colleague who knew about the AECC presentation sent me a reprint of Taylor & Twomey's (1993) article documenting damage to the spine found on autopsy in patients killed in auto accidents from non spine trauma. One of the requirements for inclusion in the study was an x-ray and an MRI read as "normal". Upon autopsy, the patients were found to have cracks in the vertebral end plates, fractures between the end plate and the disc, tears in the disc annulus, and small bulges that allowed the disc nucleus to contact the end plate or the damaged disc annulus none of which appeared on spinal imaging. She followed this up by sending two papers each from Olmarker (1993, 1995) and Ozaktay (1995, 1998) showing that the nucleus pulposus of the disc is not only inflammatory but neurotoxic. The nucleus

pulposus material did not amplify pain impulses in the spinal cord or nerves; it stopped them. The original model was wrong.

If impulses in the spinal cord pain pathways were slowed or stopped what would happen to pain signals? *Principles of Neural Science* by Kandel & Schwartz (1985) would have the answer in the section on pain processing. The text opened to the paragraph that explained what we were seeing. "Central pain can arise not only from pathologic lesions in the thalamus but also from lesions placed *anywhere* along the nociceptive pathway from the spinal cord and brain stem to the thalamus."

The next paragraph listed pain descriptors used by patients to describe central pain and they were exactly word for word the descriptors used by cervical trauma fibromyalgia patients to describe their pain. Burning, aching, stinging, stabbing, sharp, dull were all circled on the intake forms the fibromyalgia patients filled out in the office. No other patients circled all of the pain descriptors. The text commented that central pain was particularly bothersome emotionally and this matched the distress unique to this patient group. The disc injuries were damaging the pain pathways in the spinal cord and causing central pain. The questions were answered, the model fell into place and the paper was ready to present at the AECC meeting.

Speaking at NIH – presenting the model

The next week Dr. Jay Shah, a physiatrist working at The National Institutes of Health (NIH), called because he was in charge of recruiting speakers for Grand Rounds presentations at NIH and needed a speaker to replace someone who had canceled at the last minute. He asked if I was interested in presenting the data and the model for treating fibromyalgia from cervical trauma at a Grand Rounds presentation in April 2000. Dr. Shah is one of the world's experts in myofascial trigger points and he took the FSM seminar in 1999 to see if it could be effective for his patients. During that seminar he heard about the results being produced in fibromyalgia patients and wanted to expose his colleagues at NIH to this new therapy. The answer was an enthusiastic but slightly intimidated, "Yes!" The next few weeks were a whirlwind of seeing patients during the week and learning how to make Power Point slides on the weekends.

Two weeks later Dr. Jeffrey Bland called and asked for a presentation on the topic "Energy Medicine in

Clinical Practice" to be presented at the Institute for Functional Medicine International Symposium to be held in May of 2000. That talk would once again present the frequency-specific response and our outcomes in the treatment of cervical trauma induced fibromyalgia and the concept that one specific frequency combination had specific effects in treatment.

The AECC presentation went well. The next month Dr. Shah helped fine tune the presentation for the much more sophisticated and demanding audience of physicians at NIH. At the end of the NIH lecture, the assembled audience of thirty physicians and PhDs were asked to help find *something* that could be measured to document objectively what was changing besides pain as we treated this group of patients. Terry Phillips, a PhD immunochemist recently recruited from George Washington University to bring his expertise in micro immunochemistry to the NIH, came up after the lecture and said that if he had spots of the patient's blood on pieces of blotter paper taken at different times during the treatment he could tell me what was changing. He sent the blotter paper in the mail and when it arrived, the ideal patient was called.

The volunteer and the cytokine data

MK was a delightful young woman who had been treated unsuccessfully in the clinic for widespread myofascial pain, neck and arm pain for four months in 1998. She eventually had neck surgery in 1999 to fuse two herniated discs that were the source of the trouble but told us that her pain had generalized to the full body and became worse after the surgery. When she answered the phone she said yes her hands and feet did hurt and wondered why we wanted to know. Delighted but skeptical when she was told that there was a new treatment that might help her she said she would be happy to donate five drops of blood to help us find out what was happening during the treatment.

The session started with a physical examination. She had hyperactive patellar reflexes and the cervical nerve roots were hypersensitive to sharp stimulation. Her pain was a 7–8/10 and she had stopped taking narcotics because they did not help the pain. She had the 11 out of 18 tender points tender to less than 4 lbs/in^2 pressure, full body pain and disturbed sleep that are diagnostic for fibromyalgia. A finger stick from a diabetes blood tester gave us the blood spot for the first small strip of blotter paper. The microcurrent machine was set to deliver 40Hz on channel A and 10Hz on channel B, the graphite gloves were placed at her neck and feet with the current polarized positive and the treatment began. In a few minutes her neck muscles started to relax and soften, the pain started decreasing in her feet and legs and we knew the treatment would be effective.

After 30 minutes of treatment she opened her eyes sleepily and asked incredulously, "Is this legal?" The euphoric effect is something like that produced by morphine or Versed and very profound on the first treatment. Her pain was down to a 4/10 after 40 minutes and dropping fast. We took blood samples every 30 minutes. When her pain was down to 0/10, the frequency was changed to the frequency combinations that Van Gelder used to reduce "nervous tension", "emotional tension" and "concussion" for 20 minutes. The last blood sample was taken and MK went home pain free for the first time in four years. The paper strips dried overnight, went into a plastic container and were mailed to Terry Phillips at NIH the next day.

The busy weeks at the clinic flew by and the IFM Symposium was two days away when the fax machine started clattering and out slipped a page with columns of data listing the substances from each blood spot taken during the treatment. There were substances called IL-1 (Interleukin-1), IL-6, IL-8, TNF-α, CGRP (calcitonin gene related peptide), which were all inflammatory peptides called cytokines, and substance-P, endorphins, cortisol, and serotonin.

Dr. Phillips and his miraculous testing equipment had discovered in great and minute detail what was changing. The numbers, measured in nano and pico liters, changed dramatically by factors of 10–20 times between the first and last readings. The function of most of the peptides was a mystery but it was apparent that such dramatic changes had to be significant. Every pain specialist knows that substance-P is produced in the spinal cord and that the huge changes in substance-P could only mean that the treatment did indeed affect spinal cord function. The dramatic reductions in the inflammatory cytokines had to mean that the treatment reduced inflammation, and the huge increases in endorphins had to be the explanation for the induced euphoria. The treatment success was no longer subjective changes in pain scores. Objective data showed that something very real was changing (McMakin 2004).

Table 1.1 Complete listing of immunochromatography data from NIH

Sample	Date	IL-1	IL-6	IL-8	TNF-α	IFNγ	SP	CGRP	VIP	NY	β Endorph	Cortisol	Serotonin
MK1	05/11/2000	392.8	204.3	59.9	299.1	97.2	132.6	100.8	8.5	18.1	5.2	15.5	285.6
MK2	05/11/2000	288.5	200.8	47.6	265.7	99.8	127.5	97.6	10.2	13.7	7.1	12.6	309.2
MK3	05/11/2000	103.2	121.7	21.3	96.5	73.7	82.4	61.3	32.9	7.2	21.4	33.7	202.1
MK4	05/11/2000	52.6	33.9	11.4	43.4	32.6	38.2	22.4	48.4	5.1	69.1	78.3	169.5
MK5	05/11/2000	21.4	15.6	4.8	20.6	11.4	10.5	8.6	69.9	6.6	88.3	169.9	289.6

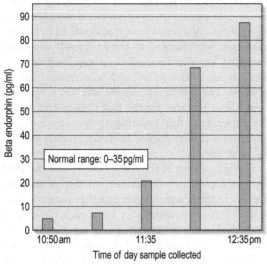

Figure 1.6 • β-endorphins increased from 5.2 to 88.3 pg/ml in 90 minutes. They had increased by four times in 40 minutes prompting the visibly affected patient to ask, "Is this treatment legal?"

Presenting the cytokine data

Dr. Bland greeted us as we arrived at the Phoenix resort where the meeting was being held. He took the offered data sheets and when his hand started to tremble, it was clear the numbers were as good as they appeared. He said, "This is going to knock their socks off."

The 2:00pm workshop lecture "Energy Medicine in Clinical Practice" the next day had to be moved twice to accommodate new registrants and the audience of more than 200 people filled every chair, sat on the floor and stood along the sides and the back of the room. The lecture was timed to the minute but

there was time to include the new data slides at the end. The room was totally silent as the bar graphs showed inflammation and substance-P plummeting and endorphins rising by factors of 10–20 times. The physicians in the audience knew better than the speaker that these rates of change had never been seen before and were not possible to create by any other known method of treatment.

The last sample taken after the pain was zero showed every parameter continuing to move in exactly the same direction except for serotonin. Serotonin dropped during the treatment that reduced the pain and when the frequency was changed to the combinations used to reduce nervous tension, emotional tension and concussion, serotonin turned around and doubled itself in 20 minutes. This was energy medicine in practice and the audience sat in stunned silence until they burst into applause.

The Australia connection

Mike Curley, the director of HealthWorld, a nutritional supplement distributor in Australia, was sitting in the back of that workshop room listening to the lecture. He decided to bring FSM to his practitioners in Australia. We made the arrangements and scheduled the first Australian FSM seminar for September 19, 2001. Mike promoted the seminar by flying all over Australia during the spring and summer (Australia's fall and winter) of 2001 promoting the course and recruiting a very large and enthusiastic group. September 11, 2001 closed US airports, changed the face of international air travel and postponed the seminar into October.

The first course, held in Sydney was presented on a white board projected to a large video screen in a huge hotel ballroom to 60 medical physicians, chiropractors and naturopathic doctors. Considering that the US course had never had a class larger than 25, teaching a group this size was a challenge. The practicum sessions were barely controlled chaos with a group this size and the Australian students proved to be exuberant and intense learners. The yearly five-day Australian seminars continued with large and enthusiastic groups each year until 2007 when Mike retired. The Australian connection led to the next big leap in FSM development.

FSM animal research

In 2002 Wayne Reilly, a research associate with HealthWorld, arranged for an experiment to be done at University of Sydney by his friend and colleague, Dr. Vivienne Reeve. Dr. Reeve studies drugs and processes that reduce inflammation in a mouse model and together they designed a study that would test the effect of frequencies to reduce inflammation. The process is simple. The researchers paint arachidonic acid on the mouse's ears, which creates inflammation at a predictable rate and then measure the swelling with a caliper in millimeters. They administer some drug before or after the exposure and see if it reduces the swelling compared to an untreated control group.

Dr. Reilly chose the frequencies to be tested in the experiment. When the first batch of ten mice was treated with 40Hz on channel A and 116Hz on channel B to "reduce inflammation in the immune system" the swelling went down by 70% in four minutes in every animal treated. Dr. Reeve stopped the study because in 18 years of research on anti-inflammatory drugs she had never seen any prescription or non-prescription drug that reduced swelling by more than 45%. She "blinded" everyone in the lab by moving each process into a separate room and not allowing anyone working on any part of the study to know whether the mouse being treated was in the active treatment group or the sham group. She turned the machine around so that the person treating the mice didn't know if it was running and she put a sham frequency in the protocol. The treated mice still had a 62% reduction in swelling compared to the untreated and the sham groups. And it was a four minute time-dependent response. Half of the effect is present at two minutes, the full effect is present at four minutes and every one of the 20 animals treated responded (Reilly 2004).

They tested three different frequency combinations from the FSM list. No other frequency combination reduced inflammation at all. They were each equivalent to placebo.

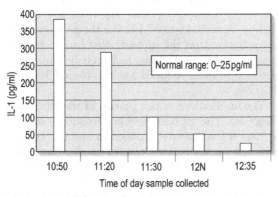

Figure 1.7 • Reduction in Cytokine IL-1. Interleukin 1 was reduced from 392.8 pg/ml to 21.4 pg/ml in 90 minutes in a peripheral blood sample. The normal range is 0-25 pg/ml. Cytokines are known to be difficult to change and change only slowly, when they change at all, making this data even more remarkable. The reduction in cytokines correlated to the reduction in pain.

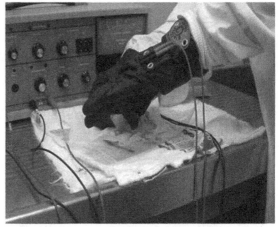

Figure 1.8 • Wayne Reilly held each mouse for four minutes as they were being treated. Notice that the gloves contact the mouse where it is being held on the back and at the tail and not on the ears where the reduction in swelling was measured.

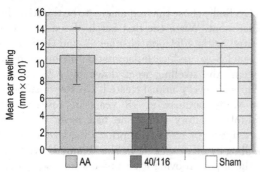

Figure 1.9 • Arachidonic acid was painted on the ears of hairless mice. 40Hz/116Hz reduced by an average of 62% in four minutes in every animal tested and the sham frequency shown on the far right had no effect on swelling.

Then they exposed the hairless mice to a measured dose of ultraviolet light, just enough to create a mild sunburn, make the ears swell and create immune system suppression. One half of the mice were treated immediately after the sunburn with 40Hz and 116Hz and the other group was treated two hours after the exposure. The group treated immediately had no decrease in swelling but the group treated at two hours had a small (0.01) but significant decrease in swelling.

Before the sunburn the mice were painted on a hind leg with a substance, called oxazolone, which they would be allergic to on the second exposure

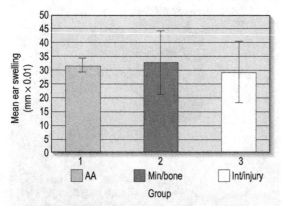

Figure 1.10 • The researchers tested three different frequency combinations including the frequency to "remove minerals" in "bone" and a group of three frequencies for injury and none of them had any effect in reducing inflammation. They were equivalent to placebo.

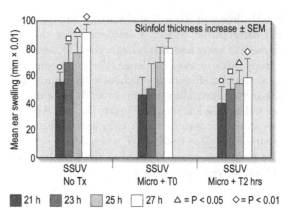

Figure 1.11 • The mice were exposed to UV light creating immune suppression and swelling. The mice treated immediately with microcurrent had no reduction in swelling but the mice treated at two hours had a small but statistically significant reduction in swelling caused by sunburn.

if the immune system was operating normally. Sunburn suppresses the immune system so mice that have been sunburned do not swell as much as normal mice when their ears are painted with oxazolone two weeks after the first exposure.

The results of the FSM study were fascinating. The untreated mice had ear swelling of 30 units (0.01 x mm) when exposed to oxazolone the second time. The sunburned, untreated mice had the swelling reduced, and the immune system suppressed by 63.4% as expected. The group treated with FSM at two hours, that had the best reduction in swelling, had their immune system suppression reduced slightly from 63.4% to 57.5%. But the group treated immediately after the sunburn, that had no significant reduction in swelling, had their immune system suppression reduced by half from 63.4% to 31.05%.

The implications of this portion of the trial were staggering. The application of one frequency combination for four minutes changed an immune system response when measured two weeks after the application of the frequency. The change to the immune system was effectively permanent.

Dr. Reeve is an established, well-published, conservative PhD in a tenured university research position. She wanted to repeat the study with a larger group of mice but would never accept funding for the project. Dr. Reilly presented a brief abstract at a medical conference but the data has never been published.

FSM seminars go national

Throughout 2000, 2001 and 2002 the practice and the US seminars continued to grow. The seminars were now two and a half days long and still presented by writing on a white board with a felt marker in a hotel meeting room in Portland, Chicago or Jacksonville Florida. The syllabus expanded to 60 typed pages and the summary of frequencies and treatment protocols filled two full columns on both sides of a laminated sheet. The conditions treated successfully with FSM continued to grow as the practice increased and the cases accumulated from practitioners around the country.

There was one frequency combination that turned out to be effective for reversing shingles and both oral and genital herpes. The pain disappeared after ten minutes of treatment and 60 minutes of treatment each day for three days would prevent the blisters from appearing if delivered in the painful pre-shingles prodrome. Sixty minutes of treatment would eliminate the pain and clear up the blisters in five days instead of five weeks if treatment started after the blisters appeared. That frequency combination was not useful for any other condition and everyone treated so far with these conditions has responded positively. In 2002, one frequency combination was found to be effective in eliminating kidney stone pain; it did nothing for the stone, it just stopped the pain within minutes in every one of the 25 patients treated that year. Some frequencies treated new injuries and accelerated the healing by three to four times if treatment was administered in the first four hours after injury. Any condition from asthma to irritable bowel syndrome that involved inflammation or scar tissue seemed to respond dramatically.

In 2002 Jeff Katke, the president and CEO of Metagenics, Inc., a large nutriceutical company providing professional grade nutritional supplements to physicians, suggested a collaboration. Metagenics would promote FSM seminars and the FSM seminar would recommend Metagenics supplements to be used to support the changes created with FSM treatment. In fact, this is how treatments were done at the clinic. Those patients with proper nutrition and a stable state to support the changes made by FSM treatment recovered more quickly and had better outcomes than patients who did not have good nutrition or take supplements. It seemed to be a reasonable way to get the FSM information out to more people.

By this time Dr. Kristi Hughes, the naturopathic physician who helped when FSM was being developed, was now a speaker for Metagenics giving lectures around the country about functional medicine approaches to health. Metagenics sponsored nine FSM seminars in 2003 and Dr. Hughes lecture series preceded the FSM seminars by six to eight weeks in most cities. Any time she talked about her results using FSM and nutrition to treat pain patients, people signed up for the FSM seminars in droves.

Travels with Dr. Bland

In addition to his position at the Institute for Functional Medicine, Dr. Jeffrey Bland was also the chief science officer for Metagenics and gave day-long lectures in 18 cities around the country in the spring of each year, describing the biochemistry and science behind nutritional approaches to improve health and prevent disease. The FSM display booth and I joined Dr. Bland on his 18 city tour from January through April. On most Fridays we traveled to the city where he would lecture on Saturday. He lectured from 8:30 to 4:30 and Saturday night we flew on to the next city. He lectured on Sunday and we traveled home either immediately afterward or on Monday morning. Tuesday, Wednesday and Thursday found me back at work at the clinic until we left again on Friday. Jeff was gracious and generous and made my first experience with national seminar travel as painless as possible.

Doctors attending the day's lecture could be treated at the FSM booth during the breaks as FSM was discussed and demonstrated. One physician had been injured 14 years previously when she rode her bicycle into a 20-foot deep unmarked construction trench on her way home from the hospital one night. She was pacing at the back room and had the facial expression of someone in pain. At the break, I asked about her history and then inquired if her hands and feet hurt. She replied that they did and agreed to sit in the back of the room and be treated. Cloth napkins from the refreshment table combined with warm water from the tea service became makeshift electrodes with the graphite gloves wrapped inside and were wrapped around her neck and feet. The experience gained from treating 25 patients a year for four years made the treatment faster and the relief longer lasting. In 60 minutes this physician was pain free for the first time in 14 years and after a few more treatments the pain was permanently eliminated. She took the FSM seminar in Detroit that year and is a skilled and successful FSM practitioner in Toronto to this day.

The FSM course began to make the transition from typed text to Power Point slides in January 2003. The first FSM seminar was scheduled for mid-February 2003 and somehow 60 pages of text became 742 power point slides in six weeks. The FSM seminars in 2003 were so well attended that the number of practitioners in the US doubled from 150 to 300 in ten months.

New equipment – new possibilities

The Precision Microcurrent had always been a two-digit specific device with two numbers set on the frequency switch and 0.1, 1, and 10 multiplier switch to turn 0.68 into 6.8, 68, and 680. The frequencies came in three digits: for example the frequency

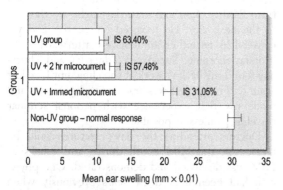

Figure 1.12 • UV exposure to the point of sunburn reduces immune system response. The mice were painted on the hind leg with a sensitizing chemical at the time of UV exposure and painted again on the ear two weeks later. Normal mice who had not been exposed to UV responded two weeks later with 30 units of swelling. The swelling is a normal response. Sunburned mice had their immune system suppressed (IS) by 63.4% from exposure to UV. Mice treated with FSM two hours after the UV exposure had the best reduction in swelling and had immune system suppression reduced from 63.4% to 57.48%. The mice treated immediately with FSM had immune system suppression reduced by half from 63.4% to 31.05%. A single four minute treatment created a change in immune system response lasting two weeks and assumed to be permanent.

for tendon is 191Hz, the frequency for the bursa is 195Hz. With only two digits the treatment could not be specific enough to target important tissues. Glen Smith, the engineer-designer and owner of Precision Microcurrent, responded reluctantly to the request for a three-digit specific machine in 1999 saying he didn't think it could possibly make a difference. It not only made a difference; it made a huge difference in the patient's response. After 1999, he made only three-digit specific devices for Frequency-specific Microcurrent practitioners.

There were now enough FSM practitioners and patients that Microcurrent Technologies agreed to develop an automated unit that would run sequences of frequencies in treatment protocols for various conditions. The first "AutoCare" allowed the standard routine protocols to be applied more efficiently in the office. The clinic staff who had been changing frequencies every two minutes on the Precision Microcurrent cheered when the first automated unit arrived. The AutoCare was upgraded in 2004 and again in 2006 to become the AutoCarePlus running 83 automated frequency protocols. The HomeCare, released in 2004 finally made it possible for a fibromyalgia patient to be treated at home under a practitioner's direction and become pain free at will. The HomeCare unit made recovery from fibromyalgia possible.

Practitioners wanted a HomeCare pocket sized unit they could program from a computer. Microcurrent technologies took the leap and developed the CustomCare in 2007. Patients with the most complex conditions can now maintain treatment and find relief at home with protocols designed for them by the FSM practitioner.

In 2003, athletic trainers came from all over the country for the first FSM Sports seminar in Phoenix in June. Because of their body size, muscle mass and injury profile, athletes require higher current levels and different frequency treatment protocols than the average person. Microcurrent Technologies developed the first SportsCare unit specifically designed for athletes in July of 2003.

Precision Distributing provides the three-digit specific Precision Microcurrent and all of the automated units to practitioners who have attended the FSM Core seminar but any microcurrent device that can deliver one frequency on each of two channels in a ramped square wave pulse can be used for a Frequency-specific Microcurrent treatment. Many students took the course and used their own equipment when they went home to practice.

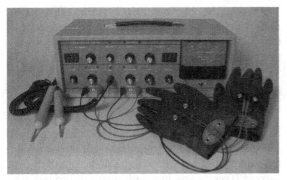

Figure 1.13 • Three Digit Precision Microcurrent. Glen Smith, the engineer who designed the original Precision Microcurrent, created the first three-digit specific Precision Microcurrent in 1999 convinced that the specificity would not make a difference. The improvement in results made such a difference that soon three-digit machines were used exclusively. Any three digit specific device can be used for treatment.

The Sports Care and the Precision Microcurrent made their NFL debut when Keith Pyne, DC arranged for us to work in the Oakland Raiders training room for the day after our July 2003 San Francisco Core seminar and we treated most of the defensive team including legendary figures such as Bill Romanowski. Buddy Prim, a private trainer for NFL athletes, heard about FSM and brought most of the offensive line from the San Francisco 49er's to a treatment room set up in an airport hotel on the next day. Reducing inflammation, scar tissue and mineral deposits in men whose job required determined performance and incredible conditioning was a real learning experience. The world of professional sports had discovered FSM.

After FSM made it possible for Terrell Owens, a well known wide receiver for the Philadelphia Eagles, to recover from surgery and heal torn ankle ligaments and a fibular fracture in six weeks instead of the predicted 18 weeks so he could play in the Super Bowl, the word spread throughout the NFL about FSM. The SportsCare, CustomCare, and Precision Microcurrent became training room standards for a few teams and hundreds of players. Through the efforts of skilled athletic trainers like Jeff Spencer, Mike Hatrack, Mark Lindsay and many others, FSM has treated US Postal and Lance Armstrong as they won the Tour de France, helped Tiger Woods recover from knee surgery, and helped Lashinda Demus heal her hamstring injury and win the US National women's 400 meter hurdles.

The first FSM symposium

The FSM Advanced Course presented new frequencies and advanced treatment concepts every fall since 1999. Students asked for a symposium where FSM outcomes and research could be shared. The 2003 FSM Advanced course was held on Friday afternoon and Saturday morning and the first FSM Symposium was held on Saturday afternoon and all day Sunday in a beautiful ballroom in a downtown Portland hotel. Ninety practitioners attended all four days and it was a joyous celebration.

Jim Oschman, PhD a bio-physicist and author of Energy Medicine; the Scientific Basis (Oschman 2000) was our guest speaker. His task was to explain why the tissue softens so dramatically and why the graphite gloves became warm when the frequency is correct for the patient's condition. "Why does it get warm; why does it go smoosh?" His explanations mesmerized the attendees and at the end of his lecture he had everyone stand and tone to demonstrate the power of a resonance field.

To complete the demonstration everyone in the room was connected to the microcurrent unit by putting the red leads contact on one side of the aisle and the black leads contact on the other side of the aisle and then having everyone hold hands on each side and across the back to complete the circuit. The frequencies to "restore joy" pulsed through 90 people and the induced euphoria in the room was an experience that everyone still talks about.

The Advanced FSM course and workshops are held every year in February. The symposium is held every two years and includes presentations from practitioners in the US, Ireland and Australia and Dr. Oschman and other speakers still join us every year to try to explain why and how it works.

The low back myofascial pain cases from the American Back Society presentation were published as "Microcurrent Therapy: A novel treatment method for chronic low back myofascial pain" in the Journal of Body Work and Movement Therapies (JBMT) in April 2004. The cytokine data and the cases of successful treatment of fibromyalgia caused by spine trauma were published as "Cytokine changes with microcurrent treatment in fibromyalgia associated with cervical trauma" in JBMT in July 2005. FSM now had three published papers and a track record of incredible case reports. And this is just the beginning.

Crohn's disease case report

The practitioner case reports at this symposium were an astonishing demonstration of the versatility of the resonance response, the ability of microcurrent to increase the rate of healing and the commitment of the FSM practitioners to patient care and clinical research.

Scott Bergman, DC took his first FSM Core Seminar in Portland in February 2003. The FSM course teaches the frequencies for the digestive system and the frequencies thought to reduce inflammation, chronic inflammation and histamine among others. At the symposium he reported the results of his FSM treatment of a 14-year-old girl with Crohn's disease. She had a history of being hospitalized with an episode of Crohn's every spring and every fall for two years in spite of ideal diet, appropriate nutritional support and the best medical care. She was on the path to her first hospitalization of the year when the gastroenterologist told her on Monday morning to collect her school work and be prepared to be hospitalized on Thursday for about one week of the standard treatment for Crohn's.

Dr. Bergman treated her on Monday afternoon when she and her mom returned from the gastroenterologist looking for some alternative to four days in the ICU. When the treatment started her abdomen was painful and distended, she was nauseous and her appetite was gone. Dr. Bergman combined his knowledge of Crohn's disease with the tools he gathered from FSM and created a treatment protocol. At the end of one hour's treatment, her abdomen was non-tender and flat, she was pain free and she was hungry. Each day for four days she was treated. Each day her symptoms were less than they were the day before. And each day when she left, the pain and bloating were gone, her abdomen was non-tender and she was hungry. She never did check into the hospital. She still gets treated once a month, her Crohn's disease remains in remission and she has never again been in the hospital for Crohn's.

This and the other case reports at the 2003 symposium were just the beginning of the "miracle stories" that FSM practitioners would document in presentations at every advanced course and symposium.

FSM and the future

At each symposium since 2003 practitioners report on successful treatment of conditions that no one would have thought of treating with frequencies and microcurrent 10 years ago. Incomplete spinal cord injuries, disc herniations and reflex sympathetic dystrophy, Alzheimer's and Parkinson's, PTSD (post-traumatic stress disorder), anxiety and obsessive compulsive disorder, sports injuries, post-operative pain and wound healing, skin anti-aging, interstitial cystitis, diabetic neuropathies, uterine fibroids and ovarian cysts and others are presented as cases by practitioners who have treated them successfully.

It has been 12 years now and there are 1200 FSM practitioners in the US, 165 in Australia and 45 in Ireland, 1 in the Netherlands, 1 in Germany, 1 in Spain, 2 in England, 1 in South Africa, and 1 in Hong Kong. The practitioners are an enthusiastic varied interdisciplinary group made up of MDs, DCs, DOs, NDs, NPs, PTs, OTs, LMTs, PhDs, and licensed acupuncturists. The treatment protocols are more refined and more efficient and attending the Core seminar is still like learning a new language in three days.

There are controlled trials planned in medical facilities to study the effects of FSM in the treatment of diabetic wounds and peripheral neuropathies, oral and genital herpes, shingles and in postoperative wound healing and pain control and in dental applications including orthodontics, periodontics and post-operative healing. There doesn't seem to be any end in sight for what can be accomplished by resonance in the hands of dedicated and caring practitioners.

Bibliography

Cheng, N., 1982. The effect of electric currents on ATP generation, protein synthesis, and membrane transport in rat skin. Clinical Orthopedics 171, 264–272.

Electronic reactions of Dr. Abrams. Republished articles from Electronic Medical Digest 1980. Borderland Sciences Research Foundation, Vista CA.

Kandel, E., Schwartz, J., 1985. Principles of neural science, second ed. Elsevier, New York, pp. 331–336.

McMakin, C., 1998. Microcurrent treatment of myofascial pain in the head, neck and face. Topics in Clinical Chiropractic 5 (1), 29–35.

McMakin, C., 2004. Microcurrent therapy: a novel treatment method for chronic low back myofascial pain. Journal of Bodywork and Movement Therapies 8, 143–153.

McMakin, C., Gregory, W., Phillips, T., 2005. Cytokine changes with microcurrent treatment of fibromyalgia associated with cervical spine trauma. Journal of Bodywork and Movement Therapies 9, 169–176.

Olmarker, K., Rydevik, B., Nordberg, C., 1993. Autologous nucleus pulposus induces neurophysiologic and histologic changes in porcine cauda equina nerve roots. Spine 18, 1425–1432.

Olmarker, K., Blomquist, J., Stromberg, J., et al., 1995. Inflammatogenic properties of nucleus pulposus. Spine 20, 665–669.

Oschman, J., 2000. Energy medicine: the scientific basis. Churchill Livingstone, Edinburgh.

Ozaktay, A.C., Cavanaugh, J.M., Blagoev, D.C., 1995. Phospholipase A_2-induced electrophysiologic and histologic changes in rabbit dorsal lumbar spine tissues. Spine 20, 2659–2668.

Ozaktay, A.C., Kallakuri, S., Cavanaugh, J.M., 1998. Phospholipase A_2 sensitivity of the dorsal root and dorsal root ganglion. Spine 23, 1297–1306.

Reilly, W., Reeve, V.E., Quinn, C., 2004. Anti-inflammatory effects of interferential, frequency-specific applied microcurrent. Proceedings of the Australian Health and Medical Research Congress.

Taylor, J.R., Twomey, L.T., 1993. Acute injuries to cervical joints, an autopsy study of neck pain. Spine 18, 1115–1122.

The theoretical foundation for frequency-specific microcurrent

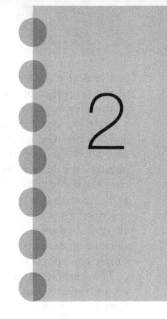

2

After 12 years of clinical use, thousands of anecdotes, hundreds of patient and practitioner testimonials, one blinded placebo-controlled trial in animals showing unprecedented reductions in lipoxygenase mediated inflammation and biochemical data in humans reporting unheard of reductions in inflammatory cytokines all in response to only very specific frequency combinations and current flow, it is clear that there is some sort of frequency-specific effect on biological tissue created by pulse trains and microamperage current.

No one who has experienced FSM either as a patient or practitioner has any question that there is some sort of frequency-specific effect. Tissues soften and change state in seconds, scar tissue appears to dissolve, inflammation disappears, injuries heal, endorphins increase and patients get euphoric all at remarkable rates. But how are these effects created? There needs to be some intellectually satisfying explanation that describes how microamperage current increases cellular energy by 500% and how one frequency combination, and only one frequency combination, reduces inflammation in a blinded placebo-controlled animal trial by 62% in four minutes.

Physics describes the electromagnetic composition and function of matter; bio-physics describes the electromagnetic structure and function of biological systems. Chemistry describes the characteristics and bonds that hold atoms and molecules together and describes the reactions that alter those bonds to create new molecules; the science of biochemistry does the same for biological systems. Physics and chemistry, and their biological-science siblings, provide the basic information and conceptual framework that explains how frequency-specific microcurrent probably creates its effects.

Biological quantum system

Physics has two branches that study in detail the structure, properties and function of matter. Classical or Newtonian physics describes the behavior of physical objects on a macroscopic scale. Classical physics describes and can predict with certainty the behavior of large collections of particles such as the metal beams, hinges and glass lenses used to construct the Hubble telescope. But classical physics is not sufficient to describe the behavior of very small systems such as the atoms, molecules, black holes and streams of energy that the telescope observes in the voids of space.

Quantum physics studies the submicroscopic forces that shape our universe at the atomic level. Quantum theory states that energy is not continuous but comes in discrete packets or quanta. These quanta behave like particles having mass at some times but they behave as waves of energy without mass at other times depending on the circumstances. Quantum physics must deal with uncertainty because the position and the momentum of a particle cannot be known at the same time and quantum phenomena, while coherent, are inherently unpredictable. Quantum physics is relevant at the atomic scale describing the behavior of atoms, molecules, electrons and protons. In the new field of quantum biology, electrons from green tea's anti-oxidant catechins have been observed tunneling instantaneously across a gap between molecules to bind and inactivate a free radical, a process forbidden in classical physics (Anderson 2009).

DOI: 10.1016/B978-0-443-06976-5.00002-2

Classical physics provides accurate descriptions of the properties of the body as a large collection of particles but only quantum physics can provide a model for our internal submicroscopic structure and function. Our bodies appear as solid objects that have all of the properties described by Newtonian physics. We have mass, momentum, inertia, and obey the law of gravity. But we are at the same time an electromagnetic system with all of the properties described by quantum physics. We are as much energy as we are matter. This is not an esoteric or spiritual appreciation of the human condition; it is simply basic physics.

The principles of both classical and quantum physics are simultaneously true for large collections of particles such as the human body. Electrons in the outer orbital of a hydrogen atom that is attached to a carbon atom in a collagen strand in your forearm are no different than the hydrogen atoms whizzing around the linear accelerator at Fermi Labs in Chicago, Illinois. Electrons may have different energy states because of their relationship to nearby atoms but the electron itself has the same basic structure. A proton is a proton but the resonant frequency of a proton, for example, depends on a property known as the Larmor frequency, which will be different for protons in different tissues due to the proximity of other nearby atoms. If your body represented the nucleus of a hydrogen atom, the nearest electron would be one quarter mile away and would appear as a potential in space into which the energy of the electron could materialize as a charged particle under appropriate conditions. We, our bodies, are in fact more space than they are matter. And all of that space and all of that matter is electro-magnetic and electro-biochemical in nature.

Using frequencies and current to successfully modify the structure and function of biological tissue brings the FSM practitioner to a practical appreciation of this quantum reality. One of the basic principles of science is that you cannot throw out the data because it doesn't match the model of how the system was thought to operate. When new data appears then the model has to change to allow for it. The first time one specific frequency combination and 100µamps of pulsed direct current caused scarred muscles to elongate and soften permanently; the author's model for how biological systems operate changed forever.

The model that follows is an attempt to explain in fairly simple terms how it is that the observed affects of FSM are created. It is a rough approximation and by no means complete or thoroughly understood but it is what can be proposed given our current level of knowledge.

Four factors operating

There are at least four factors operating simultaneously to create the effects seen with the use of Frequency-specific Microcurrent.

1. **Current**: The microamperage direct current alone produces specific well documented and predictable effects.
2. **Frequencies**: Two frequencies are used simultaneously, one from each channel, and produce specific effects that are independent of the current applied.
3. **The Human Biological Semiconductor**: The electromagnetic nature of biological tissue provides a semi-conductor tissue matrix that mediates the response to both the current and the frequencies.
4. **Stable State**: And finally the patient's general physical and emotional health, conditioning, diet, hydration and history create an environment that will either support or erode the changes created by the frequencies and the current in any given treatment or any course of treatments.

1. Effects of the current

Trial and error and clinical experience has shown that appropriate current levels, contact placement and current polarity are essential to successful FSM treatments, especially when treating pain. Larger and more muscular patients require higher current levels. Children and frail patients require smaller current levels. When treating the viscera or the central nervous system, current flow doesn't seem that important; the treatment appears to affect the target tissue whether the contacts are positioned so the current flows through it or not. How does the current facilitate the treatment?

All matter, living and non-living, is ultimately an electromagnetic phenomenon (Becker 1985). All atoms are bonded electrically and all bonds are ultimately electromagnetic because the electrons creating the bonds are in constant motion and moving electrons create a magnetic field. The material world is a collection of atomic structures held together by electromagnetic forces.

Biological tissue is made up of complex combinations of atoms and molecules creating the membranes, organelles and cells that determine physical structure and physiologic function. Every cell and tissue membrane has an electrical potential or charge difference between one side of the membrane and the other (Kirsch 1998). Furthermore, the body as a whole has an electromagnetic field created by charge differentials between one area and another. The human system is more positively charged at the top near the head and along midline at the spine and more negatively charged in the periphery. Becker established that the bioelectric field produced by these linked electrical potentials is responsible for intracellular communication and tissue repair and eventually he proposed that the electromagnetic field controls all life processes (Becker 1985).

All living systems have an electrical component whose existence is now well established but whose function is still not completely understood. The following basic principles of electronic circuitry apply to all biochemical, bio-electric living systems.

Current is created by the movement of electrons from one point to another using some conducting medium. The electron is a negatively charged particle that moves in, or is likely to be found in, a particular volume, called an orbital around the positively charged nucleus of an atom. Electrons have mass when measured as a particle but have only energy when measured as a wave. Energy and matter are actually interchangeable in all matter. For our purposes the electron is the basic unit of charge that moves in any circuit including the human bio-electric circuit.

Amperage describes the number of electrons moving past a fixed point in a unit of time; it is the amount of current flowing. Current is measured in amperes or amps.

Voltage is the measure of pressure or push behind the electrons flowing in a circuit and is measured in volts.

Resistance to current flow is measured in ohms and is determined by factors that inhibit current flow.

Circuit: To have current flow you need a circuit. Current is introduced in one spot, flows through a conductor and eventually gets back to the generator by way of some conductor.

Water flowing through a garden hose is the classic analogy used to describe these circuitry concepts. The amount of water flowing through the garden hose corresponds to the amperage or current, how many gallons per minute come out of the end of the hose. The water pressure corresponds to the voltage, how much water pressure is there behind the stream driving the water out of the hose. The size of the hose or any impediment to the flow of water corresponds to the resistance. A smaller hose, or even a larger hose with a tangle of fiberglass webbing in the line, will have more resistance to water flow.

In the garden hose circuit analogy, water is made available by the municipal water district and conducted through a series of pipes to the garden hose. The garden hose delivers some total amount of water to the lawn that is determined by the water pressure, the size of the hose and the amount of time spent watering. Some of the water is absorbed by the grass and, combined with sunlight, turns into the energy that makes the grass grow; some of it evaporates, goes into the clouds and returns to the municipal water district in the form of rain; and some of it percolates through the ground into the aquifer and returns to the wells used by the water district. The water or current is produced someplace, travels to someplace and does something and then returns to the source to complete the circuit.

This relationship between voltage, current and resistance is described in Ohm's law, Voltage = Current × Resistance ($V = I \times R$). If the voltage stays the same and the resistance goes up then the current will go down. If the current must be kept constant then the voltage must increase if the resistance increases. If one parameter changes it automatically changes at least one other parameter.

Microcurrent devices used in FSM treatments are "constant current generators". The machine increases the voltage automatically as needed, up to a maximum of about 30 volts, in order to keep the current constant and push the desired amperage through the body's resistance.

Resistance to current flow is created by anything that interferes with conductivity or that acts as an insulator. Blood, water, collagen and lymph all conduct electricity; oil, scar tissue and inflammation resist current flow. Total resistance in a human body is determined by fluid content or lack of it, general health and inflammation, muscle mass, amount of oil on the skin, adipose and hydration.

Current increases ATP energy

Current flowing through the body fuels all biological process. Gnok Cheng (Cheng et al 1982) and his associates demonstrated that applying additional current

Box 2.1

The direct relationship between voltage (V), resistance (I) and current (C)

$V = I \times C:$

Microcurrent devices are constant current generators. The voltage will increase as needed to maintain the current level that has been set as long as the resistance is low or stays constant. Eventually if the current requirement is increased enough the voltage will not be able to increase sufficiently to maintain current levels and the percent conductivity shown on the machine will decrease.

$V = I \times C:$

If the resistance (I) increases, for example when a patient is dehydrated or when the conducting medium has too much resistance, the voltage (V) must increase to keep the current (C) constant at the level the machine has been set to deliver. If the resistance increases past a certain point, the voltage will not be able to increase sufficiently to maintain the current level. And the percent conductivity shown on the machine will decrease. The percentage of current conducted will return to 100% if the current level set on the machine is reduced or if the resistance decreases.

$V = I \times C:$

If the current is set to very high levels of 300–400µamps, as it is when treating athletes, the voltage can compensate as long as the resistance stays low. This need to reduce resistance may explain why athletes need to be more hydrated than the average patient. It also suggests that the combination of graphite gloves wrapped in wet towels may be a very low resistance conducting medium since it is so effective in conducting the higher levels of current required for athletes and heavier patients.

to a biological system could increase both protein synthesis and energy production dramatically as long as the current was *small enough*. Direct current levels of 50 to 1000µamps applied across rat skin increased glycine (amino acid) transport by 75% compared with untreated controls and current levels of 500µamps increased aminoisobutyric acid (amino acid) uptake by 90% indicating a dramatic increase in protein synthesis. But current levels above 1000µamps decreased protein synthesis by as much as 50%.

ATP (adenosine triphosphate) is the chemical energy molecule that fuels every biological process. Direct current levels between 100 and 500µamps applied to rat skin increased ATP levels by three to five times (300% to 500%). Current exceeding

1000µamps caused ATP production to level off and currents above 5000µamps reduced ATP levels as compared to untreated controls. Once the external current was discontinued the ATP production and amino acid transport levels returned to baseline; there was no residual effect in rat skin.

Cheng and his colleagues hypothesized that the increased number of electrons from the DC current flowing along the mitochondrial membranes increased the proton gradient across the membrane thereby increasing ATP production. Oschman (2009) has proposed that the electron transport chain in mitochondria can become electron-deficient, and that microcurrent provides more electrons that are semiconducted through the living matrix to the mitochondrial membranes. In either case, the additional ATP available is probably responsible for the increase in protein synthesis. There have been no studies that demonstrate increased ATP production in a living system but the increases in healing seen with microamperage current are usually attributed to this increase in ATP production and protein synthesis. Cheng and colleagues did not attempt to explain why current levels over 1000µamps reduced ATP production and protein synthesis. It is worth noting that all electrical stimulation devices except microcurrent use current levels above 1000µamps and may be decreasing ATP production, although that has not been demonstrated.

It has been proposed that Voltage Gated Ion Channels (VGICs) may also be affected by the current flow along or across the membrane but no one has measured changes in these transport proteins in response to externally applied microamperage current. VGICs transport ions such as sodium, potassium, calcium and others across the cell membrane and control virtually all cellular processes. VGICs require ATP activation to change configuration allowing them to transport their ion across the cell membrane. There has been some suggestion that microcurrent and the voltage pushing it along or across membranes has a direct affect on the VGICs but there is no data to support this hypothesis. The current could be altering VGIC function simply because it increases ATP production.

Current has a clinical effect

Whatever the mechanism, current clearly has an influence on treatment. Clinical trial and error has determined that the current must be polarized positive with the positive leads at the spine and the negative leads at the distal end of the nerve for the

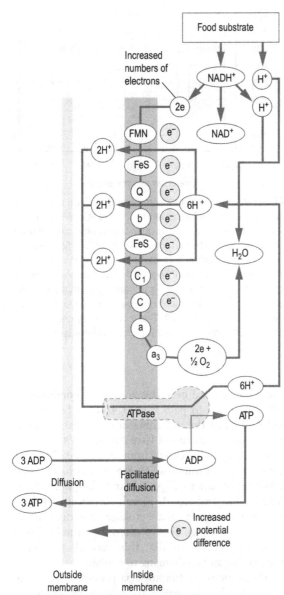

Some patients respond better to polarized positive current for all applications and some patients do better with pulsed alternating DC current. In any FSM course, roughly half of the students being treated during a practicum session respond better to polarized current and the other half respond better to alternating DC current. No explanation is offered for this observation but any model for the biological effects of pulsed DC current must be able to explain the observations.

Current levels must be appropriate to the patient's size and muscle mass for successful treatment of muscle pain and scar tissue. A larger or more muscular person requires higher current levels than a smaller, deconditioned or frail person. If the current levels are too low, response to treatment is slow or equivocal. There is almost no detectable response when 100µamps are used to treat a 250 pound professional football player but increasing the current to 400µamps creates an immediate positive response to the same frequencies. A small frail deconditioned patient will respond well to 100µamps and will find 400µamps irritating and bothersome. A very ill patient may find anything more than 20µamps irritating or too stimulating.

These observations dictate the treatment parameters discussed in this text but there is nothing specific in microcurrent theory or research to explain these phenomena.

2. The effects of frequencies

Current flow alone creates some positive effect but the most dramatic effects of FSM occur in response to specific frequencies. The frequency to neutralize a condition is delivered on one channel. The frequency for the tissue being addressed is delivered simultaneously on a second channel. In a blinded placebo controlled trial in mice, one frequency combination, 40Hz on channel A (reduce inflammation), and 116Hz on channel B (the immune system) reduced arachidonic acid induced lipoxygenase (LOX) mediated swelling in the mouse's ear by 62% in four minutes. The ear swelling was measured with mechanical calipers and recorded in millimeters. Three unrelated frequency combinations (new injury, remove mineral from bone, and .3Hz) tested in the same model had no effect on inflammation or swelling. According to the researcher who performed the tests, no prescription or non-prescription drug has ever reduced inflammation in this animal model by more than 45% (Reilly et al 2004).

Figure 2.1 • ATP is produced when electrons, stripped off of food substrate, flow through an electron transport cascade and also flow along the cell membrane creating a difference in charge between one side of the membrane and the other. The charge gradient pulls protons across a membrane and ATP is produced. Increased current flow up to 500µamps increases ATP production. Current flow above 1000µamps overwhelms the system and decreases ATP production.

successful treatment of nerve pain. The treatment for fibromyalgia associated with spine trauma and for post-stroke central pain is most successful when the current is polarized positive with the positive leads at the neck and the negative leads at the feet.

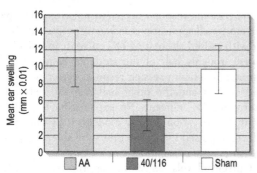

Figure 2.2 • The bar on the left is the normal swelling at 11 units seen when arachidonic acid is painted on a mouse ear and measured with calipers. The bar in the center represents the reduction in swelling to 4 units seen when the mice were treated with 40Hz and 116Hz for four minutes. The bar on the right is the swelling at 10 units seen when a sham frequency was applied for four minutes. This is a time-dependent response; half of the effect is present at two minutes and the full effect is present at four minutes.

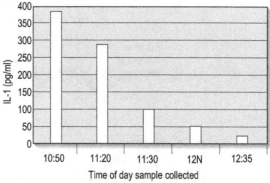

Figure 2.3 • Interleukin 1 normal range is 0–25 pg/ml. IL-1 started at 392 and dropped to 21.4 in 90 minutes in response to one specific frequency combination, 40Hz on channel A and 10Hz on channel B in patient MK. For five patients the average IL-1 of 330 ± 39 reduced to 80 ± 31pg/ml. IL-6, TNF-α, IFN-γ, CGRP all changed at similar rates. Medical cytokine researchers report that cytokines are difficult to change and change slowly when they can be made to change at all. This is a time-dependent response taking 60–90 minutes for the full effect to be achieved.

In a subsequent trial measuring reductions in COX mediated inflammation, 40Hz (reduce inflammation) and 116Hz (immune system) reduced swelling and inflammation by 30% which is identical to the prescription injectable anti-inflammatory Toridol when it was tested in this same mouse model. But 40Hz on channel A (reduce inflammation) and 355Hz (skin) on channel B had no anti-inflammatory effect and was equivalent to placebo (Reilly 2005). This suggests that the pattern created by both frequencies used is responsible for the anti-inflammatory effect, as long as one of the frequencies is 40Hz. The frequency from the second channel has a definite impact.

The response in mice was time dependent – one half of the response was present at 2 minutes and the full response was present at 4 minutes. Further time spent on the frequency had no additional positive effect. Why and how is the reduction in inflammation time dependent?

In a clinical setting, fibromyalgia patients whose fibromyalgia was associated with spine trauma responded only to the frequencies 40Hz on channel A (reduce inflammation) and 10Hz on channel B (the spinal cord), even when they didn't know what treatment was being done and had no expectations that anything would help them. This frequency combination, and only this frequency combination (40/10), reduced pain from 7.4/10 to 1.4/10 and reduced all of the inflammatory cytokines at logarithmic rates by factors of 10 to 20 times in 90 minutes. Interleukin 1 decreased from 392pg/ml down to 21pg/ml in 90 minutes, TNF-α was reduced from 299pg/ml down to 21pg/ml, and IL-6 went down from 204pg/ml to 15pg/ml. Medical cytokine researchers report that cytokines are difficult to change and change slowly when they can be made to change at all, making this data all the more remarkable and challenging to explain.

The response in fibromyalgia patients is also time dependent. Roughly half of the effect is present at the end of 45 minutes and the full effect is present at 90 minutes. Treating for more than 90 minutes doesn't improve the outcome. Treating for less than 60 to 90 minutes is unsatisfactory. Why and how is the reduction in inflammation and pain time dependent?

Scar tissue responds only to specific frequency combinations that cause the tissue to elongate and soften dramatically allowing increases, even doubling, of range of motion within 10 to 20 minutes. If the scar tissue is very dense or very chronic the process requires more time and repeated treatment but is usually successful. The frequency to reduce inflammation does nothing for scar tissue; the frequency for

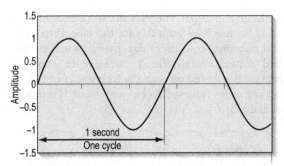

Figure 2.4 • 1Hz as a sine wave is a single cycle passing a point in space every second. A 1Hz square wave with the same amplitude or height contains high frequency harmonics to create the single pulse but it still represents only one cycle per second. The amplitude is measured from the peak to the valley. Larger amplitude waves have more energy than smaller amplitude waves.

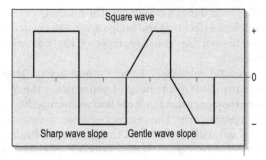

Figure 2.5 • Square waves that deliver the current in microcurrent devices are actually ramped square waves. The leading edge of the wave can have a steep slope giving it more "impact" when it encounters the target tissue or it can have a gradual increase to the peak amplitude creating a gentle wave slope. The sharp waveslope is more effective in chronic conditions but can be irritating on newly injured tissue. The gentle waveslope is more comfortable in acute injuries presumably because the current increases gradually giving the injured membrane time to incorporate the additional current flow.

removing scar tissue does nothing to reduce inflammation. Regardless of the condition being treated, when the frequency is correct the patient and the practitioner can often feel a sensation of warmth underneath the skin contact as the tissue begins to soften.

How could a frequency create these observed changes? Why does the area being treated get warm just before the tissue changes? Why and how is the reduction in inflammation time dependent?

First let's define some basic terms and concepts.

Frequency: Frequencies refer to the number of pulses of sounds or electrons moving through a conducting medium in one second. Frequencies are measured in hertz. One hertz is a single waveform or cycle passing a fixed point in one second. In engineering terms, the word "frequency" should only be used when referring to the pulse produced by a sine wave which has no harmonics. Microcurrent devices usually output square wave pulses containing a large number of high frequency harmonics instead of using sine waves because the clinical effects were found to be better with square waves. A square wave frequency of 40Hz is technically a *pulse train* of 40Hz – 40 square waves that pass a point in space every second.

Even though it is a pulse train and not a sine wave the word frequency still accurately describes the number of pulses per second regardless of the high frequency harmonics in the pulse. A middle C note played on the piano will sound different than middle C played on a violin or a flute because of the difference in harmonics but the note played is still middle C.

Amplitude: The size of a wave as measured from the peak to the valley. Larger amplitude waves have more energy than smaller waves.

Waveslope: Waveslope describes the shape of the leading edge of the wave form. The FSM microcurrent devices use a ramped square wave to deliver the current and form the frequency pulse because it was thought to overcome skin resistance more effectively. The leading edge of the square wave may be more acute forming a sharp edged wave form or it may be a more gradual slope allowing the current to build up more slowly. A sharp waveslope is used to treat chronic pain but is irritating in new injuries. A gentle waveslope is more comfortable in new injuries. This observation has not been explained.

Resonance

The frequencies create tissue changes by resonance. Resonance is the tendency of a system to oscillate at larger amplitudes in response to some frequencies and not others. Every mechanical system and every chemical bond has a resonant frequency. At the resonant frequency even small driving forces can produce very large amplitude vibrations. These large amplitude vibrations can cause the system to oscillate so violently that it comes apart. Mechanical resonance destroyed the Tacoma Narrows Bridge when the resonant frequency of the bridge was matched by the frequency of oscillations in the bridge caused by the wind during a rain storm. The resulting violent pendulum effect tore the bridge apart and created a most memorable visual example of the power of resonance.

Acoustic resonance shatters a lead crystal glass when the musical note being played matches the resonant frequency that binds the lead atoms together in the crystal matrix. The resonance causes the atomic bonds to oscillate, like the Tacoma Narrows Bridge, and the glass comes apart. Resonant phenomena occur with every type of vibration or wave and every type of bond and structure.

If every chemical bond and every physical structure has a binding energy that holds it together and has a resonant frequency that will cause it to oscillate, then it is possible to imagine that a resonant frequency exists for every bond that will cause oscillations sufficiently violent to weaken or break the bonds that hold the structure together.

As the bonds began to vibrate, the fluids in the surrounding area would become warm from the friction of the vibration much as your hands become warm when you rub them together on a cold night. This warming response to vibration could explain why the tissue being treated feels warm when the frequency is correct and appropriate.

Think of scar tissue as a physical structure made of collagen that is wound up tight and coiled in on itself like a rubber band that has been twisted to operate the propeller of a toy airplane. The coiled scar tissue is held together in this configuration by cross linked bonds that keep it shortened and tight. Think of the collagen coil cross-links as the bonds in the lead crystal glass. When the frequencies are used that seem to dissolve scar tissue, the scarring begins to soften almost immediately and over the next few minutes the tissue elongates and continues to soften until it feels almost normal and the range of motion has increased. Once the bonds break that hold the coils tight, the collagen unwinds and as it elongates the cross-link binding sites are separated and cannot reconnect. In general, once scar tissue dissolves it doesn't return.

When scar tissue dissolved in one particular burn patient, this meant that he could bend his fingers enough to hold a coffee cup for the first time in the three years since his injury. Patients who have been burned develop severe scar tissue that limits range of motion and activity and is resistant to every other type of therapy. Range of motion was measured in seven patients by occupational therapists at Mercy St. John's Medical Center in Springfield Missouri on

a Monday in 2003. The patients were treated with FSM for one hour each day for the next three days and measured again on Friday. Every patient treated had statistically significant increases in range of motion that lasted through the four weeks of follow-up and were assumed to be permanent (Huckfeldt et al 2003).

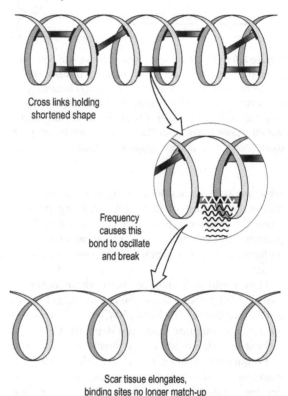

Cross links holding shortened shape

Frequency causes this bond to oscillate and break

Scar tissue elongates, binding sites no longer match-up

Figure 2.6 • The collagen in scar tissue is wound tight in coils that are cross linked to hold them in place. It is possible that the frequencies resonate with the bonds holding the cross links in place and break them allowing the collagen to elongate and the scar tissue to soften and lengthen. Once the scar tissue elongates the binding sites don't match up and the scar tissue doesn't reform. This model attempts to demonstrate one possible mechanism by which the observed effects could be created.

Think of Interleukin 1 and the other inflammatory cytokines as the Tacoma Narrows Bridge. The frequency may resonate with one or more crucial bonds that hold inflammatory peptides together in the crystalline structure that makes them act as a mediator of inflammation. The resonant vibration and oscillations from the frequency could weaken and eventually change or break the bond that holds the cytokine in its shape causing the peptide to change configuration. The changed conformation means that the peptide no longer fits into the receptors in the cell membrane that create the effects of inflammation. The de-configured peptide would not be recognized as a cytokine by immunochromatography and the levels would drop dramatically as they did in the fibromyalgia study.

This would account for the rate and degree of reductions in cytokine levels. Any other mechanism that has been considered doesn't explain the rate of reductions in measurements of cytokine levels in blood or in mean ear swelling in mice. The time required to shatter the bonds could account for the time dependent nature of the response seen in the mouse research. The vibration of the bonds during the oscillation phase could account for the warmth felt as the frequency begins to create an effect.

All that is required for resonant phenomenon to operate in a biological system is bonds that resonate and a conducting medium to convey specific frequency patterns. We are immersed in a sea of electromagnetic signals that form environmental electronic white noise from television and cell phone signals to light bulbs and 60 cycle wall current. While Becker makes a good case for their general negative effects on the immune and autonomic nervous system they don't appear to have immediate specific effects on specific conditions (Becker 1990).

But coherent frequency patterns delivered in conjunction with current that increases cellular energy production could reasonably be expected to create a resonant effect. "Living matter is highly organized and exceedingly sensitive to the information conveyed by *coherent* signals" (Oschman 2000). There are protein receptors in the cell membrane that mediate all of the functions of the cell. Cellular biologist Bruce Lipton points out that even when the nucleus is removed cells can still perform their normal functions perfectly for up to 30 days through the actions of the membrane proteins embedded in the cell wall operating in a co-ordinated self-directed fashion in response to environmental signals. These membrane proteins are sensitive to electromagnetic signals, as well as neurotransmitters, hormones, nutrients, toxins and oxidative stress and even emotions or thoughts (Lipton 2008). Drugs and nutrients act like a key in a lock to change the configuration of cell membrane proteins and thereby change cell functions. A coherent frequency pattern could change cell membrane protein configuration and cellular function like the key beeper that opens your car door lock from 20 feet away.

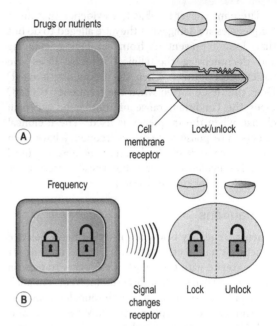

Figure 2.7 • Cell membrane proteins carry out all basic cellular activities and can be influenced by medications or nutrients acting like keys in a lock to change protein configuration and function. The membrane proteins can also be influenced by frequencies acting like the "key beeper" that opens the lock at a distance with an electromagnetic signal.

Limitations

This model doesn't explain why the reductions in inflammation stop when the levels get into the normal range. It doesn't account for why the patients with spinal cord inflammation only responded to 40Hz (reduce inflammation) and 10Hz (spinal cord) but did not respond to the frequencies to reduce inflammation (40Hz) in the immune system (116Hz) that reduced inflammation in the mice. But it is a start and provides something that can be tested when the research opportunity presents itself.

These two frequencies "reduce inflammation" and "reduce scarring" are easy to conceptualize and it is relatively easy to measure scar tissue and inflammation and changes created by treatment. But there are other frequencies presented in this text that are less amenable to measurement and may be difficult for some to even conceptualize. How does one measure the "fact of trauma", or "toxicity" or "allergy reaction" or the "emotional component" of a patient's condition? There are frequencies in this text for each of these pathologies or conditions that might affect any given tissue.

There may never be objective evidence that these frequencies are doing what they are alleged to do but that doesn't prevent us from employing, enjoying and documenting the clinical effects. Does the patient feel warmth when the frequency is used? Does the tissue soften when the frequency is used? Does the condition, range of motion or the pain change when the frequency is used? These clinical effects in response to a correct frequency have been observed consistently in different settings and until objective evidence is available these observations form a basis for future research.

Precautions

When a frequency is applied it either has a positive effect or it has no effect at all. If there is nothing for it to resonate with the frequency appears to pass on through the tissue with no discernible effect. The analogy of unlocking your car door with your electronic key beeper illustrates this phenomenon. When your car is parked in a crowded parking lot, it is only your car door that unlocks when you press the button that sends the electronic signal from your key fob to open the lock. The frequency from your car key resonates with your car only, and not with any others. In a similar fashion, the frequency chosen to treat a particular condition in a particular tissue appears to do that and nothing else. So, in general, there is no harm in trying a frequency for a particular condition / tissue combination.

But the response to certain frequency effects has been sufficiently powerful that the entire process must be approached with both humility and respect. For all of the disclaimers and caveats included in this text the author has learned through experience that the frequencies actually do what they are alleged to do (in a hydrated patient).

For example the body uses inflammation to control infection. The frequency to "reduce inflammation" does indeed reduce inflammation and when this frequency is used in a patient who has an infection that the doctor does not suspect, the infection will become more symptomatic in a very short time when the frequency is used. The bad news is that the infection becomes precipitously worse; the good news is that this predictable response is diagnostic and leads to appropriate treatment of an infection that was previously occult.

And good intentions will not prevent a frequency from having its effect. When Dr. Hawks left the clinic in 1997 and started her practice in Minnesota, it was thought that the frequency 81 Hz described on Van Gelder's list as "secretions" would *normalize*

secretions. Dr. Hawkes spent an hour treating a young girl for the lung congestion of cystic fibrosis and at the end of the hour the patient's lungs were completely clear. Thinking that 81 Hz would "normalize" the lung secretions Dr. Hughes used it at the end of the treatment. The lungs became re-congested in less than 10 seconds. Knowing that they needed to explore this affect, they took a short break, repeated the original treatment and cleared the lungs again. At the end of this treatment the frequency 81 Hz was not used and the child's lungs stayed clear for about two weeks. Dr. Hughes' called the clinic immediately to report this new understanding; 81 Hz was found to *increase* secretions rather than normalize secretions.

It is worth noting that the intention to normalize secretions did not prevent the frequency from increasing secretions. Experiences such as these have created profound respect for the effect of the frequencies. It is safest to assume that the frequencies will do what they are alleged to do and think ahead to what will happen when the effect occurs.

Science starts with observation

All science starts with observation. This is what we observe. The condition changes; the glove gets warm; the pain is reduced. Then science has to ask, "Is it reproducible or just a coincidence?" In any hydrated patient with the same symptoms and physical examination, treated by any practitioner with knowledge, skill and the correct diagnosis will the treatment produce the same response? So far experience suggests that the affects are reproducible. Then science asks if the response is predictable. If you know the appropriate diagnosis and the treatment can you predict the patient's response? If you use the treatment response as a diagnostic indicator will the patient response to treatment help clarify the diagnosis? Once again experience suggests that the response is predictable.

Still, it must be said that the descriptions for the frequency effects are just a model for what the frequency is thought to do and appears to do. Until there is more research to document that the observed change corresponds to removal of the pathology specified by the frequency and that it happens in the tissue specified by the frequency, any claims must be approached with caution. This caveat should not deter the thoughtful practitioner from taking advantage of the apparent effects. Medicine used aspirin as an anti-inflammatory and anti-pyretic for hundreds of years before its mechanism of action and effects on prostaglandin chemistry were known.

3. The human biological semiconductor

In order for the current and frequencies to have an effect on living tissue there has to be some conductor that conveys the current and the frequencies and mediates the observed responses. The human body is that conductor.

Insulators: Insulators do not conduct current and serve to stop its flow. In the garden hose circuit analogy the plastic exterior of the hose itself is an insulator – the water stays inside the hose. The plastic coating on electrical wire or the ceramic stand-off separating the wire and the pole are insulators as long as the voltage and current are appropriate to the material in the insulator.

Conductors: To continue with the garden hose analogy for current, voltage and resistance, the different types of conductors can be thought of as being different types of garden hoses. Water, copper wire, metal foil and graphite are all conductors we use every day.

Metallic conductors conduct current as a cloud of electrons moving rapidly along the surface of a metal wire providing the electricity for light and power to our homes.

Ionic conductors use positively and negatively charged inorganic ions to create current. Ions are charged particles released when a salt like sodium chloride dissolves in water creating positively charged sodium ions and negatively charged chloride ions. The charged ions dissociate from the parent molecule and flow through a medium or across a membrane to create balance and a net zero charge. Even water, H_2O, ionizes to some extent creating H^+ and OH^- ions that balance out to a net zero charge in its liquid form.

Living organisms create ion gradients by actively pumping charged ions to different sides of a membrane using voltage gated ion channels (VGICs) to make one side of the membrane positively charged and the other side relatively negative in charge. Organisms use these ionic gradients and the difference in charge between one side of the membrane and the other to power certain cellular processes.

Three sodium ions are pumped from the inside of the cell to the outside of the cell for every two potassium ions that are pumped from outside the cell to the inside to maintain a charge difference across the membrane. The negatively charged proteins inside the cell combine with the smaller number of positively charged potassium ions to make the inside of the cell −70 mV more negative than the outside of the cell. Each transfer of sodium and potassium across the membrane consumes one ATP molecule.

This voltage gradient is maintained at some physiologic expense and is used to power numerous cellular functions.

Ionic currents die out after short distances and travel just across the distance of the membrane making them unsuitable for long distance transmission. The ionic potential across a cell membrane can depolarize and reverse temporarily and then repolarize, creating a wave that moves along the neuron (the action potential). This creates a form of long distance communication but the ionic current itself at any given moment travels only the short distance across the membrane.

Semiconductors are halfway between conductors like metal and insulators like plastic, rubber or ceramic. Semiconductors are materials having an orderly molecular structure like crystals in which electrons can move easily from the electron cloud around one atomic nucleus to the cloud around another, carrying small currents instantaneously over long distances. Crystalline semiconductors, like silicon and germanium in computer chips, are arranged in neat geometric lattices where electrons can move easily through the space in the lattice where there is no electron. Semiconductors are useful because current flows through them instantaneously over long distances without losing energy and can be used to transmit information depending on the flow pattern through the lattice matrix.

Albert Szent-Györgyi (1941, 1988) determined that the water molecules lining cell membranes, proteins and collagen form such a lattice matrix, sharing electrons and making "holes" that allow current to flow instantaneously through the body as in a semiconductor. In this water–protein semiconductor matrix, electrons and holes can carry energy and information much more rapidly than the energy and information stored in chemical bonds in slowly diffusing molecules such as ATP and hormones. The semiconductor matrix can also transfer information much faster than nerve impulses.

Types of current

Direct or DC current

Direct or DC current is a unidirectional steady flow of current (electrons) that travels from the source through a conductor or semiconductor to the load

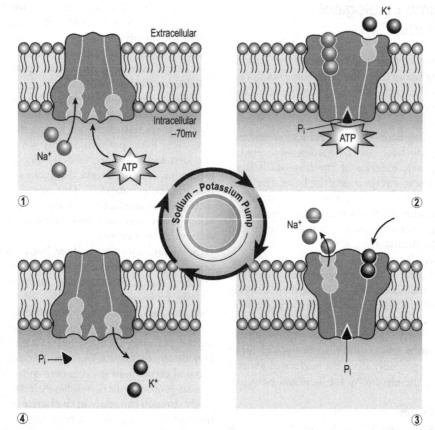

Figure 2.8 • The sodium potassium pump that maintains cell membrane potential is an example of an ionic current. Three sodium ions are pumped to the outside of the membrane and two potassium ions are pumped to the inside of the membrane where they combine with the more negatively charged intracellular proteins to make the inside of the membrane −70mV more negative than the outside. This charge differential drives many cellular processes.

and back again to the source forming a DC circuit. Direct current is used to charge batteries and in nearly all electronic systems as the power supply because it is simple and direct.

Analog versus digital

Analog systems take into consideration the whole gradient of intensity of information available to them. They therefore can detect and transmit a broader spectrum of information than digital systems. However, analog systems are slower than digital systems, which only sample information in bits that are strong enough to reach a certain pre-set threshold. Digital systems can transfer information longer distances without loss or distortion, and can process information in a wide variety of ways, as in a digital computer. Analog computers were used before digital computers, and were much slower and had much less functional flexibility. When a voice is recorded in an analog

system all of the vibrations are impressed on the tape in a continuous stream of information which can be reproduced in the same continuous stream. No decoding is required. The perineureum, the glial membranes surrounding the nerves, carry continuous and complete information as well as pulsing direct currents in an analog system from the brain to the periphery and in the opposite direction (Becker 1985).

Digital systems use on/off–all-or-none signals to encode information and they can be very precise. Digital recordings take the continuous stream of the human voice and break it into tiny on/off impulses that can be manipulated and decoded to provide information we call sound. The brain and nervous system are the best example of a biological digital system. Nerve impulse action potentials are on/off digital pulses which encode signals between the brain and the periphery for rapid information transfers seen in thought, movement and sensation.

Alternating or AC current

Alternating or AC current as delivered in the United States builds up voltage which is positive on top of the wave form and negative on the bottom pushing current through the system. The voltage source falls off and then changes direction back and forth – as long as current is moving in one direction or the other the object being powered will operate. The cycle repeats itself endlessly with the wave-form reversing polarity 60 times a second in the US to create what we know as "60 cycle house current". Alternating current has advantages over direct current for distribution that make it a better choice for transporting large amounts of power over long distances and it is the type of current used to power our homes.

Nerve impulses are a good example of AC current in the body. The action potential is an on/off spike carrying an impulse down a nerve that then repolarizes to be ready for the next discharge. The AC action potential allows the nervous system to operate like a computer, transferring and interpreting large amounts of information very rapidly by using a digital on/off data transfer and storage system.

Practical applications of DC current and the living semiconductor

In his 1985 book, The Body Electric, Robert Becker described his experiments on limb regeneration in salamanders. He concluded that the perineureum or glial membrane covering nerves serves as a primitive analog, direct current semiconducting information system that facilitates tissue repair and regeneration.

The normal difference between the more positively charged salamander's head (think of the brain as a battery) and his front leg is $-10mV$; the leg has more electrons than the head and is more negatively charged. When the salamander loses the limb to a predator (or to an orthopedic surgeon researcher such as Becker), the injured limb immediately becomes more positive, the current changes direction and electrons flow away from the injured site making it $+20$ mV more positive than the salamander's head. This reversal of current was called the "current of injury". Within a few days the current flow changes direction again and gradually becomes more negative as electrons flow into the injured area, presumably from the brain as battery, until it reaches $-30mV$. By the time the limb is completely regenerated at 25 days the charges are back to their baseline difference of $-10mV$ between the head and the leg.

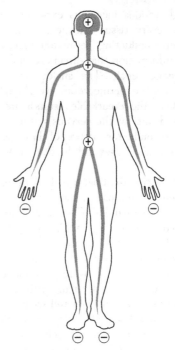

Figure 2.9 • Robert Becker demonstrated that the salamander and the human body are charged DC current systems. Humans and salamanders are more positively charged at the head and along the spine and more negatively charged distally at the ends of the arms and legs (adapted with permission from Becker & Seldon 1985).

Frogs and mammals do not regenerate severed limbs in their normal state and Becker discovered that they do not show the same changes in current flow and polarity as the salamander. In frogs and mammals, the site of injury remains positively charged, and electron deficient, until scarring and healing have been completed. Becker was able to create limb regeneration in frogs and rats by using a battery attached to the head to artificially induce the same pattern of electron flow in these animals that exists in the salamander. The DC current flow was the key to limb regeneration as long as the perineureum was intact. If the perineureum was removed regeneration would not occur.

He was also able to facilitate repair of experimentally induced spinal cord injuries in cats by using direct current to keep the electrical potential negative, electron rich, in the injured spinal cord. The untreated cord goes into "spinal shock", becomes electron deficient and electropositive and the normal course leads to a paraplegic outcome.

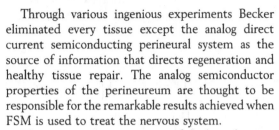

Through various ingenious experiments Becker eliminated every tissue except the analog direct current semiconducting perineural system as the source of information that directs regeneration and healthy tissue repair. The analog semiconductor properties of the perineureum are thought to be responsible for the remarkable results achieved when FSM is used to treat the nervous system.

The semiconductor nature of biological tissue creates some advantages and disadvantages for FSM treatments.

A head injury patient became dizzy in response to the frequency combination for "removing trauma" (94) from "the medulla" (94) when the contacts were placed at her neck (see Chapter 10). The dizziness resolved in a few minutes and when she felt normal again, she was asked to participate in an experiment. The contacts were placed at her knees and she was treated while sitting with the machine turned away so she could not tell what frequencies were being used. Four different combinations were tried for one minute each and each time the patient was asked how she felt. Each time she said she felt fine. As soon as the frequency combination 94Hz/94Hz was used, with the contacts at her knees, she became immediately dizzy and her eyes began to oscillate in a saccadic movement.

This response was interpreted to mean that the frequency for "removing trauma" from the "medulla" made this patient dizzy no matter where the contacts were placed but more importantly it meant that the frequency for "removing trauma" from "the medulla" would resonate with the medulla no matter where it was applied in the semiconductor matrix. The reaction to this frequency combination only occurs in a small percentage of patients who have a certain type of vestibular injury and its mechanism is not understood, but the reaction is so specific and characteristic that it is diagnostic. The implications of this discovery made it possible to treat the brain, through the semi-conductor matrix, by placing the contacts at the abdomen and back.

The disadvantages of this phenomenon dictate some of the precautions recommended in treatments discussed in the following chapters. The frequencies for removing scar tissue cannot be used any place in the body for six weeks after a new injury even if the current does not flow through the newly injured area. The body requires scar tissue to form in order to heal a new soft tissue injury. But, if the frequency to "remove scar tissue" will cause collagen cross links to vibrate and weaken by resonance, they will do

so no matter where they are applied in the semiconductor matrix that is the body.

4. The stable state

The patient's general physical and emotional health, conditioning, diet, hydration and history create an environment that will either support or erode the changes created by the frequencies and the current in any given treatment.

"Stable state" is a term from thermodynamics meaning the ability of an energy system to maintain equilibrium and implies a state of balance. In a state of equilibrium there are no unbalanced driving forces within the system and the system can maintain its energy state. For example water is completely stable as ice as long as the surrounding environment is 0°C. If you add energy to the system so that the water becomes a liquid it is completely stable as a liquid as long as the surrounding environment is between 0°C and 100°C. If you add energy to the system so that the water becomes steam it will remain in a vapor state as long as the surrounding temperate is above 100°C. But if the surrounding atmosphere doesn't support that state then the water molecules will drop back into the energy state that the system supports. It is the same with people; it is just more complicated.

In the human system the equilibrium is complex and dynamic and consists of physical, nutritional, biomechanical, emotional, neuro-endocrine, circulatory, neuromusculoskeletal and immunological factors that are affected by toxicity, allergies, chronic infections, disuse, misuse, trauma, scarring and other factors to mention what is certainly only a partial list.

Two stable state cases

Two patients presented to the clinic in the same week and their stories are the perfect illustration of the power of the stable state.

The first patient was a 54-year-old woman who worked as an executive secretary in a very high pressure company who presented with neck, shoulder and upper back pain of six years duration. She was a smoker of normal weight and height, eating a varied "normal" diet and did not enjoy exercise. She seemed tense, had a negative attitude about most things but did not consider herself to be depressed and was not being treated for depression. She presented with reduced cervical spine range of motion, multiple myofascial trigger points in all of the neck and shoulder muscles and pain of a 6–7/10 on a visual analog scale.

She was treated with FSM twice a week for six weeks. At the end of each treatment her pain was reduced from a 6/10 down to a 2/10. At the end of each treatment she was encouraged to drink more water to support tissue health and detoxification. She refused saying that she didn't like water and preferred coffee or tea. She was encouraged to change her posture at work and take hourly brief breaks to do shoulder shrugs and upper body stretches. She refused saying that she did not have time to stretch in her high pressure job and no time or attention to spare for such frivolous things. She was asked to purchase a magnesium supplement either from the clinic or a nutrition center to help the muscles relax. She replied that she knew for sure that supplements were a useless waste and only helped the manufacturers and retailers make money.

For six weeks she left every treatment session with her pain reduced from a 6/10 to a 2/10 and every post-treatment conversation was a repeat of the last one and her pain always returned within two days. FSM could change the muscles and reduce the pain but when she left the treatment room there was nothing in her body or emotions to maintain the changes. The ice that melted during treatment and became liquid was plunged back into the frigid environment of her life style and turned back into ice within two days.

The contrast between this patient and a 48-year-old man who came in for treatment at about the same time was striking. The man was a student at the National College of Naturopathic Medicine, a very demanding medical training program in Portland, who presented with pelvic and hip pain of 30 years duration acquired when he ran hurdles in high school track competitions. He meditated daily and did Tai Chi and Qi gong regularly in spite of his sedentary student lifestyle, had a vegetarian macrobiotic diet, took supplements regularly and drank at least two quarts of filtered water per day. He glistened with health and seemed happy and content. He presented with reduced range of motion in the right hip, multiple myofascial trigger points in the hip and pelvic floor muscles and pain of a 5–6/10 on a visual analog scale.

His pain was reduced from 6/10 to 0/10 at the end of the first treatment. He returned for the second treatment with pain of a 2/10 and was again pain free at the end of the treatment. He canceled his third

appointment because he had no remaining symptoms. We happened to meet in a grocery store one year later and he reported that his pain had never returned. His pain and muscle injury were more chronic than the secretary's but he responded more quickly because of his overall health, attitude and life style. The ice in his muscles melted and remained permanently liquid in the balmy environment of his life.

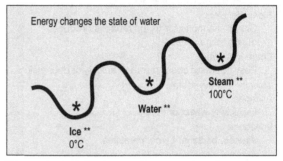

Figure 2.10 • Water is used as an analogy for a human "stable state". Water is completely stable as ice as long as the surrounding temperature is 0°C. It is stable as a liquid as long as the environment is between 0 and 100°C and stable as steam at 100°C and above. If the surrounding atmosphere doesn't support the state then the water molecules will drop back into the energy state that the system supports. People are the same way; it's just more complicated.

The stable state is the fourth component of any FSM treatment. The treatments described in this text predictably create remarkable changes in tissue, pain and function. But those changes have to be supported by the lifestyle, mental, physical, emotional and even spiritual milieu that is the patient's life if they are to become permanent.

The rapid improvement in symptoms and function create not only pain reduction but hope and can encourage patient compliance because the exercises, lifestyle and diet modifications that seemed futile before now seem worth the effort.

The practitioner is encouraged to pursue any training in nutrition, biomechanics, exercise, reconditioning, emotional support, motivation, detoxification strategies and allergy management that seems useful and interesting. This information will bear fruit in creating a stable state that allow changes produced by FSM treatments to persist.

Box 2.2

Stable state factors

Biomechanical factors
    Instability, disc bulges, leg length inequality
Deconditioning
General health
    Co-morbidities such as diabetes, obesity, asthma,
    irritable bowel
Nutritional deficiencies
    Insufficiencies
    Anti-oxidants and minerals
Sleep deficiency
    Growth hormone for tissue repair is produced
    during stage 4 sleep
Emotional stress
    Post-traumatic stress disorder, anxiety or depression
Toxicity – heavy metals
Allergies
    Especially wheat or milk
Infections
    Viruses, bacteria, Lyme, parasites

Box 2.3

Factors operating in each treatment

- The CURRENT increases in ATP and changes
  membrane protein function
- The FREQUENCIES resonates with pathologies and
  tissues to create changes
- The human SEMICONDUCTOR system that conveys
  information instantaneously throughout the body
- The STABLE STATE allows the changes to happen
  and helps them to persist

In every treatment each of these factors operates simultaneously and must be taken into consideration to some degree depending on the situation and the patient. The current increases ATP and changes protein synthesis and membrane protein function. The frequencies resonate with pathologies and tissues to create very specific predictable changes. The semiconductor matrix that conveys information throughout the body allows the effects of the frequencies to travel throughout the system. The stable state allows the changes to happen and helps them to persist and become permanent.

The model

One of the basic principles of science is that you cannot throw out the data because it doesn't match the model of how the system was thought to operate. When new data appears then the model has to change to allow for it. A new model for how the universe operates was required to explain the consistent, reproducible, and ultimately predictable changes observed with the application of frequencies and current to the human system.

This chapter is an incomplete model of the electromagnetic reality of human experience and should not be confused with the reality itself which is complex beyond imagining. It will take years to test, confirm or clarify the model and longer than that to appreciate the reality within which it operates, but in the meantime it aims to provide an intellectually satisfying framework that allows the practitioner reassurance in using the technique until a more complete understanding can be achieved.

Bibliography

Anderson, M., 2009. Is quantum mechanics controlling your thoughts? Discover Magazine, February 2009.

Becker, R.O., Seldon, G., 1985. The body electric: electromagnetism and the foundation of life. Quill, William Morrow, New York.

Becker, R.O., 1990. Cross currents. Jeremy Tarcher/Penguin, New York.

Cheng, N., et al., 1982. The effect of electric currents on ATP generation, protein synthesis, and membrane

transport in rat skin. Clinical Orthopedics 171, 264–272.

Huckfeldt, R., Mikkelson, D., Larson, K., et al., 2003. The use of micro current and autocatalytic silver plated nylon dressings in human burn patients: a feasibility study. Pacific Rim Burn Conference.

Kirsch, D.L., Lerner, F.N., 1998. Electromedicine: the other side of physiology. In: Weiner, R.S. (Ed.), Pain management, a practical guide

for clinicians, vol. 2. CRC Press, LLC Boca Raton Florida.

Lipton, B., 2008. The biology of belief: unleashing the power of consciousness, matter and miracles, second ed. Mountain of Love Productions, Hay House, Inc, Carlsbad, CA.

Oschman, J., 2000. Energy medicine, the scientific basis. Churchill Livingstone, Edinburgh.

Oschman, J.L., 2009. Mitochondria and cellular aging. In: Klatz, R.,

Goldman, R. (Eds.), Anti-aging therapeutics, vol. 11. American Academy of Anti-Aging Medicine, Chicago IL, pp. 185–194.

Reilly, W., Reeve, V.E., Quinn, C., 2004. Anti-inflammatory effects of interferential, frequency-specific

applied microcurrent. Proceedings of the Australian Health and Medical Research Congress.

Reilly, W., Reeve, V.E., 2005. Private communication – unpublished data from mouse study.

Szent-Györgyi, A., 1941. Towards a new biochemistry? Science 93, 609–611.

Szent-Györgyi, A., 1988. To see what everyone has seen, to think what no one has thought. Biol. Bull. 174, 191–240.

Treating neuropathic pain

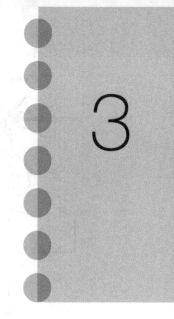

3

Although resistant to most medical treatment approaches neuropathic pain responds exceptionally well to frequency-specific microcurrent. The challenge for the practitioner is to recognize that the pain is neuropathic based on history, mechanism of injury, examination findings and response to previous therapies.

Neuropathic pain is typically difficult to treat medically and does not reduce significantly in response to narcotic or opiate medications. This characteristic can be useful in diagnosing pain as neuropathic and distinguishing neuropathic pain from other potential pain generators in the same area. Patients are usually asked to report pain on a 0 to 10 visual analog scale. Nerve pain tends to be moderate to severely painful and is commonly rated between a 5 and 9/10. If the pain is still reported as a 5–7/10 while the patient is being treated with narcotics the pain almost certainly has a strong neuropathic component.

Epidural injections at the nerve root with one of the "caine" class of anesthetics plus an anti-inflammatory steroid can reduce neuropathic pain. These injections, while done routinely, are invasive and expensive, require very specialized training and equipment, have significant risks and are not universally effective or permanent. But if an epidural injection has reduced the patient's pain, even temporarily, then it is almost certainly neuropathic pain.

Unlike acute pain from trauma which is mediated by the firing of primary afferent nociceptors, chronic neuropathic pain is mediated by inflammation in the nerves through the action of the inflammatory cytokines IL-1, IL-6, TNF-α, and substance P (Meyers 2006, Zieglgansberger 2005, Tal 1999).

FSM has been shown to reduce inflammatory cytokines while treating the pain of fibromyalgia associated with cervical spine trauma which is thought to be neuropathic. One specific frequency combination has been shown to reduce IL-1 (330 to 80pg/ml, $p = 0.004$), Il-6 (239 to 76pg/ml, $p = 0.0008$), TNF-α (305 to 78, $p=0.002$), and substance P (180 to 54pg/ml $p = 0.0001$) and to increase endorphins (8.2 to 71.1pg/ml, $p = 0.003$) Pain scores were reduced from an average of 7.3 ± 1.2 to 1.3 ± 1.1 in 45 of 54 patients ($p = 0.0001$) (McMakin 2005). The treatment that reduced the pain also reduced cytokines.

Studies have shown an association between induction of Cox-2 increased prostaglandin release and enhanced nociception in neuropathic pain. Expression of Cox-1 and Cox-2 in primary afferents and in the spinal cord suggests that NSAIDs act there by inhibiting synthesis of prostaglandins (Zieglgansberger 2005, Tal 1999, Bennett 2000).

A controlled trial using a mouse model for lipoxygenase (LOX) mediated inflammation demonstrated 62% reduction in ear swelling in mice treated with frequency-specific microcurrent (FSM) using 40Hz and 116Hz when compared with the controls. COX mediated inflammation was reduced in the same mouse model by 30% which was equivalent to the prescription anti-inflammatory injectable Toridol when it was tested using the same mouse model. FSM experimentation demonstrated the result to be reproducible, application time dependent, and specific as other FSM frequencies had no effect on the model (Reilly 2004).

An unpublished retrospective study of 20 neuropathic pain patients with a mean chronicity of 6.7 years showed reductions in pain from an average 6.8 ± 1.8 to 1.8 ± 2.1 ($p < 0.001$) during the first treatment. Pain was reduced from 4.8/10 to 0.97/10 during the second treatment ($p < 0.001$). 13 of the 20 patients had disc

© 2011, Elsevier Ltd.
DOI: 10.1016/B978-0-443-06976-5.00003-4

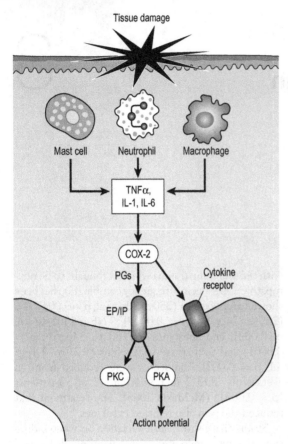

Figure 3.1 • Tissue damage stimulates the immune system to produce inflammatory cytokines (IL-1, IL-6, TNF-α) and prostaglandins cyclo-oxygenase (COX) and lipoxygenase (LOX) causing an action potential in a pain nerve.

injuries as the source of their neuropathic pain, two had nerve traction injuries and the other five patients had dermatomal nerve pain of unknown etiology. 65% (n = 13) of the patients recovered fully in an average of 4.6 treatments. 25% (n = 5) terminated care prior to recovery. One patient required an epidural and one patient uses a HomeCare microcurrent unit for palliative care (Precision Distributing Inc, Vancouver, WA) (McMakin, unpublished work, 2007). The only frequency combination observed to reduce dermatomal neuropathic pain is the frequency to reduce inflammation, found to be effective in the mouse model combined with the frequency for the nerve as a target tissue.

When the nerve becomes inflamed calcium ions flow into the nerve through voltage gated ion channels (Winquist 2005). The open channels create impulses interpreted as pain, the pain impulses travel up the nerve to the spinal cord and up the spinal cord to the pain processing centers in the brain.

Any inflamed tissue eventually experiences calcium influx and then fibrosis. Inflamed neural tissues are no exception. The concept of mobilizing fibrosed neural tissue and the surrounding fascia or dura has been well explored by Butler (1989a,b, 1991). FSM has well documented success in modifying scar tissue (Huckfeldt 2003) and its use in neural mobilization provides dramatic improvements over manual mobilization techniques both in comfort and in speed of response. The only frequency combinations observed to have an effect on neurofibrosis are those for scar tissue, sclerosis and fibrosis combined with the frequency for the nerve as a target tissue. The frequency to reduce pain does not reduce fibrosis or increase range of motion. If the nerve is traumatized by too vigorous stretching only the frequency to reduce inflammation will reduce the resulting pain.

When treating neuropathic pain with FSM, the practitioner must consider the mechanism of injury to the nerve, the relationships between the nerve and the surrounding or associated tissues, the patient's general state of health and overall inflammatory status and the possibility of central pain sensitization.

FSM is clinically derived. The frequencies were chosen through 10 years of experience according to the patient's clinical presentation and response to treatment and not as a result of exploration of the literature describing the pathology of neuropathic pain. It was convenient but not inevitable that the mechanisms of neuropathic pain derived by medical research match the frequencies found to be effective in relieving it.

It is important to remember that the patient is entitled to more than one pain generator and more than one diagnosis. It is not uncommon for a patient to have pain coming from the nerve, from trigger points in the muscles, from inflammation in the spinal facet joints or discs and from inflammation in the peripheral joint such as the shoulder or hip simultaneously and in any combination or proportion. Any and all of these pain generators can cause local pain as well as referred pain in the arms or legs. Being able to make the distinction between overlapping pain generators becomes important when deciding what to treat and assessing prognosis and setting expectations. If the neuropathic component can be treated quickly and easily and removed from diagnostic consideration, it simplifies the challenges of diagnosing and treating all chronic pain.

Frequency-specific microcurrent is low risk, cost effective and widely available – making it an ideal tool for treating neuropathic pain. The preliminary clinical data, cytokine data and collected anecdotal reports suggest that more formal controlled trials should be done to confirm FSM's benefits in neuropathic pain. Until such studies are completed, considering the low risks associated with its use, FSM can be a valuable adjunct in the treatment of neuropathic pain.

Types of nerve pain

Nerves come out of the spinal cord as nerve roots and describe sensory patterns known as dermatomes; cutaneous nerves are branches of dermatomal nerves and provide sensation to specific areas of the skin. Nerves become pain generators when they are injured. A complete description of all types of neuropathic pain and their mechanisms is beyond the scope of this text and the reader is referred to Neurology in Clinical Practice (Bradley 2000) for a comprehensive treatment of the subject.

This chapter will cover the diagnosis and treatment of dermatomal nerve pain due to spinal disc injuries and traction injuries, two of the compression neuropathies – carpal tunnel syndrome and thoracic outlet – and peripheral neuropathies due to diabetes. Information on more advanced strategies in the treatment of other types of neuropathic pain is available in an FSM seminar setting.

The treatments for different kinds of neuropathic pain are different and the key to successful treatment is an accurate diagnosis. The following sections are intended to help the reader arrive at an accurate clinical diagnosis.

Basic physical examination to evaluate nerve function

A skilled and thoughtful physical examination can reveal almost as much about nerve function as the most sophisticated imaging or electrodiagnostic testing. Sensation for sharp reveals the state of sensory nerve function and spinal cord facilitation. Muscle strength reveals the state of motor nerve function and deep tendon reflexes reveals the relationship between the nerves, the spinal cord, the muscles and the brain. Most practitioners reading this text have been trained to perform a physical examination to evaluate the nervous system. This brief description is meant to be a reminder and a guide to interpretation rather than a comprehensive instruction. The reader who desires more complete instruction is referred to a text on physical examination.

Sensory examination

The sensory nerves and spinal cord pathways for sharp also carry pain information. Gentle stroking of the nerve distribution with a pin or sharp object such as a paper clip or making light contact with a pinwheel as it rolls across the skin is sufficient stimulation to assess sensation for sharp and pain. Test one side and then the other being careful to use the same pressure on both sides. Evaluate the non-painful side first. Check all of the cervical, thoracic and lumbar dermatomes in a similar fashion at both the proximal and distal ends of the nerves. All dermatomes, not just those in the painful area should be tested during the initial evaluation. Any painful area should be tested for cutaneous nerve sensation and sensitization.

The examination can be done in any order that flows well and allows the organized gathering of information. The author starts with the patient seated facing the examiner with hands facing palms up on the thighs and tests the C6 dermatome on the thumb and forearm first and then proceeds to the other cervical dermatomes. Ask the patient to report whether the sensation caused by the sharp object feels "normal – just prickly or sharp", "dull – it feels like pressure but it doesn't feel sharp", or "icky or unpleasant". The patient may ask what "icky" feels like but most patients react strongly to sensory hyperesthesia, which is the medical term for an "icky" sensation. Most male patients cannot bring themselves to say "icky", but they will react in some way when the hyperesthetic nerve is stimulated. For these patients the distinction becomes sharp, dull and ouch (!). When nerves become inflamed they first become hypersensitive and then progress to numbness.

Occasionally a patient will describe an area as feeling numb but the sensory testing shows an appropriate appreciation of sharp. The patient is describing "paresthesia" or "feels as if it should be numb but it is not". Paresthesia often appears in the referred pain area for myofascial trigger points and can be mistaken for a description of neuropathic dysfunction.

If nerve function is impaired, the sensory examination may show either hyperesthesia or reduced sensation to sharp in a dermatomal nerve root, cutaneous nerve or in the glove/stocking pattern characteristic of a peripheral neuropathy. Record the findings on the dermatome chart as shown below. The record is a useful way to document progress as the nerves return to normal function with treatment.

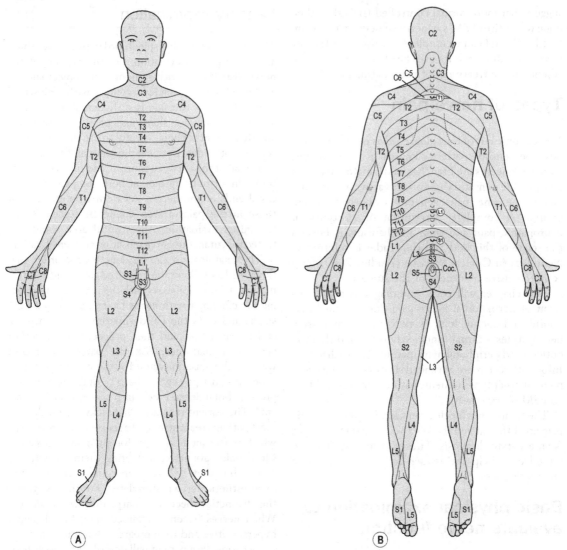

(A)   (B)

Figure 3.2 • This dermatome chart is only one of several versions of dermatomal sensory distribution commonly used. There are individual differences among patients and the sensory diagram is an approximation of nerve distribution in any given patient. Record the findings from the sensory examination on the dermatome diagram noting hyperesthesia, normal findings and reduced or absent sensation.

Reflex testing

Reflexes are tested with a quick strike of a reflex hammer or the examiner's rigid flexed fingers used to create a brisk tendon stretch of a muscle innervated by the nerve root being interrogated. The tendon stretch stimulates a reflex arc in the spinal cord and causes a brisk immediate muscle contraction in the stimulated muscle.

Deep tendon reflexes are rated from +1 to +4 to describe the strength of reflex muscle contraction

created by the tendon stretch. A +4/4 reflex involves clonus or rapid repeating involuntary muscle contractions due to complete loss of central descending inhibition in either the brain or the cord.

A normal reflex is graded as +2/4 and is characterized by a small brief brisk muscle contraction.

A reflex will be hyperactive and graded as +3/4 if the spinal cord is inflamed above the level being tested. A normal +2/4 reflex depends on descending inhibitory impulses from brain reaching the tested segment in time to dampen the reflex. Inflammation in the spinal cord slows the descending inhibitory impulses so they cannot reach the stimulated level in time to dampen the muscle contraction but not so much as to create clonus. The muscle contraction will be stronger than it should be and there may be simultaneous contraction of a muscle on the opposite side innervated by the same nerve root. The patellar reflex will be hyperactive if a disc bulge is inflaming the spinal cord above L3. If the cord is sufficiently inflamed the adductors (innervated by L3) will contract on the side opposite the one being tested.

A reduced reflex has little or no contractile amplitude or force and is graded as +1/4. Reduced reflexes may be a sign of nerve compromise caused by disc injury or some other segmental pathology. Reflexes are also reduced in hypothyroid patients and in all patients as they age. If a patient older than age 65 has a +2/4 (normal) patellar reflex it raises suspicion of some spinal cord inflammation above L3 since the patellar reflex is usually reduced in patients of this age.

An absent deep tendon reflex suggests a serious compromise of nerve function as the reflex arc is interrupted and the stretch response is either not conducted to the spinal cord from the tendon or from the spinal cord to the motor fibers.

Note: If the patient has engaged in some sport such as martial arts, racket ball, or sprinting that trains the quick twitch muscle fibers in the legs the patellar reflex may be reduced or absent without pathology. The quick stretch in the tendon should activate the neural arc and cause the quick twitch muscles to reflexively contract. If the quick twitch fibers have been sufficiently trained, they effectively "beat" the reflex arc and the quadriceps muscles do not contract in response to the tendon stretch. In this case the reflex findings must be evaluated in the context of the clinical presentation, the complete physical examination and history.

Muscle testing

To test motor function the examiner isolates a muscle associated with specific cervical and lumbar nerve roots and asks the patient to apply resistance to pressure. The muscle strength is graded from complete paralysis +0/5 to full strength +5/5. For complete instruction in the techniques and interpretation of manual muscle testing the reader should refer to a physical examination text such as Hoppenfeld's (1976).

If a weakened muscle is innervated by the same nerve root level that has hypersensitive or missing sensation and hypoactive reflexes it completes the clinical picture indicating significant neural compromise.

Clinical example

This basic clinical neurological examination can give a fairly detailed assessment of the condition of the spine and nerves and when combined with the patterns found in the history and the mechanism of injury eventually create a clear picture when all of the elements are analyzed.

For example if the patient was a 44-year-old right handed non-smoking male who exercises regularly and works as a computer programmer, complains of severe right shoulder and midscapular pain rated as 7/10 of two weeks duration that started after he used a pick to dig a trench in hard soil in the back yard, how would the source of his pain be discovered? Is it simply an injury to the shoulder or are the nerves, discs and neck involved?

History and mechanism of injury

The history gives basic parameters and a proposed mechanism of injury. The pain complaints are in the right shoulder in a right handed man and there is pain between the scapulae. Consider the mechanism of injury. The mechanism of injury comes from the ballistic forces of the pick striking the soil while the patient has the neck flexed looking down at the target. The ballistic forces from the impact translate into compressive forces on the disc when the cervical muscles contract forcefully to stabilize the spine. The shoulder muscles and joint structures are also challenged by the impacts. Neck flexion and rotation while the arms are raising the pick for the next impact create additional stress on the disc annulus. Eventually it becomes a "strength of materials" problem when the forces exerted simply overwhelm the structural integrity of the traumatized tissues.

The hypothesis is formed during the history and by observation of the pain diagram: the disc annulus fails, develops small fissures and the inflammatory chemicals in the disc nucleus become exposed to the nerve and the cord. The shoulder joint may also be compromised by the same forces.

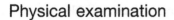

Physical examination

The basic physical examination will disclose the condition of the nerves and joints and either confirm or contradict the hypothesis.

In our computer programmer, sensation in the right and left C4 dermatome, and the right C5 and C6 dermatomes were hyperesthetic. All other dermatomes had normal sensation for sharp.

The patellar reflex was hyperactive bilaterally and striking the right patellar tendon caused the left adductors to contract, indicating spinal cord inflammation above L3. The biceps (C5) and brachioradialis (C5–6) reflexes on the right were slightly reduced, and the triceps reflex on the right was slightly more brisk than the triceps on the left. All other deep tendon reflexes were +2/4 or brisk and considered "normal".

Muscle testing revealed slight weakness in the right biceps and forearm flexors; all other muscles were full strength and rated +5/5.

Palpation of the muscles in the cervical spine and shoulder revealed trigger points and tenderness in most of the shoulder muscles and in the muscles of the anterior cervical spine especially at the C5–6 level.

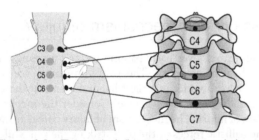

Figure 3.3 • The cervical disc annulus refers pain in between the shoulder blades stepwise down the spine according to the levels injured. The presence of mid-scapular pain helps diagnose the presence of an injured disc as the cause of neuropathic pain. It should be kept in mind that there are nine muscles, seven thoraco-costal joints and seven cervical facet joints that also refer to the midscapular area (adapted with permission from Cloward 1959).

Interpretation and diagnosis

The physical examination suggests that he had a small contained right, paracentral disc herniation at C5–6 brushing the thecal sac at the spinal cord that was not large enough to compress the nerve root since nerve functions were altered but not eliminated.

The central portion of the disc inflamed the cord enough to create hyperactive patellar reflexes

bilaterally, crossed adductor contraction and the hyperactive right triceps reflex. The reflex can be hyperactive at any level below the inflammation. The disc was close enough to the nerve and the cord at C5 and C6 on the right to reduce the right C5 and C5–6 reflex arcs and create slight muscle weakness in the biceps. The sensory nerves at C4, C5 and C6 were inflamed by the disc material and became hypersensitive. Muscle palpation revealed myofascial trigger points in the anterior scalenes over the C5 and C6 disc levels and trigger points in most of the shoulder muscles, which are innervated by the C5 and C6 nerve roots.

The history and reported pain pattern suggested a disc injury at C5–6. The ballistic compression damaged the disc annulus which inflamed the nerves and the cord. The midscapular pain is consistent with referred pain from the disc annulus (Cloward 1959).

The MRI confirmed the findings suggested by the history and physical examination. FSM treatment and a home exercise program resolved the pain and normalized the neurological examination in 8 treatments over four weeks.

Dermatomal nerve pain due to disc injuries

Spinal nerve roots most commonly become painful because of exposure to the inflammatory chemicals released by the spinal discs. The central part of the disc, or nucleus pulposus, is rich in a highly inflammatory substance called phospholipase-A$_2$ (PLA$_2$). PLA$_2$ has the ability to turn ordinary membranes into the cellular equivalent of battery acid, damages the nerve and eventually impairs its ability to conduct impulses (Ozaktay 1995, 1998). If the disc ruptures and releases a piece of nucleus material it is said to herniate. If the disc nucleus is injured but remains contained within the disc annulus it is said to be a contained herniation. If the herniated disc material forms a fragment and compresses the nerve it can create serious damage to the nerve including complete loss of sensory and motor function and compromise of deep tendon reflexes which may become permanent if not treated appropriately. A surgical consult is prudent if reflexes or muscle strength is lost even if the patient is to be treated with FSM.

It is possible for the disc to be minimally damaged with a small tear in the annulus that allows the PLA$_2$ in the nucleus to leak out and create chemical inflammation in the nerve (Olmarker 1993, 1995). This has been called "chemical neuritis" (Marshall 1977).

Inflammation in the posterior joints of the spine called facet joints can diffuse out to the nerve roots and create neuropathic pain and osteophytes from the facet joints can both inflame and mechanically compress dermatomal nerves. Any condition or pathology that creates an inflammatory response in the vicinity of the nerve can contribute to or cause neuropathic inflammation and pain.

Diagnosing neuropathic pain from disc injuries

The history will include a mechanism that would explain a disc injury usually involving flexion, flexion combined with rotation, a whiplash movement from an auto accident or a fall with ballistic compressive impact to the spine. Lifting or postural strain involving repetitive flexion of the neck or trunk, especially when flexion is combined with rotation, can injure a disc. Prolonged static position that places the weight loaded spine in combined flexion and rotation, such as falling asleep for four hours with the head on chest, can weaken the disc annulus through connective tissue creep. A disc does not have to be herniated to cause neuropathic pain. When there is a temporal association between onset of dermatomal pain symptoms and some trauma or change in activity that involves flexion and rotation, common sense suggests the connection and the need for treating both the nerve and the disc.

Diagnosing dermatomal nerve pain due to nerve traction injuries

Nerves can be injured mechanically by forces that cause traction or pull on the nerve, damaging the nerve membrane, creating inflammation from glial activation, pain, sensory changes and even motor weakness. Look for a mechanism of injury that involves one end of the nerve being held stationary while the other end of the nerve is stretched or pulled away.

Nerve traction injuries are typically created in auto accidents, falls, and contact sports and by positioning or procedures during surgery. The brachial plexus is particularly vulnerable to traction injuries since the C5 through C8 nerves are tethered to the vertebra as they leave the spine by ligaments while the distal ends of these nerves are free to move. Patient position

during a surgery in which the nerve is statically stretched for a prolonged period such as a cardiac bypass procedure or a cervical tumor dissection can create nerve traction injuries. Surgery in which the nerve is stretched acutely along with the soft tissue to make room for a knee or hip replacement can also create persistent neuropathic pain. Nerve traction injuries may heal without treatment over time as the nerve lining slowly repairs itself but many nerve traction injuries remain painful for years after the trauma and never become pain free on their own.

The diagnosis of a nerve traction injury is made on the basis of the pain pattern, the history and the neuro-sensory examination. The patient will describe pain that matches one or more dermatomal nerves. The history will include a mechanism of injury that could stretch a nerve. The physical examination will show sensory hyperesthesia or sensory loss in a dermatome that matches the patient's pain complaint. The reflexes will be +2/4 or brisk and considered normal unless the mechanism of injury included a flexion and rotation component that caused a disc bulge as well as the nerve traction injury. The patient, as always, is entitled to more than one complaint.

Examples of nerve traction injuries

The auto accident patient holding the steering wheel with both hands when the air bag deployed into her chest rapidly stretching the thoracic nerve roots, had nerve traction injuries to the thoracic intercostal nerves. She was diagnosed with "costochondritis" for 20 months following the accident. The sensory examination showed hyperesthesia from T2 to T6 nerve roots and the "costochondritis" resolved permanently in a single 60 minute treatment for neuropathic pain from a nerve traction injury.

The police officer who landed on the ground under the suspect with his trunk left rotated and his right arm stretched around the torso of the DCS (drunken combative suspect) was diagnosed with a "chronic thoracic sprain strain" for three years following the injury. In all that time no one had done a sensory examination. The sensory examination revealed hyperesthesia in the right T4 through T7 dermatomes and the patellar reflex was hyperactive on the right only. The MRI showed a small disc bulge (contained herniation) at T5. The injury resolved in three 60 minute treatments for the nerve and an additional three treatments for the disc.

The patient was the seat-belted driver with her trunk turned to the right at the time of a side impact collision. The car spun to the left creating traction of the left side of her neck and left arm. Fourteen months after the accident she still complained of left shoulder and chest pain, left arm weakness, tingling in her fingers and lower arm. She had been diagnosed with thoracic outlet syndrome. Her sensory examination showed hyperesthesia of the left C5 through T1 nerve roots and completely normal reflexes at all levels. Her pain was reduced from 6/10 to 2/10 with the first 60 minute treatment and she was pain free with full strength and range of motion after six treatments.

Once it becomes possible to resolve nerve traction injuries the clinician is more likely to diagnose and treat them.

Treating nerve traction injuries with FSM

FSM treatment for nerve traction injuries uses the frequencies to reduce inflammation, reduce fibrosis between the fascia and nerve and to improve secretions in the nerve. Nerve traction injuries respond very well to FSM as long as the nerve is not torn because there is no perpetuating factor. The sensory distribution of the injured nerves may be hypersensitive or it may have reduced or absent sensation to sharp as tested with a pin or a pinwheel. If the nerve is not torn the pain and sensory changes should resolve in two to four treatments. Motor weakness may require more treatments and may take longer to resolve than pain and sensory changes.

In one case involving a professional football player who lifted a tackle off of his back using his neck, the pain and sensory changes resolved with treatment for the nerve traction injury created by the forceful lateral flexion of his neck. But the motor weakness in the external rotators would not resolve even after three treatments. The weak muscles were all innervated by the subscapular nerve which travels through a small foramen on the scapula immediately adjacent to the attachment of the levator scapulae. It became apparent eventually that the swelling caused by the muscle strain injury to the levator was compressing and inactivating the motor nerve. Treating the injured muscle and using Russian stim to make it contract and then treating the motor nerve resolved the muscle weakness in less than an hour.

If the nerve root is torn the area of sensory loss may become smaller during treatment but the numbness does not resolve. If the nerve is torn, the pain will be reduced but not eliminated during treatment and returns within hours. The treatment is so consistently effective that a lack of response to FSM treatment suggests that the nerve root is torn and suggests the need for a neurology consult and medical management.

Note on the C2 nerve root

The C2 nerve root exits the spine at C1–C2 and innervates the posterior portion of the scalp up to an imaginary line drawn across the top of the head between the ears and provides sensation along a thin stripe on the lower portion of the jaw and upper neck. This nerve can be tractioned or crushed during whiplash injuries. The key to diagnosis will be complaint of an intense headache at the back of the skull. If the patient says, "I have had a migraine every day since the accident that doesn't respond to migraine medication", check sensation in the C2 nerve root. In cases such as this the C2 dermatome will be strongly hyperesthetic. If C2 should happen to be numb it usually means that the nerve has been crushed and may not respond well to treatment. Treat with the protocols for any nerve traction injury. The prognosis is guarded if the nerve is numb initially and optimistic if the nerve is hyperesthetic.

Treating dermatomal nerve pain

 Hydration

- The patient must be hydrated to benefit from microcurrent treatment.
- Hydrated means 1 to 2 quarts of water consumed in the 2 to 4 hours preceding treatment.
- Athletes and patients with more muscle mass seem to need more water than the average patient.
- The elderly tend to be chronically dehydrated and may need to hydrate for several days prior to treatment in addition to the water consumed on the day of treatment.
- *DO NOT* accept the statement, "I drink lots of water"
- *ASK* "How much water, and in what form, did you drink today before you came in?"
- Coffee, caffeinated tea, carbonated cola beverages do not count as water.
- Water may be flavored with juice or decaffeinated tea.

Channel A: condition frequencies

The frequencies listed are thought to remove or neutralize the condition for which they are listed except for 81 and 49 / which are thought to increase secretions and vitality respectively. They are listed alphabetically not in order of use or importance. Frequencies rationale is explained in the treatment protocol.

- Calcium ions   91 /
- Chronic inflammation   284 /
- Emotional shock   970
- Histamine   9/
- Inflammation   40 /
- Paralysis   321 /
- Scarring   13 /
- Sclerosis   3 /
- Secretions (Increase)   81 /
- Trauma   94 /
- Vitality   49 /

Channel B: tissue frequencies

- Dermatomal or Peripheral Nerve: ___ / 396
  - Any nerve outside the spinal cord
- Fascia: ___ / 142
  - Fascia is the thin connective tissue covering surrounding the muscles and virtually all visceral tissue. Nerves travel in a fascia–nerve–fascia sandwich. Any time a nerve is inflamed or injured the fascia becomes inflamed to some extent and adhesions will develop between the nerve and the fascia.
- Disc Annulus: ___ / 710
  - The well innervated disc annulus is the most pain sensitive and most easily injured portion of the disc. It consists of coiled layers of sturdy connective tissue wrapped around the gel like nucleus.
- Disc Nucleus: ___ / 330
  - The gel like disc nucleus fills the center of the disc and absorbs water to become a cushion for the vertebral bodies in the spine. It is very high in PLA_2 and very inflammatory.
- Disc as whole: ___ / 630
  - This frequency is thought to address the entire disc structure.

- Muscle Tissue as a tissue type: ___ / 46
  - This frequency is rarely used and is thought to possibly represent the sarcomere or some contractile portion of the muscle. Combining the frequency to "increase secretions" in the nerve and "muscle tissue" has been observed to eliminate neuropathic atrophy in numerous cases. This protocol has no effect on disuse atrophy.

Treatment protocol

Channel A condition / Channel B tissue

Reduce the pain

40 / 396

- Reduce inflammation / in the nerve
- 40 / 396 polarized positive is consistently effective in reducing nerve pain.
- Current polarized positive +
- Positive leads at the spine – Negative leads at the distal end of the nerve. See photos for details of set up.
- *Treatment time.* Use 40 / 396 until the pain has been reduced to approximately 2/10 on a 0 to 10 VAS scale. In most cases of dermatomal nerve pain this will take approximately 20–30 minutes but it may take up to an hour. Pain reduction usually begins distally and progresses proximally. If the patient is on narcotics or is dehydrated or has low essential fatty acid levels due to poor diet or lack of supplementation, response may be slow or poor. See the notes on what to do if response to treatment is slow.
- It is essential to reduce the pain by using 40 / 396 before treating the nerve for any other pathology.

 Stenosis precaution

If there is dense scar tissue or bony stenosis of the nerve root or spinal cord or if a disc fragment is compressing the nerve root or cord at the involved level the patient's pain may increase when polarized positive current is applied. If the patient is positioned comfortably, it is the only time the pain will increase during polarized positive treatment for nerve inflammation. It may increase in the dermatome or at the spine or both. Assess patient position to determine whether it is contributing to the pain increase.

Continued

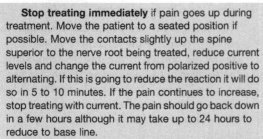

Stop treating immediately if pain goes up during treatment. Move the patient to a seated position if possible. Move the contacts slightly up the spine superior to the nerve root being treated, reduce current levels and change the current from polarized positive to alternating. If this is going to reduce the reaction it will do so in 5 to 10 minutes. If the pain continues to increase, stop treating with current. The pain should go back down in a few hours although it may take up to 24 hours to reduce to base line.

This reaction is diagnostic. If physical examination findings of reduced sensation and deep tendon reflexes at the involved level or hyperactive deep tendon reflexes below the involved level are present this reaction suggests the need to x-ray or perform an MRI to confirm the presence of compression.

Remove the basic pathologies / from the nerve

970, 94, 321, 9 / 396

- Remove the emotional component, remove nerve trauma, restore function, and remove histamine / from the nerve
- This sequence comes from Van Gelder's concept of concussion as discussed in Chapter 10. In Van Gelder's model, emotional shock and trauma leads to "paralysis" which leads to "allergy reaction" and reduction in secretions and vitality.
- "Emotional shock" from an injury or trauma changes tissue function; 970 / takes the "fact of" this emotional shock out of the membrane.
- "Trauma" stuns the nerve, overloading it rather like a power surge that trips a circuit breaker causing it to switch into something like a "safe mode." The "safe mode" preserves the most important critical functions and allows for repair and recovery at some later time.
- "Paralysis" does not refer to complete loss of function or true medical paralysis. The analogy to the loss of function when a computer "locks up" and loses the ability to move to the next step is most apt. The fact of the trauma interferes with the smooth transfer of information within the tissue that allows it to know what to do next. The frequency to remove "paralysis" is Van Gelder's conceptual equivalent of the computer command "control–alt–delete" that reboots the computer system.
- "Allergy Reaction" refers to the body's first response to any dysfunction which is to release histamine as a way of starting the inflammatory

cascade. Removing the allergy reaction allows the tissue to complete the return to normal function.
- *Note*: These four frequencies are known collectively as "The Basics". They are usually used in sequential order as a group combined with the channel B frequency for the injured tissue but each can be used individually as needed based on the patient's condition.
- Treatment time. Use each frequency for 1 to 2 minutes each. Current polarized positive.

Remove pathologies from the nerve

284 / 396

- Chronic Inflammation / Nerve
- Treatment time: Use 284 / 396 for 2 to 5 minutes after treating with 40 / 396 when the pain is down to a 2–3/10 and when the nerve pain has been present for longer than 3 months. Acute and chronic inflammation coexist and 284 / has a different but complementary affect on chronic nerve pain.

 Precaution: induced euphoria

Treating inflammation and chronic inflammation in the nerve has a curious effect on affect and cognitive function. Most, but not all, patients will experience an "induced euphoria" that is characteristic of this treatment. It is most pronounced while using 40 / 396 and the practitioner may want to reassure the patient that it is a normal effect as it begins. The first sign will be a reduction in the rate of blinking, respiration and speech that starts within 10 to 15 minutes. Some patients fall asleep and some get so "stoned" that they do not wish to or simply cannot speak.

This is a temporary effect and will wear off as the other frequencies are used.

The patient will remain relaxed but will come to full function within an hour or so after treatment. Most patients are in full possession of their faculties by the time they are dressed and ready to leave the clinic. The practitioner should take care to ensure that the patient is safe to drive. In extreme cases patients have been warned against making important financial decisions until the effect has worn off. The effect is most profound in the first few treatments.

Treat the disc – if nerve pain is discogenic

40 / 330, 630, 710

- Remove inflammation / in the disc nucleus, the disc as a whole and the disc annulus

- If the pain is from a nerve traction injury it is not necessary to treat the disc
- Treatment time: 4 minutes each

Soften the tissue

91 / 396
- Remove Calcium Ions / from the Nerve

91 / 142
- Remove Calcium Ions / from the Fascia

The frequency 91Hz was originally thought to remove calcium from "stones" in the kidney or bile duct as indicated by its description on Van Gelder's list of frequencies. In July 2003, it was used for the first time to treat "hardening in the fascia" in the legs of a professional football player because his muscles and fascia felt like "stones" as they were being treated; 91Hz produced remarkable softening in the fascia. Its usefulness in treating nerve pain was a late accidental discovery and its effectiveness was a pleasant surprise.

As it turns out, calcium ions flow into nerve and fascial membranes during nerve depolarization and inflammation (Winquist 2005). Using 91/396, 142 seems to remove the calcium influx that perpetuates nerve pain and hardens the fascia around the nerve although there are no biopsy findings to confirm this. Clinically these frequency combinations produce profound softening of the tissue and reductions in pain and the exact mechanism of these changes is yet to be discovered.

- Treatment time: Use these combinations for 2 to 5 minutes each or until the softening response slows or stops. Current Polarized Positive +.

Treatment application

Current level

- 100–300µamps for the average healthy patient.
- Use lower current levels of 20–60µamps for very small or debilitated patients. Current levels above this will be irritating and may make the patient restless or agitated.
- Use higher current levels of 300–500µamps for larger or very muscular patients.
- In general, higher current levels reduce pain more quickly and improve response.
- Do not use more than 500µamps as animal studies suggest that current levels above 500µamps reduce ATP formation.

- Current Polarized Positive +: Current is polarized positive for most nerve treatments except for shingles (see Chapter 9) and peripheral neuropathies which require alternating DC current. Nerves respond very well and very quickly to polarized positive current.
- Waveslope: The waveslope refers to the rate of increase of current in the ramped square wave as it rises in alternating mode from zero up to the treatment current level every 2.5 seconds on the Precision Microcurrent and the automated family of FSM units. Other microcurrent instruments may have slightly different wave form choices. A sharp waveslope has a very steep leading edge on the square wave shape indicating a very sharp increase in current. A gentle waveslope has a very gradual leading edge on the waveform indicating a gradual increase in current.
  - Use a moderate to sharp waveslope for chronic pain.
  - Use a gentle waveslope for acute pain or new injuries. A sharp waveslope is irritating in new injuries.

Lead placement

- Positive leads. The positive leads contact wraps around the neck or is placed along the spine at the exiting nerve root. The positive contact must cover at least the foramenal area where the nerve exits the spine
- Negative leads. The negative leads attached to an adhesive electrode or wrapped in the warm wet fabric towel are placed at the end of the dermatome or nerve being treated. The placement is shown in the photographs.
- Electrode Contacts. FSM typically uses graphite gloves to conduct the current but any conductor can be used as long as it has low resistance and can be wrapped around the spine at the exiting nerve root and have good contact with the distal end of the nerve being treated.
- Adhesive electrode pads can be used if they are long enough (3 inches) to encircle the foramenal area where the nerve exits the spine and to give good contact at the distal end of the nerve.

The graphite gloves need to be kept moist so they conduct the current comfortably. The current will prickle and irritate if the gloves become dry.

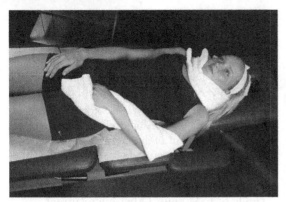

Figure 3.4 • The positive leads are placed in a warm wet towel wrapped around the neck. The fabric contact does not have to encircle the neck as long as the neural foramen are covered.

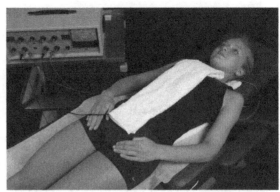

Figure 3.7 • The negative leads are placed in a warm wet towel at the terminus of the thoracic nerve roots. Adhesive electrode pads would be placed lengthwise at the end of the involved thoracic nerve root.

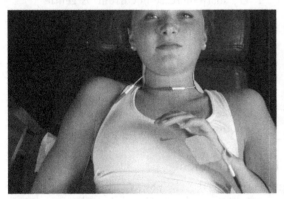

Figure 3.5 • Low resistance, silver adhesive electrode pads (2 inches × 3.5 inches) can be used for treating dermatomal nerve pain. The positive leads are attached so they cover the neural foramen. The negative leads are placed at the end of the affected nerve root. The set up for the C6 dermatome is shown in the photograph.

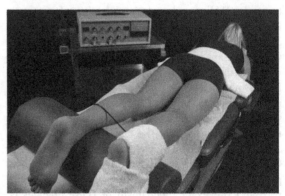

Figure 3.8 • The positive leads are placed in a warm wet towel placed across the low back so the contact covers the lumbar nerve foramen. The negative leads are placed in a warm wet towel wrapped around the foot for L4, L5 and S1. Adhesive electrode pads would be placed at the end of the dermatome being treated.

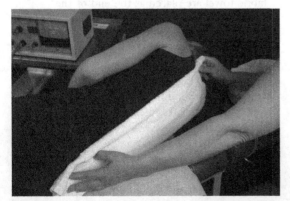

Figure 3.6 • Positive leads are placed in a warm wet hand towel positioned lengthwise down the spine. Adhesive pads would be placed lengthwise at the spine at the level of the affected nerve roots.

The graphite gloves can be wrapped in a warm wet hand towel or leads can be attached to the fabric using alligator clips.

Treatment of cranial nerve pain such as trigeminal neuralgia and Bell's palsy in the facial nerve is challenging because these nerves originate inside the brain and running current through the brain is not recommended. There is some success in treating these two nerves by placing one contact inside the external ear canal and the other out on the face at the end of the nerve distribution but it is by no means as successful as treating spinal and peripheral nerves.

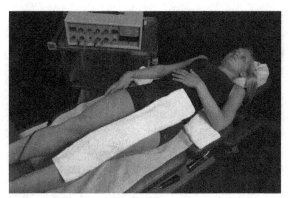

Figure 3.9 • The negative leads contact is placed at the end of the L1, L2 or L3 nerve roots. This placement would be useful for femoral nerve traction injuries due to hip replacement surgery or sports injuries.

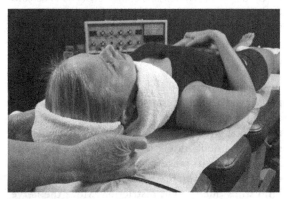

Figure 3.10 • The positive leads are placed in a warm wet towel wrapped around the neck. The negative leads are placed on the top of the head at the end of the C2 nerve root. This nerve cannot be treated with adhesive electrode pads. To move the nerve through its range have the patient tip the chin gently downward and then back to neutral.

Patient position

The patient can be placed prone or supine or in any comfortable position in which the body is well supported. Patients can become very relaxed during this protocol and may fall asleep so the head and trunk should be well supported. Positioning a patient in a way that increases pain (by putting a disc patient in flexion or putting a patient with facet joint problems in extension) can confound interpretation of treatment results.

Improve motion in the nerve

13 / 396
* Remove scarring / from the Nerve
13 / 142
* Remove scarring / from the Fascia
3 / 396
* Remove sclerosis / from the Nerve
3 / 142
* Remove sclerosis / from the Fascia
* Current Polarized Positive

When nerve pain improved after treatment, the patient usually increased activities and would report that the pain returned when activities required an increase in range of motion. Experience with treatment revealed the mechanism of the increased pain and suggested its remedy. Nerves travel in a fascia–nerve–fascia sandwich. When the nerve has been inflamed it adheres to the surrounding fascia and restricts motion when the patient attempts to move the limb through its normal range of motion during return to normal activities, exercise or physical therapy (Lewis 2004, Butler 1991). Treating with frequencies to remove scarring and sclerosis between the nerve and the fascia improves range of motion during the treatment, creates longer lasting pain relief and immediately improves function.

Treatment time – manual technique

13 / and 3 / while having subtly different effects on tissue are similar enough in reducing adhesions between the nerve and fascia that the reader may try either one for increasing range of motion in the nerve.

13 / seems to be more affective in changing dense scar tissue. 3 / changes a stiffer "stringier" kind of adhesion. The practitioner will eventually be able to palpate the difference in response to the two frequencies and after some experience will be able to determine by the feel of the tissue before treatment which frequency is most likely to produce the optimal change.

Slowly and **carefully** move the nerve through its range either actively or passively while treating with 13 or 3 / 396.

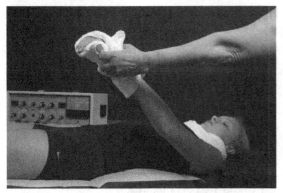

Figure 3.11 • #1 Arm movement of cervical nerve through its range while running 13 / 396. While using the frequencies 13 / 396 move the arm until the patient reports the first sign of discomfort or sense of tightness and then stop and return the arm to neutral.

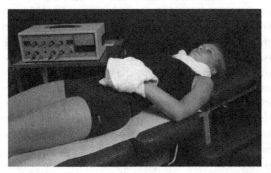

Figure 3.12 • #2 Arm movement of cervical nerve resting in neutral while running 13 / 396. Allow the arm to rest in neutral for one to two minutes as the frequencies 13 / 396 are being used.

To improve motion in extremity nerves move the involved limb in such a way as to stretch the nerve until the patient reports some slight sensation of pressure or pain. To stretch and treat thoracic nerves have the patient expand the chest and move the intercostals nerves by taking a deep breath or by rotating the torso until the patient experiences a sensation of pressure or slight discomfort. To stretch and treat the suboccipital nerves have the patient gently tip the chin towards the chest while the contacts are held at the neck and at the top of the head at the end of the C2 nerve root.

Take care to stop at the first sign of pressure or discomfort.

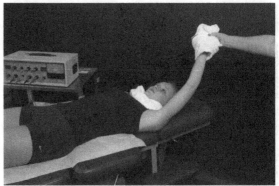

Figure 3.13 • #3 Arm movement of cervical nerve towards its end range while running 13 / 396. Move the arm through its range and stop when the patient reports the first sign of discomfort. The range should have increased. Return the arm to neutral and repeat the process until the range of motion in the affected limb is full and pain free. It may take several repetitions of this sequence to achieve full range. Be aware of joint restrictions and the anatomical limits of the joint and nerves being treated.

When the patient experiences a sense of tightness or the beginnings of pain, stop the nerve stretch and move the nerve back to a neutral pain free position. Treat with 13 or 3 / 396 for 1 minute and then slowly and deliberately have the patient move the nerve through its range again. The range of pain free motion usually increases by 20–30% unless the limb stops due to joint restriction. Move the nerve back to its pain free position and continue to run either 13 / 396 or 3 / 396 for one to two minutes. Move the nerve again to the edge of comfort and continue this process until the range is normal and pain free. It normally takes three to five repetitions over 5 to 10 minutes to achieve pain free full range of motion.

Use 40 / 396 to reduce any increase in pain created during this process.

If pain increases during this process because the nerve has been stretched too far or too fast change the frequency and treat with 40 / 396 until the pain is eliminated. Resume the process of increasing the range of motion with 13 / 396 once the pain is reduced to 0–2/10. Be aware of joint restrictions to motion and reasonable anatomical limits of motion for the nerve and joints being treated.

This process usually requires 10 to 15 minutes but can occasionally require as much as 30 minutes or as little as 5 minutes to normalize nerve function.

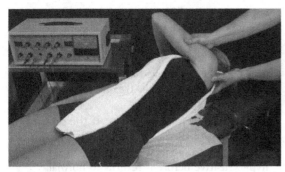

Figure 3.14 • #1 Trunk movement to increase range of motion in thoracic nerve roots. Move the thoracic and intercostal nerves by rotating the torso or by having the patient take a deep breath to increase range of motion in the thoracic nerve roots while running 13 / 396.

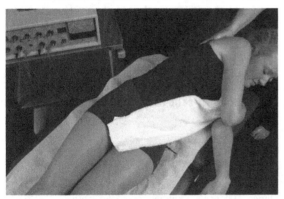

Figure 3.15 • #2 Trunk movement to increase range of motion in thoracic nerve roots. Rotate the torso in both directions to move the thoracic and intercostals nerves to increase range of motion in the thoracic nerve roots while running 13 / 396.

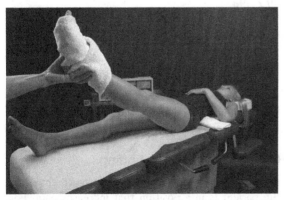

Figure 3.16 • #1 Leg movement to increase range of motion in L4, L5 or S1 nerves. While running 13 / 396 raise the involved leg until the patient reports slight discomfort or sense of tightness. Stop movement and return leg to rest position. Wait 1 to 2 minutes and then repeat leg raise.

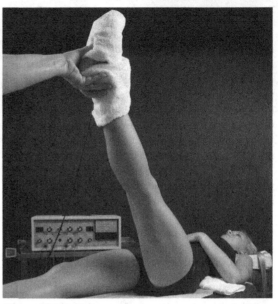

Figure 3.17 • #2 Leg movement towards end of range. While still using 13 / 396 raise the leg again and the motion should be freer and the range should be increased. If full range has not been achieved repeat the process until leg has reached a range limited not by nerve pain but by muscle tightness or joint limits.

Note: Practitioners are advised to operate within the limits of their training in physical medicine and to be careful and prudent while moving joints and nerves with this protocol.

Improve sensation restore function
81 / 396, 46

- Current polarized positive
- Increase secretions / in the nerve and the muscle: Once the pain is eliminated or reduced to the 0–2/10 range, and sensation is normal and the motion is close to full and pain free it is important to restore normal secretions in the nerve.

Precaution: Only use 81/396 when pain is reduced to 0–2/10. 81 / increases secretions and when pain is moderate one of the secretions increased appears to be substance P. Pain has been known to increase if 81 / 396 is used while pain remains moderate. Use 40 / 396 to reduce pain. Use 81 / 396 only when pain is 0–2/10

Treatment rationale and case experience

81Hz had been observed to increase secretion in various organs whose secretions can be easily measured. In a postmenopausal woman whose salivary estrogen measured 1.4 only the frequency to "increase secretion in the ovary" (81 / ovary) increased salivary estrogen from 1.4mg/ml to 37.1mg/ml in 30 minutes. Once the frequency was changed away from 81 / ovary, the estrogen levels dropped back to normal pre-treatment levels within 30 minutes.

81Hz was first used to treat the nerve and muscle when a professional body builder presented with atrophy in the distal five inches of the vastus lateralis muscle in the thigh. He had torn the quadriceps muscle away from the patella by doing a squat with 800 pounds on his shoulders and his 18 months of postoperative rehabilitation had restored all but the last five inches of the muscle. This section of muscle was atrophied and flat in contrast to the rest of his very well-developed quadriceps. Treating with 40 / 396 and polarized positive current, from the low back to the knee and treating to remove the scar tissue from the nerve and fascia restored muscle tone – the last five inches of the muscle popped up to normal conformation. But the muscle became flat again after one or two contractions.

When this pattern continued after three repetitions of treatment and test, it seemed obvious that there was some secretion between the nerve and the muscle that was adequate for two contractions but insufficient for full function. This treatment in March 2003 was the first time that 81 / 396, 46 was used clinically. We have no data to show what "nerve or muscle secretions" might be increasing but acetylcholine is a reasonable guess given the change in function that occurred. Treating with 40 / 396 caused the muscle to plump up and return to its normal conformation in approximately 5 minutes. Upon using 81 / 396 for 5 minutes, the muscle contracted normally and had full strength for repeated contractions. The patient was instructed to recondition it carefully and the improvement was reported to be permanent in a one year follow-up. This effect has been duplicated in numerous patients. The mechanism by which the change in muscle tone and conformation occurs is not known. This protocol has no effect on muscle tone or function caused by disuse atrophy.

- *Treatment time for restoring motor function*: Treat with 81 / 396 and 81 / 46 for five minutes each while the muscle is at rest. Change in muscle

appearance should become apparent after 10 minutes. Alternate use of the two combinations for five minutes each for up to 30 minutes until normal function has returned. If no positive effect has been achieved after 30 minutes then it is unlikely that further treatment will be helpful.

- *Treatment time for sensory loss*: If the sensory distribution of the nerve was numb, it is normal for the area to progress from numb to hypersensitive before it returns to normal sensation. The period of hyperesthesia is temporary and treatment with 81 / 396 using polarized positive current for two minutes alternating with 40 / 396 used for five minutes should continue until the sensation returns to normal. Be patient with this phase of treatment; it may take up to 30 to 60 minutes to restore a nerve from numbness to normal sensation. If no positive effect has been achieved after 30 to 60 minutes then it is unlikely that further treatment will restore function and the possibility that the nerve has been torn should be considered.

Note: If clinic scheduling requires shorter treatment times, successful treatment may take more appointments but is still possible.

Improve vitality/ in the nerve
49 / 396

- Treatment Time: Once sensation is normal use 49 / 396, vitality / nerve for 1 minute
- 49 Hz is thought to restore "vitality" to the tissue treated. While vitality is hard to quantify it is intuitively obvious that restoring normal function of a tissue would increase vitality. Use 49 / 396 for one minute at the end of the treatment once pain is down and motion is normalized.

Caution: patient positioning

It is not possible to reduce pain with treatment while the patient is in a position that increases pain. For example, if the patient is lying prone and has low back spinal facet joint pathology, low back pain will increase. If the neck is positioned in extension cervical facet pain may increase. Patients with disc pathology may have increased pain when lying in a position that flexes the spine at the affected levels. Patients may have pathologies that allow comfort in only very restricted positions. Modify the patient's position as needed to permit comfortable treatment. Beware of the stoic patient who doesn't say anything until the end of the treatment. Ask the patient if the position is comfortable before starting treatment.

What to do if response to treatment is slow

Nerve pain responds so predictably that if the pain has not started decreasing in 10–15 minutes consider the following causes and remedies.

Dehydration

Question the patient again regarding hydration status. If the patient has not had sufficient water, have the patient drink 8 to 16 ounces of water while on the treatment table. Try treating again once the patient has hydrated. Dehydration is especially prevalent in patients over 60. Do not accept the patient's statement, "I drink lots of water." Ask specifically how much water they have had to drink that day and in what form. One patient who had a poor response to several treatments swore each time that he had consumed 32 ounces of water during the morning before the treatments. Upon close questioning at the fourth appointment he described the "water" as being caffeinated iced tea or cola.

Narcotics

If patients are taking opiates for pain or have had multiple injections with anesthetics it is sometimes necessary to run the frequencies to "remove" narcotics and anesthetics. It is not thought that these frequencies actually remove the narcotic or anesthetic. It is much more likely that they somehow influence the membrane proteins making them somehow more receptive to treatment with 40 / 396.

43, 46, 19 / 396
- Remove opiates and anesthesia / from the nerve
- The current application and lead placement are the same as for the nerve treatment.

Nerve may not be the source of the pain

The response to treatment for nerve pain is so predictable that it may be used diagnostically. If the patient is not dehydrated and is not taking large

doses of opiates and 40 / 396 applied properly does not change the pain, then it is very likely that the nerve is not the source of the pain. Check for myofascial trigger points in the muscles that cause referred pain in patterns similar to dermatomal pain. Glute medius and minimus referral patterns mimic sciatica and anterior scalenes mimic C6 arm and hand pain. Treat the involved muscle and see how it affects the pain.

Treatment interval

Nerve pain can be treated as often as needed to keep the patient comfortable. Aside from the induced euphoria, which lessens after repeated treatments, there have been no side effects or ill effects from nerve pain treatment except for breakdown in small areas of skin under the negative electrode pads that appear with use of a home unit for more than 6 hours a day.

If the patient has a disc injury or some inflammatory condition perpetuating the nerve pain and needs frequent or daily treatment until the cause can be repaired the patient may be treated daily or as needed for palliation. Prescription and purchase of a preprogrammed small portable microcurrent unit may be more economical than in office treatment. TENS devices are not effective in nerve pain. The microcurrent device for home use must deliver microamperage current and must approximate the appropriate frequencies.

Adjunctive therapies

There are no adjunctive recommendations for treating neuropathic pain except to do whatever is necessary to correct the cause of the nerve pain particularly rehabilitation of the disc. When treating dermatomal nerve pain caused by disc injuries treat the disc with 40 / 330, 630, 710 and exercises appropriate to restore disc function. See Chapter 4 for details.

Nutritional support

Omega 3 Essential fatty acids EPA/DHA reduce inflammation and DHA is an important component of neural membrane tissue. These lipids are found in lipid rich animal sources such as salmon and halibut. Tuna must be consumed with care

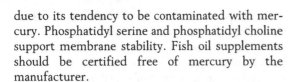

due to its tendency to be contaminated with mercury. Phosphatidyl serine and phosphatidyl choline support membrane stability. Fish oil supplements should be certified free of mercury by the manufacturer.

Treating central pain amplification

All parts of the brain are affected by neuropathic pain. The cortex interprets the pain and modifies behavior that is affected by pain. The normal function of the midbrain is pain suppression. A bump on the shin increases pain quickly and strongly in response to the acute soft tissue injury. But within minutes the pain is suppressed by the midbrain even though the injury to the soft tissue is progressing on its inflammatory path to stimulate repair.

When pain comes from chronic peripheral pain generators, the midbrain thalamic pain processing centers can change from their normal pain suppression function to a pain amplification function. To further complicate things, the pain transmission tracts in the spinal cord are "plastic" or adaptable and become facilitated in transmitting pain impulses. Facilitated segments in the spinal cord transmit pain messages more easily than they would in a normal cord.

Early childhood trauma or pain, anxiety and elevated stress levels can all affect the pain processing centers and increase the likelihood of central sensitization and amplification. While pain, especially nerve pain, is felt as a local phenomenon it has unavoidably systemic affects which need to be addressed in order for the patient to recover full function. There are frequencies included in the treatment protocols to address central sensitization in the midbrain and spinal cord.

Channel A: condition frequencies

The frequencies listed are thought to remove or neutralize the condition for which they are listed except for 81, 49 / which are thought to increase secretions and vitality respectively.

- Inflammation   40 /
- Chronic inflammation   284 /
- Increase secretions   81 /
- Restore vitality   49 /

Channel B: tissue frequencies

- Spinal cord: ___ / 10
   ○ Conducts impulses from the nerves to the brain
- Mid brain, Thalamus: ___ / 89
   ○ Pain impulses travel from the nerve up the spine and are processed in the thalamus which for FSM purposes is located in the midbrain.

Treatment rationale and experience

When FSM reduces chronic nerve pain in a 30 or 40 minute treatment, if the patient's midbrain is in pain amplification mode, there is suddenly nothing to amplify creating "pain amplification dissonance", translated as "it feels as if I should be in pain but I am not". The patient may look puzzled or report feeling disoriented. Quieting facilitation in the spinal cord and the amplification in the midbrain appears to reduce the central sensitization and reduces the dissonance the patient is experiencing.

Reduce facilitation and central amplification

Channel A condition / Channel B tissue
40, 284 / 10, 89
- Reduce inflammation, chronic inflammation / Cord, Midbrain

Treatment time and technique

Leave the patient set up as they were for treating the dermatomal nerves with the red (positive) leads contact at the spine and the black (negative) leads contact at the end of the nerve being treated. When the pain is 0–2/10 and the treatment to increase range of motion and secretions is complete check in with the patient.

If cord facilitation and central amplification are features, there will be some indication from the patient either by word or facial expression that being out of pain feels odd. Confirm for the patient that this is a normal phenomenon and explain the mechanism if this seems appropriate.

Change the frequencies to 40 / 10 for three to five minutes and follow that by treating with 40 / 89 for approximately 5 minutes. The patient should respond with a change in facial expression and a relaxation response when the dissonance is relieved.

The difference in state is usually obvious to the observer. The patient can be asked a neutral question such as, "How does it feel now?" to confirm the observation. Continue to use these two frequency combinations 40 / 89 and 40 / 10 for 5 minutes each until the state of being pain free feels "normal."

Caution: If the patient has pain that is **NOT** from central amplification and the midbrain is performing its normal function of pain suppression, using frequencies to reduce the activity of the midbrain reduces central pain suppression and causes the pain to increase temporarily.
- The 40 / 89 protocol is only effective for central pain amplification.
- Do not use 40 / 89 for other types of pain.
- If use of 40 / 89 increases pain switch back to 40 / 396 until the pain is reduced or use 81 / 89 for one to two minutes or until pain is reduced.

Precaution: induced euphoria

The euphoric state produced while treating with 40 / 396 usually decreases during the treatment to improve motion and restore motor and sensory function. The patient may experience an increase in the euphoric state when 40 / 10 and 40 / 89 are used. This is completely normal and is seen quite commonly. Euphoria should decrease again within 20 to 30 minutes and the practitioner is urged to use prudence and good judgment as to when to allow the patient to drive and operate in society.

Treating carpal tunnel syndrome

Compression neuropathies such as carpal tunnel syndrome, tarsal tunnel, and thoracic outlet are created by a combination of mechanical compression and inflammation of the nerves and blood vessels by shortened muscles and inflamed tendons in a confined anatomical space to create neuropathic pain. The key to successful treatment of carpal tunnel syndrome with FSM is to treat the nerve and also the tendons, tendon sheaths and muscles that are inflamed, taut and compressive. In general treatment with FSM is successful although response to treatment will depend on chronicity, general nutritional and hydration status and complicating factors such as diabetes and disc injuries.

Box 3.1

Summary for dermatomal nerve pain

- Current Polarized +
Reduce Pain
- 40 / 396
Remove Pathologies from Nerve
- 970, 94, 321, 9, 284 / 396
Soften Tissue
- 91 / 396, 142
Treat the Disc (If nerve pain is discogenic)
- 40 / 330, 630, 710
Improve Motion
- 13, 3 / 396, 142
- (With Motion – See Precautions)
Improve Sensation – Restore Function
- 81 / 396, 46
- 49 / 396
If slow response
- 43, 46, 19 / 396
Reduce Central Pain Amplification
- 40, 284 / 10, 89

Carpal tunnel syndrome

Carpal tunnel syndrome is a compression syndrome affecting the median nerve caused by inflammation and swelling of the tendon and tendon sheath within the fibrous retinaculum at the wrist. It is usually associated with overuse of the forearm flexor muscles from activities such as gardening, guitar playing, knitting, computer work, or combined gripping and lifting. It can be exacerbated by disc injury in the neck combined with tight muscles in the compartments along the path of the nerve from the neck to the wrist, creating a so called "triple crush" involving the scalene muscles, the pectoralis minor, and the forearm flexors.

Diagnosis

Carpal tunnel syndrome can be diagnosed by nerve conduction studies or by physical examination and history. Nerve conduction studies in carpal tunnel syndrome may be virtually identical to those seen with C6 nerve traction injury and care should be taken to distinguish between the two with careful history and physical examination.

Physical examination

Gentle tapping over the area of the carpal tunnel syndrome in the wrist will produce pain, paresthesia or tingling in the wrist, palm, or fingers. Physical compression of the nerves in the wrist created by asking the patient to hold a position with the hands together and the wrists extended at 90 degrees as if in prayer will produce pain or numbness in the hands, fingers, wrists or forearms. Physical compression of the carpal tunnel syndrome by flexing the wrists to 90 degrees and holding the backs of the hands together will produce similar symptoms if the carpal tunnel syndrome is inflamed.

Sensory examination: Sensory examination with a pin or a pinwheel will show hyperesthesia or sensory loss in the distribution of the median nerve but the proximal portion of the C6 nerve may have normal sensation.

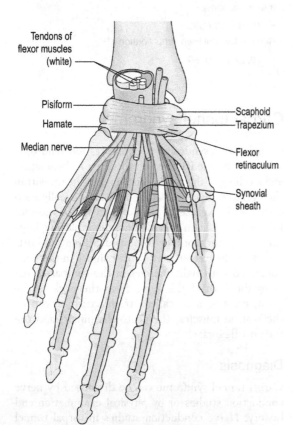

Tendons of flexor muscles (white)
Pisiform
Hamate
Median nerve
Scaphoid
Trapezium
Flexor retinaculum
Synovial sheath

Figure 3.18 • Carpal tunnel syndrome is created by inflammation and swelling of the tendon and tendon sheath at the retinaculum causing compression of the median nerve as it travels through the confined space.

Channel A: condition frequencies

The frequencies listed are thought to remove or neutralize the condition for which they are listed except for 81, 49 / which are thought to increase secretions and vitality respectively

• Inflammation	40 /
• Chronic inflammation	284 /
• Congestion	50
• Calcium ions	91 /
• Scarring	13 /
• Sclerosis	3 /
• Increase secretions	81 /
• Restore vitality	49 /

Channel B: tissue frequencies

- Dermatomal or Peripheral Nerve: ___ / 396
  - Any nerve outside the spinal cord
- Fascia: ___ / 142
  - Fascia is the thin connective tissue covering surrounding the muscles and virtually all visceral tissue.
- Artery and Elastic Tissue in the Muscle Belly: __ / 62
  - / 62 is the frequency used both for the artery and the elastic tissue in the arterial walls. The muscle belly responds to this frequency either because it is full of small arteries or because the elastic tissue in the muscle belly is somehow related to the artery wall.
- Connective tissue:___ / 77
  - This frequency appears to influence the connective tissue that creates the matrix for the muscles and fascia and the retinaculum that encloses the carpal tunnel syndrome.
- Tendon: ___ / 191
  - The tendon is a specialized fascia that connects the muscle to bone by interweaving with the periosteum.
- Tendon Sheath, bursa: ___ / 195
  - The tendon sheath surrounds the tendons in the wrist at the carpal tunnel syndrome and cushions the tendons with small lubricating sacs or bursa anyplace that tendons lay over each other or over the bone.

- Periosteum: ___ / 783
  - ○ The periosteum lines the outside of the bone, interweaves with tendinous and ligamentous attachments and is very well innervated and pain sensitive.
- Disc Annulus: ___ / 710
  - ○ The well innervated disc annulus wraps around and contains the nucleus.
- Disc Nucleus: ___ / 330
  - ○ The gel like disc nucleus fills the center of the disc and absorbs water to become a cushion for the vertebral bodies in the spine. It is very high in PLA_2 and very inflammatory.
- Disc as a whole: ___ / 630
  - ○ This frequency is thought to address the disc as a unit.
- A/B Pair 40 / 116
  - ○ Reduce inflammation in the immune system.

Treatment protocol for carpal tunnel syndrome

Channel A condition / Channel B tissue

Reduce inflammation

40 / 116
- Reduce inflammation / in the immune system
- This frequency combination reduced inflammation in the mouse model regardless of the tissue involved or the chemical pathway by which the inflammation had been produced in a 4-minute time-dependent response. It is used for reducing general inflammation in any tissue.
- Treatment time: Treat for 4–10 minutes

40 / 396
- Reduce inflammation / in the nerve
- Reducing inflammation in the nerve will begin to reduce the pain
- Treatment time: Use 40 / 396 for 5 to 10 minutes

Treat associated tissues

50, 40, 284, / 191, 195, 77, 62
- Reduce congestion, inflammation, chronic inflammation / in the tendon, the tendon sheath, retinaculum, and the blood supply
- Use 40 / with each tissue frequency for two to four minutes each. Use 50 and 284 / for 2 to 5 minutes with each tissue frequency, depending

on response. If the frequency is effective the pain will decrease and the tissues will begin to soften.

Improve motion

13, 91, 3 / 191, 195, 77, 62
- Reduce scarring, hardening, sclerosis / in the tendon, the tendon sheath, the retinaculum and the blood supply
- Use 13, 91, 3 / with each tissue frequency for 1 to 2 minutes each while gently mobilizing the wrist in flexion and extension or while using gentle manual pressure to separate the tissues. Move the wrist only to the point where a sense of discomfort or pressure starts; stop and return the wrist to neutral. Run 40/396 for 1 to 2 minutes if the pain increases and then return to 13 / 396 with movement. The range of pain free motion should increase with each repetition.

Treatment application

- Current level: 100–300μamps. Use lower current levels for very small or debilitated patients. Use higher current levels for larger or very muscular patients. In general higher current levels reduce pain more quickly. Do not use more than 500μamps as animal studies suggest that current levels above 500μamps reduce ATP formation while current levels below 500μamps increase ATP.
- ± Alternating DC Current: Current is used in alternating mode for local treatment at the wrist in carpal tunnel syndrome.
- Wave slope: Use a moderate to sharp wave slope for chronic pain. Use a gentle wave slope in acute injuries.
- Lead placement:
  - ○ The positive leads from channel A and channel B should be attached to one graphite glove placed in a small wet cloth laid on one side of the wrist or wrists.
  - ○ The negative leads from channel A and channel B should be attached to a graphite glove placed in a small wet cloth on the other side of the wrist or wrists so the current flows through the wrist from dorsal to the ventral side.

OR
- The positive leads from channel A and B can be placed at the elbow.
- The negative leads from channel A and B can be placed at one or both hands.

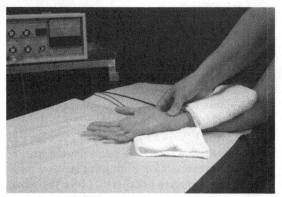

Figure 3.19 • The positive contact should be near the elbow and the negative contact at the wrist. Modify the treatment if both wrists are to be treated simultaneously so the positive leads at upper contact covers both forearms and the negative leads in the lower contact is resting on both wrists. If the hands are supinated as shown the wrists can be mobilized during treatment by having the patient move them gently into flexion and extension. Stop at the first sign of discomfort, keep the wrist in neutral for a few minutes and then move again. Repeat as needed until range of motion is full and pain free.

- Both wrists may be treated simultaneously if necessary. Care should be taken to ensure that the two contacts do not touch each other directly. Current will follow the path of least resistance and it will flow through the wet contacts instead of the patient if the wet contacts are touching.

Change application

Once the wrists are pain free it is prudent to treat the dermatomal nerves from neck to hands. Move the positive leads contact from the forearm and wrap it around the neck. Leave the negative leads contact on the fingers of the involved hand. Polarize the current positive for the final 10 minutes of treatment.

Treat the nerve from neck to wrist

40 / 396 – Polarized positive
- Reduce inflammation in the nerve.

81, 49 / 396 – Polarized positive
- Restore secretions and vitality in the nerve.
- Patient Position: The patient can be treated in any comfortable position that allows access to the neck and the wrists. This protocol does not usually produce profound induced euphoria but the patient should be in a well supported position in the event that it does.

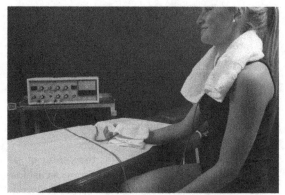

Figure 3.20 • Once the wrist pain is decreased, it is prudent to treat the dermatomal nerves with polarized positive current from neck to hands especially if inflammation from a cervical disc complicates the carpal tunnel syndrome. Move the positive leads contact from the forearm and wrap it around the neck. Leave the negative leads contact on the fingers of the involved hand. Polarize the current positive for the final 10 minutes of treatment.

Box 3.2

Carpal tunnel syndrome treatment summary

Reduce Inflammation
- 40 / 116 (alternating current ±)

Reduce Inflammation in Nerve
- 40 / 396 (alternating current ±)

Treat Associated Tissues
- 50, 40, 284, / 191, 195, 77, 62 (alternating current ±)

Improve Motion
- 13, 91, 3 / 191, 195, 77, 62 (alternating current ±)

Treat the Nerve from Neck to Wrist
- 40, 81, 49 / 396 (Current Polarized Positive +)

Adjunctive therapies

- Supplements: Carpal tunnel syndrome patients seem to benefit from vitamin B6 at the dose of 100mg per day for 4 to 6 weeks. Prolonged high level dosages of B6 are not advisable.
- Avoid provocative activities: Patients should be advised to avoid activities that use or stress the forearm flexor muscles at the wrist such as typing, computer work, gardening, guitar playing, using shears or scissors and gripping or repetitive lifting.
- Treat the disc: Consider treating the cervical discs (see Chapter 4: Treating Discogenic Pain). It is

not uncommon for the nerve to be irritated or inflamed when it leaves the neck if the C5–6 or C6–7 disc is inflamed. If disc involvement is suspected, or if the local wrist treatment is not producing improvement within two sessions, consider treating the disc when the positive leads contact is moved to the neck.

- Add 40 / 330, 630, 710 to the polarized positive protocol at the end of treatment and treat each tissue for 4 minutes.

Treating thoracic outlet

Thoracic outlet

Repetitive activities such as typing, computer or manual assembly work that place the neck in chronic forward flexion or flexion and rotation while the extended arms are being used in front of the body are associated with the onset of thoracic outlet syndrome.

Thoracic Outlet Syndrome (TOS) patients complain of pain, cold and numbness in the arms and hands, loss of pulse and sometimes weakness in the muscles. Think of the mechanism involved in TOS. Tight hardened muscles compress the neurovascular structures in the supra-clavicular space between the neck and the chest where the major blood vessels and the cervical nerve roots as the brachial plexus travel from the neck into the chest, arms and hands.

The compression of the blood vessels and the nerves reduces circulation, causes ischemia in the nerve, neuropathic pain and ultimately loss of circulation in the arms and hands. The tight muscles include the deep muscles that flex and rotate the cervical spine – the scalenes, the longus coli, and the sternocleidomastoid – and the muscles that roll the shoulders forward – the pectoralis major and minor. The poor posture that most people assume when they work at a desk, on a computer or on almost any piece of equipment involves constant cervical flexion and rotation as they sit still and attend to the work at hand.

Constant flexion and rotation compress the spinal discs causing them to become dehydrated and inflamed and to bulge posteriorly (see Chapter 4 – Treating Discogenic Pain). The disc nucleus contains the inflammatory substance PLA_2, and is dislodged posteriorly when the posterior disc annulus weakens from constant compression during flexion. The connective tissue in the disc annulus "creeps" or stretches under the constant load, bulges and eventually weakens forming small tears. The small tears allow the

inflammatory substance in the nucleus to leak out, inflaming the nerves that are just adjacent to the part of the disc annulus most likely to be damaged by compressive forces. The inflamed nerves cause the muscles to tighten forming taut bands and trigger points which compress the nerves creating neuropathic pain and myofascial pain in the chest, shoulders and arms.

The C5–6 disc is the axis of rotation for flexion in the cervical spine; the C5 and C6 dermatomal nerves are most impacted by any damage to the C5–6 disc. The C5 and C6 nerve roots innervate the scalenes, longus coli, pectoralis major, and the major stabilizing muscles in the cervical spine.

The C6–7 and C7–T1 discs are usually the next to weaken impacting the C7, C8 and T1 dermatomal nerves. The C7, C8 and T1 nerve roots innervate the pectoralis major and pectoralis minor, known as the "neurovascular entrapper" (Travell 1983). The constant muscle tightness compresses discs causing more bulging and nerve inflammation which causes more muscle tightness and neurovascular compression.

Medical sources have broken the condition into vascular TOS, neuropathic TOS and non-specific TOS but some debate whether TOS even exists. The debates about causation and diagnosis make identifying prevalence very difficult but the symptoms effect millions of patients based on work and disability claims. After physical therapy, the most common therapy is surgical resection to remove the first rib which is known to have disastrous side effects and sequellae. It is most common in females in the fourth decade.

The simplest most effective therapeutic solution would be some therapy capable of treating inflammation in the blood vessels, the disc and nerve and relaxing the tight, hardened muscles and their attachments to the ribs at the periosteum without causing further trauma. FSM fits this description and performs this function successfully in clinical settings on a routine basis.

Treat the nerve, the blood vessels, the muscles and the disc pathologies.

Treat the nerve
40 / 396
- Polarized positive +
- Positive leads at the neck

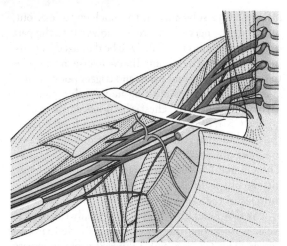

Figure 3.21 • The nerves leaving the cervical spine at the thoracic outlet travel between muscles that become tight from postural strain and the inflammation associated with overuse and disc injuries.

- Negative leads at the hands or on the chest
- Treatment time: 20 minutes

Treat the blood vessels

40, 284 / 62
- Polarized positive + current
- Positive leads at the neck
- Negative leads at the hands or on the chest
- Treatment time: 10 minutes

Treat the disc

40 / 330, 630, 710
- Remove inflammation, chronic inflammation in the disc nucleus, the disc as a whole and the disc annulus
- Polarized positive + current
- Positive leads at the neck
- Negative leads at the hands or on the chest
- Treatment time: 4 minutes each, 12 minutes total

Treat the muscle

58/00, 02, 32
- A/B pairs to remove scar tissue and adhesions
- Polarized positive + current
- Positive leads at the neck
- Negative leads at the hands or on the chest
- Treatment time: 1 to 2 minutes each

Caution: 58 / 00, 01, 02, 32
- Do not use these frequencies on injuries newer than 5 to 6 weeks old.
- Newly injured tissue must form scar tissue in order to repair itself.
- Removing the scar tissue seems to undo the healing by weeks in a new injury.
- The "58's" can be used very briefly (15 seconds) to modify scar tissue as it is forming after the first four weeks.
- Never use this combination before the injury is 4 weeks old.

40 / 142, 62, 191, 783
- Remove inflammation / from the fascia, blood vessels, tendons, periosteum
- Polarized positive + current
- Positive leads at the neck
- Negative leads at the hands or on the chest
- Treatment time: 2 to 4 minutes each

91 / 142, 62, 191, 195, 783
- Remove calcium / from the fascia, muscle belly, tendon, periosteum
- Polarized positive +
- Positive leads at the neck
- Negative leads at the hands or on the chest
- Treatment time: Use for 2 to 3 minutes each depending on tissue response. These frequencies usually produce significant tissue softening and if the practitioner is sensitive to this change in texture the frequency can be used until the softening stops.

13, 3 / 142, 396, 62
- Remove scarring, sclerosis / from the fascia, the nerve and the blood vessels
- Polarized positive +
- Positive leads at the neck
- Negative leads at the hands or on the chest
- Treatment time: Use for 2 to 3 minutes each depending on tissue response. These frequencies usually produce significant tissue softening and if the practitioner is sensitive to this change in texture the frequency can be used until the softening stops.
- Precaution: The goal is to soften and relax the muscle and reduce the compression on the disc, nerve and blood vessels and to tease the nerves and

fascia apart so they can move independently. The manual technique for this portion of the treatment requires care and respect for the delicacy and pain sensitivity of the tissues involved.

- Treat the nerve **VERY** respectfully; **GENTLY** tease it away from the fascia.
- Use 40 / 396 to reduce any increase in pain created by manipulations.

81, 49 / 396

- Increase secretions, vitality / in the nerve
- Treatment time: Use each frequency combination for one to two minutes each as long as the pain has been reduced to the 0–2/10 range. If pain is still present do not use 81 / 396. 49 / 396 may be used even if pain is still present.

Treatment application for thoracic outlet

- *Current level*: use Polarized positive + current, 100–300µamps. Use lower current levels for very small or debilitated patients. Use higher current levels for larger or very muscular patients. In general higher current levels reduce pain more quickly. Do not use more than 500µamps as animal studies suggest that current levels above 500µamps reduce ATP formation.
- *Lead placement*: Positive lead attached to a graphite glove wrapped in a warm wet hand towel and wrapped around the neck to reach the cord as well as the nerve roots on both sides and the discs. Negative leads attached to graphite gloves wrapped in a small warm wet towel that has been placed just below the pectoralis muscle on the chest to focus the current on the cervical and pectoralis minor muscles. Lay the hand and forearm on the lower portion of the towel to allow current flow to the C6 through T2 nerve roots.
- *Waveslope*: Waveslope should be set at medium. The injury is chronic but the nerves are so irritable that a sharp waveslope may increase irritation. A gentle waveslope may not be enough to break up the fibrosis and calcification in the fascia and muscle.
- *Patient position*: The patient can be treated supine or seated in a comfortable well supported position. The treatment involves treating the nerves which can create an induced euphoria and the patient may become drowsy or even fall asleep.

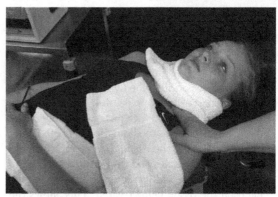

Figure 3.22 • Place the positive leads in a wet towel around the neck and the negative leads in a wet towel draped across the upper chest and down the arm to the hand. Use polarized positive current and treat the nerve, the muscle and the disc. Use the fingers of a relaxed hand to gently tease the nerves away from the fascia and muscles.

Box 3.3

Thoracic outlet treatment summary

- Current Polarized +

Treat the Nerve
- 40 / 396

Treat the Blood Vessels
- 40, 284 / 62

Treat the Disc
- 40 / 330, 630, 710

Treat the Muscle
- 58/00, 02, 32
- 40 / 142, 62, 191, 783
- 91 / 142, 62, 191, 195, 783
- 13, 3 / 142, 396, 62

Treat the Nerve
- 40, 81, 49 / 396

- *Treatment interval*: TOS patients can and should be treated twice a week for 4 to 6 weeks with at least one day separating the treatments. If progress is being made treatment can be increased to every other day. The intervening day allows time for the muscle and the patient to adjust to the new mechanics and adjunctive activities and gives the patient time to begin doing the exercises that will help correct posture and prevent recurrence.

- *Manual technique*: For those trained in manual therapies using the hands while using FSM requires some adjustment of technique. The key is to let the frequency do the work and to use the hands with very gentle pressure and complete relaxation, especially when the nerves are inflamed and exquisitely painful. The hands should be almost limp with just enough tone in the distal finger muscles to allow the fingers to gently assess the state of the tissue. The therapist should use shoulder muscles and the serratus anterior to advance the arm and increase the pressure of the hand on the tissue being treated. This allows the hand to remain relaxed while the arm muscles provide the pressure required for treatment.
- The hands are sensing change and softening in the muscles not forcing it. The thought of "asking permission" from the body to treat the muscles seems to be an effective mental strategy that promotes the right amount of palpation pressure. The patient's muscles will relax and allow deeper palpation if the practitioner's hands are relaxed and will defensively tense if the contact is too firm or if the palpating fingers are too tense.
- *Let the frequency do the work*: If possible, move the fingers to the tissue being treated when the frequency for that tissue is running. When the frequencies to affect "hardening in the tendon" are being used move the fingers to where "tendons" are known to be and feel if they are changing.
- *Learning curve*: As the tissues change, let those changes guide you in treatment and tell you when to change off of one frequency or its pathology. When the frequencies are softening scar tissue or mineral deposits use gentle but firm finger pressure to assist and assess the process. When the frequencies are "dissolving scar tissue" use the soft fingers to very gently tease apart the nerve from the fascia to which it is adhered. Let the patient's response guide your learning process. If the patient flinches or the muscle tightens use lighter pressure. If they soften quickly and are pain tolerant, gently creep the fingers in and around the SCM, in between the scalenes, the nerves and the discs.

What tissue is it? What is wrong with it?

As proficiency with FSM increases the practitioner using a manual microcurrent device can become more specific with the choice of frequencies for tissues to be treated and pathologies to be removed from them. This process usually occurs gradually as the skilled practitioner becomes more familiar with palpating the local anatomy and more sensitive to the effects of the frequencies on the structures being treated.

With an illustrated anatomy text such as the Atlas of Illustrated Anatomy (Netter 1991) as a visual guide, palpation can become very specific as to tissue. Following the recommended "relaxed hand" palpation technique allows the sensing fingers to become quite sensitive. When the finger tips encounter a painful tissue it can be identified by the tension in the muscles surrounding the area, by the patient's verbal response or by the subtle sense that the tissue is simply "different" from the less painful tissue in the area. If the practitioner will attend to the subtle awareness that the tissue is simply "different" this distinction alone is sufficient to create a very skilled palpation sense. This level of skill is within the grasp of every practitioner given time, practice and patience.

Precaution: increased segmental pain from ligament laxity

If tight myofascial tissue has been acting as a splint to stabilize a joint with lax ligaments and the FSM treatment loosens the muscles and increases the range of motion, the lax joint is no longer splinted or stable. The joint will translate instead of gliding properly, as described in Chapter 6, allowing the facet joints to crash into each other, creating stress on the discs and causing local inflammation. The patient will feel wonderful for about 2 to 4 hours following treatment but will report point tenderness over one or more joints at the spine and possibly increased nerve pain after that.

The patient will often comment that the "treatment made my pain worse" in these cases. The practitioner who has recorded a reduced pain score at the end of the treatment (see Chapter 11) will be able to remind the patient that the pain was reduced at the end of the treatment. The reply should be, "When and where did your pain increase?" This reply reassures the patient that there is a reason for the pain which can be determined by knowing exactly when and where it increased. If the pain increased within 2 to 6 hours of the treatment and palpation localizes the tender area to the posterior joints or ligaments of the spine it is diagnostic of ligamentous laxity.

The suspicion should be confirmed by performing a stress x-ray view such as a flexion extension x-ray in the cervical spine. Measurement is taken from the line of the anterior and posterior vertebral body of the segment above compared to its position relative to the vertebral body below in neutral versus flexion and extension. The vertebral bodies should remain aligned as the spine curves with motion. If the line of the vertebral body moves forward or back relative to the vertebral body below, the segment is said to translate. The x-ray report may or may not comment on slight to moderate translation and the practitioner is advised to examine the films personally. If ligamentous laxity is present treat for that in addition to treating the TOS.

Adjunctive techniques

Postural training: The patient must be schooled in the proper posture for the desk related activities that created the problem in the first place: Sit in a proper position that avoids cervical flexion and rotation. Sit upright with the belly out and the low back arched in slight extension so the neck stays in neutral with the ears over the shoulder until the posture becomes habit. Take breaks and shrug shoulders, extend the neck to pump and re-hydrate the discs and go for a short walk with arms swinging. Do corner stretches to specifically stretch the pectoral and anterior cervical muscles at a level of comfort several times a day for four or five times.

Psychological support: Patients are not only in physical pain but they may be in emotional pain as well from not being believed or not being treated seriously or at all for their complaint. The possibility of work related litigation or bureaucracy may complicate the emotional tension and providing some emotional support whether it is relaxation therapy or tapes, breathing exercises, walking recommendation or community support groups.

Strengthen the extensors and deactivate the flexors with gentle specific exercises. Strengthen the lower trapezius, latissimus and the rhomboids to stabilize the trunk posture. Relax the upper trapezius and levator scapulae.

Supplements: EPA/DHA – fish oils that have been screened to remove any mercury contaminants by a professional grade supplement manufacturer, dosed at 1–8grams/day, reduce inflammation in the nerve and the disc and help soften the muscles by supplying flexible lipid compounds to rebuild both nerve and muscle membranes.

B6, B12, and folic acid help restore nerve function during the repair process.

Magnesium malate or magnesium glycinate dosed at 500mg a day help muscles to relax and supports the softening of tight muscles.

Treating peripheral neuropathies

Peripheral neuropathies

Peripheral neuropathies differ from dermatomal neuropathic pain in that the pain and sensory changes appear in a stocking and/or glove distribution.

The factors responsible for the development of diabetic peripheral neuropathy (DPN) are vascular occlusion causing ischemia to the nerve and surrounding tissues and secondary infection. The ischemia involves small arteries in all cases. However, in up to a third of the cases, pedal pulses are palpable, indicating the sparing of medium-sized and larger arteries. The pain and numbness appear in a glove and stocking pattern and is seen more often in the feet than the hands in diabetics. It is beyond the scope of this text to detail the exact mechanisms by which the deficiencies in the blood supply compromise nerve function or every cause of every type of peripheral neuropathy. The reader is referred to Bradley for a more complete discussion of the pathologies involved in peripheral neuropathies (Bradley 2000).

The history may include chronically elevated blood sugar, hemoglobin A_1C above 6.0, history of cancer or use of chemotherapy agents or other medications known to cause peripheral neuropathies, history of prolonged sitting in a position that compresses the blood supply to the lower extremity. Check the prescribing information for details of medication side effects for **any** drug the patient was taking in the 12 months prior to the onset of the neuropathy. Peripheral neuropathies can also be caused by prolonged nutritional deficiencies of B12 or folate. Peripheral neuropathies create damage to the peripheral nerves by various mechanisms but the glove and stocking pattern is characteristic regardless of the underlying cause.

Treatment of diabetic peripheral neuropathies with FSM involves use of frequencies to reduce inflammation, chronic inflammation and fibrosis in the arteries that nourish and support the nerves and use of frequencies to reduce inflammation of the nerve. The protocols were developed through trial

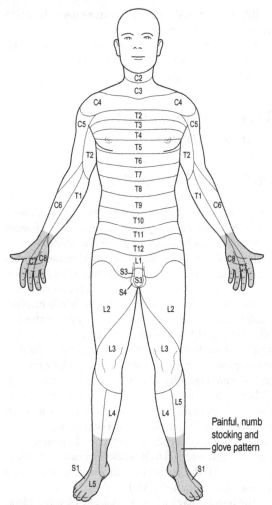

Figure 3.23 • Peripheral neuropathies create damage to the peripheral nerves by various mechanisms but the glove and stocking pattern is characteristic regardless of the underlying cause. Pain and reduced sensation are found from the foot up the lower leg towards the knee.

to treatment with FSM. There are no case reports documenting treatment response in chemotherapy neuropathies caused by other agents.

Peripheral neuropathies due to nutritional deficiencies do not respond well to FSM; the cure seems to be to correct the deficiency although FSM may be useful as an adjunct to enhance the recovery.

The protocols described below have been shown to be consistently effective in treatments in clinical settings for diabetic peripheral neuropathies. Controlled trials are planned but will not be completed for several years. There have been no reports of adverse reactions to treatment and given the dismal alternatives, a 4-week trial of three treatments each week should be considered.

Channel A: condition frequencies

The frequencies listed are thought to remove or neutralize the condition for which they are listed except for 81, 49 / which are thought to increase secretions and vitality respectively

- Chronic inflammation   284
- Calcium ions   91
- Inflammation   40
- Sclerosis   3
- Toxicity   57, 900, 920
- Increase secretions   81
- Restore vitality   49

Channel B: tissue frequencies

- Artery, Elastic tissue   62
  - This frequency is used to address the artery and the elastic tissue and blood supply in the muscle belly.
- Peripheral nerve   396
  - Any nerve outside the spinal cord

Treatment protocol

Channel A condition / Channel B tissue

Treat the blood supply and the nerves
40 / 62
- Inflammation / Artery
284 / 62
- Chronic inflammation / Artery
91 / 62
- Calcium ions / Artery

and error over a one year period and were not at all successful when only the nerve was treated. It was only when the frequencies for the artery were added that the treatments became consistently successful.

Treatment of peripheral neuropathies associated with chemotherapy agents has not been universally successful. The treatments for chemotherapy neuropathies add the frequencies to "remove toxicity from the blood vessels and nerves" to the standard diabetic protocols. These protocols have been effective for vincristine-induced neuropathies in various clinics but cisplatin neuropathies have so far been resistant

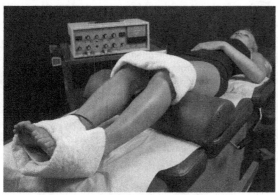

Figure 3.24 • To treat diabetic and chemotherapy induced peripheral neuropathies place the positive leads at the knees and the negative leads at the feet.
Use alternating current for the first portion of the treatment and polarize the current positive for the last portion of the treatment.

3 / 62
- Sclerosis / Artery

40 / 396
- Inflammation / Nerve

284 / 396
- Chronic inflammation / Nerve

91 / 396
- Calcium Ions / Nerve

3 / 396
- Sclerosis / Nerve
- Treatment time:
- treat with each frequency for 5 minutes
- ± alternating DC current.

For chemotherapy neuropathies add

57, 900, 920 / 62
- Toxicity / in the blood vessels

57, 900, 920 / 396
- Toxicity / in the nerve
- Treatment time:
- treat with each frequency for 5 minutes
- ± alternating DC current.

Application
- Current level: 100–300µamps. Use lower current levels for very small or debilitated patients. Use higher current levels for larger or very muscular patients. In general higher current levels reduce

pain more quickly. Do not use more than 500µamps.
- ± Alternating DC current: The current is used in "alternating" mode for treatment of peripheral neuropathies. In "alternating" DC current the pulsed DC square wave alternates from positive to negative.
- Waveslope: moderate to gentle. The waveslope refers to the rate of increase of current flow on the leading edge of the square wave. Treating peripheral neuropathies requires a moderate waveslope. If there are open wounds use a gentle waveslope to ensure that the current will be comfortable.

Lead placement for peripheral neuropathy

Positive leads from channel A and channel B are attached to a graphite glove which is wrapped in the center of a warm wet towel that has been folded in thirds lengthwise. The positive leads may also be attached to alligator clips that are attached to the warm wet towel. The positive leads towel is wrapped around the knees from back to front. If the patient is large enough that the towel won't reach around the knees, two towels can be linked together at the ends to make one longer contact.

Negative leads from channel A and channel B are attached to a graphite glove which is wrapped in the center of a warm wet towel that has been folded lengthwise. The leads may also be attached to alligator clips that are attached to the warm wet towel. The negative leads towel is wrapped around the feet including the toes. If the skin is too fragile to be wet for up to an hour have the patient place their feet on top of a warm wet towel or place adhesive electrode pads connected to the negative leads on the soles of each foot near or on the toes.

Using adhesive electrode pads

The positive leads can be attached to adhesive electrode pads placed just above the knee on the lower thigh and the negative leads can be placed on the plantar surface of the foot near or on the toes. The adhesive electrode pads are placed so the channels cross forming an "X" with the area to be treated in the middle of the "X".

If the channel A positive lead is placed on the right thigh; the channel A negative lead is placed on the ball or toes of the left foot. If the positive lead from channel B is placed on the left thigh; the negative lead from channel B is placed on the ball or toes of the right foot.

Box 3.4

Peripheral neuropathy treatment summary

Treat the Blood Vessels and the Nerves
• 40, 284, 91, 3 / 62, 396

For Chemotherapy Neuropathies Add
• 57, 900, 920 / 62, 396

Polarize Positive and Treat the Nerve
• 40, 81, 49 / 396

Note: This treatment protocol will not be effective for neuropathies from some chemotherapy agents, heavy metal toxicity or from nutritional deficiencies. Careful history will help to distinguish the cause of the neuropathy. The treatment will not make these neuropathies worse and it may be worth a trial to determine if treatment can produce any improvement. The FSM advanced course provides protocols to help address these types of peripheral neuropathies.

Change the current application to treat the nerve

After treating with the protocols above, polarize the current positive (+) leave the leads set up in the same position with positive leads at the knees and negative leads at the feet and treat with:

40 / 396
• Inflammation / nerve
• Treatment time: 10 minutes
• Current Polarized Positive +

81 / 396
• Increase secretions / nerve
• Treatment time: 2 minutes
• Current Polarized Positive +

49 / 396
• Increase vitality / nerve
• Treatment time: 2 minutes
• Current Polarized Positive +

This treatment takes approximately 60 minutes. At the end of the treatment time foot pain should be reduced and sensation may be improved. More severe disease requires more treatments to show improvement but in general some additional improvement should be obvious at the end of each treatment.

The practitioner is advised to perform a sensory examination at the beginning and end of each treatment to track progress. The author measures the levels with a tape measure or actually makes small ink marks on the patient's leg (with permission) before and after treatment. The area of altered sensation should be reduced to some extent at the end of each treatment. Even the most resistant patient should have restored sensation and reduced pain within 10 to 12 treatments. This treatment will also help heal peripheral wounds and diabetic ulcers unless they are infected. More complete information on the topic of treating wounds with potential infections is provided in the FSM Core and Advanced seminars.

Adjunctive therapies

Diabetic patients should attempt to maintain good sugar control during the treatment period by modifying diet. EPA/DHA, essential fatty acids, will help reduce inflammation and provide proper lipids for membrane repair. B12, folic acid and B6 are easily available and helpful in restoring nerve function.

Treatment interval

Patients should be treated two to three times a week until pain has been eliminated and sensation restored. Diabetics with well controlled blood sugars will require re-treatment once a week or less to maintain the gains achieved in the 10 weeks. Improvements will last longer if the blood sugar is at optimal levels.

Case reports

Thoracic nerve traction injury case report

"I Have My Life Back"

After 7 months of constant pain that increased while trying to do daily life's chores, I now feel a sense of relief and can see the light at the end of the tunnel. I owe this feeling of relief to a procedure called Frequency-specific Microcurrent Therapy. After two sessions using this therapy my intense nerve injury pain in my chest wall, rib pain and breast pain due to scar tissue around my incisions, range of motion in my arms and shoulders are gone and I feel 90% pain free. I look forward to resuming my life again, working in my classroom, going for walks, swimming and living life as it was 7 months ago.

My story begins 7 months ago when I was told that I had an abnormal mammogram and would need to have a surgical biopsy to see if I had cancer. From my 2-hour needle location done during a mammogram on my right breast, another quicker mammogram on my left breast, to two excision biopsy surgeries on my right breast and one excision biopsy surgery on my left breast I have suffered daily intense pain. It hurt to breathe, lift my arms, reach, carry anything, take care of myself and try to work. After all the surgeries my final diagnosis was abnormal ductal hyperplasia in my right breast only and all the other tissue looked clean. Six months later I went for my follow-up mammogram and have no abnormal cells or cancer.

My journey to find an answer to why I had so much pain and how it could be fixed, took me back to my breast surgeon, oncologist, naturopath, dietician and internist. All of whom could not explain my pain. The only recommendation I received during those 7 months was to go to a physical therapist. After several treatments at the physical therapist, involving light massage, lifting light weights and stretching, my pain became worse.

Determined to try to work on women's issues that arose due to the lack of estrogen which I was told I could not take due to my diagnosis, I pursued a recommendation for a new gynecologist. When I told her about my chest wall, rib and breast pain she said," This is out of my league." When I asked her whose league it was in she referred me to a functional medicine OB/GYN doctor, who referred me to Carolyn McMakin, MA, DC Chiropractic Physician at Integrated Pain Solutions in Portland Oregon. My pain was reduced from the very first treatment and after only three treatments I went home pain free, able to breathe freely, lift my arms and move normally. I needed two more treatments one month later when I increased my activity but I have been pain free since then with all my activities.

Without this treatment, I would still have the kind of pain that made daily life very difficult. So my advice is never give up looking for an answer, trust your own feelings and thoughts about yourself and your pain and give frequency-specific microcurrent therapy a try. It worked for me when nothing else did. It's hard to express the gratitude I feel to having found a caring practitioner and a process that worked. I am writing this in hopes that others who find themselves in a similar situation will not have to suffer as long as I did and will know that there is an end to nerve injury pain. Thanks, MR

Peripheral neuropathy case report

- Submitted by Norri Collier, DC, Houston, Texas

The patient was a 57-year-old chronic diabetic who presented with the following examination findings:

- Ulcer 7 cm in length on the medial aspect of left leg
- Edema in both legs and feet +3 (sustained pitting), the right leg being worse than the left
- Ankle motion in dorsi-flexion and plantar flexion reduced by 60%
- Right foot is mostly gray in color
- Left foot is mottled gray
- Right distal second digit has significant area of necrotic tissue
- Left distal third digit has some necrotic tissue
- Sensation is lost 7/10 test areas on plantar surface

The patient was treated twice a week for 6 weeks for 45 minutes at each treatment. Both lower legs and feet were wrapped in wet towels with the gloves enclosed in one towel on each leg to make them conductive. The current was applied to both the left and right leg and both feet. The diabetic ulcer was healed in 3 weeks after six treatments. Full sensation was restored in 5 weeks after 11 treatments (7-2-02 to 8-02-02). Range of motion in the left ankle was full and pain free in five treatments. Range of motion was full and pain free in the right ankle in 11 treatments. Necrosis was completely gone in the left distal third digit in seven treatments. Necrosis was completely gone and regeneration of the right second digit was 70% complete after 11 treatments in 6 weeks.

Carpal tunnel syndrome case reports

Carpal tunnel syndrome case report #1

The patient was a right-handed 39-year-old janitor at a local high school whose job description had changed in the previous 2 months to include lifting heavy wet garbage sacks from the kitchen daily. When he presented for the initial evaluation his pain was rated as a 7–8/10 and the left wrist was visibly swollen. There was no sensation for sharp in the palms of both hands and the distribution of the median nerve. Gentle tapping at the ventral wrist (Tinnel's sign) produced strong pain into wrists and fingers on both hands. Grip strength was 8 pounds in the left hand and 16 pounds in the right hand. He was referred to an orthopedic surgeon who decided that he was not yet a candidate for surgery and referred him for FSM and conservative treatment measures.

He was treated with the FSM carpal tunnel syndrome protocol three times a week for 2 weeks and twice a week for 2 weeks. He took 100mg of B6 per day, wore wrist splints at night and did wrist stretches twice a day for 4 weeks. At the end of 4 weeks he was pain free with normal sensation. Grip strength was 100 pounds in the left hand and 110 pounds in the right and Tinnel's sign was negative. His returned to work at his normal duties and the carpal tunnel syndrome symptoms did not return.

Carpal tunnel syndrome case report #2

• Submitted by Marty Freeman

We treated our first carpel tunnel patient who is a construction worker. The nerve conduction velocities prior to the FSM Carpel Tunnel Protocol showed the median nerve to be 7.4. He was treated with the carpal tunnel syndrome protocol from the course and was tested again immediately following the treatment. The nerve conduction velocities had dropped to a 6.8. 7.4 represents very advanced disease and surgery is usually done above a 5.

Immediate improvement is never seen in the NCV because the nerves only recover at 1mm a day. So, while it may not look like much, the change between 7.4 and 6.8 represents a huge change for one 80 minute treatment. He will be tested again in 2–3 weeks and we will continue to treat his hand once a week for a few weeks. He will be tested again at 6 weeks as well. Most physicians don't even bother to retest until 6 weeks after surgery because typically there are no changes prior to 6 weeks. The patient also reported that he had no pain that night for the first time in over a year.

Bibliography

Bennett, G.A., 2000. Neuroimmune interaction in painful peripheral neuropathy. Clin. J. Pain 16, S139–D143.

Bradley, W.G., Darhoff, R.B., Fenichel, G.M., Marsden, C.D., 2000. Neurology in clinical practice, third ed. Butterworth Heinemann, Boston.

Butler, D.S., Gifford, L.S., 1989a. The concept of adverse mechanical tension in the nervous system. Part 1: testing for dural tension. Physiotherapy 75, 622–629.

Butler, D.S., Gifford, L.S., 1989b. The concept of adverse mechanical tension in the nervous system. Part 2: Examination and treatment 75, 629–636.

Butler, D.S., 1991. Mobilization of the nervous system. Edinburgh, Churchill Livingstone.

Cloward, R.B., 1959. Cervical discography: mechanisms of neck, shoulder and arm pain. Ann. Surg. 150, 1052–1064.

Hoppenfeld, S., 1976. Physical examination of the spine and extremities. Appleton-Century Crofts, Division of Prentice Hall, New York.

Huckfeldt, R., Mikkelson, D., Larson, K., et al., 2003. The use of micro current and autocatalytic silver plated nylon dressings in human burn patients: a feasibility study. Pacific Rim Burn Conference.

Lewis, C., 2004. Physiotherapy and spinal nerve root adhesion: a caution. Physiother. Res. Int. 9, 164–173.

Meyers, R., Campana, W., Shubayev, F., 2006. The role of neuroinflammation in neuropathic pain: mechanisms and therapeutic targets. Drug Discov. Today 11, 8–20.

McMakin, C., Gregory, W., Phillips, T., 2005. Cytokine changes with microcurrent treatment of fibromyalgia associated with cervical spine trauma. Journal of Body Work and Movement Therapies 9, 169–176.

Marshall, L.L., Trethewie, E.R., Curtain, C.C., 1977. Chemical radiculitis. A clinical, physiological and immunological study. Clinical Orthopedics 129, 61–67.

Netter, F., 1991. Atlas of human anatomy. Ciba-Geigy, Plate 159, New York.

Olmarker, K., Rydevik, B., Nordberg, C., 1993. Autologous nucleus pulposus induces neurophysiologic and histologic changes in porcine cauda equina nerve roots. Spine 18, 1425–1432.

Olmarker, K., Blomquist, J., Stromberg, J., et al., 1995. Inflammatogenic properties of nucleus pulposus. Spine 20, 665–669.

Ozaktay, A.C., Cavanaugh, J.M., Blagoev, D.C., 1995. Phospholipase A_2-induced electrophysiologic and histologic changes in rabbit dorsal lumbar spine tissues. Spine 20, 2659–2668.

Ozaktay, A.C., Kallakuri, S., Cavanaugh, J.M., 1998. Phospholipase A_2 sensitivity of the dorsal root and dorsal root ganglion. Spine 23, 1297–1306.

Reilly, W., Reeve, V.E., Quinn, C., 2004. Anti-inflammatory effects of interferential, frequency-specific applied microcurrent. Proceedings of the Australian Health and Medical Research Congress.

Tal, M., 1999. A role for inflammation in chronic pain. Curr. Rev. Pain. 3, 440–446.

Travell, J.G., Simons, D.G., 1983. Myofascial pain and dysfunction: the trigger point manual. Williams & Wilkins, Baltimore.

Winquist, R.J., 2005. Use-dependent blockade of Cav 2.2 voltage-gated calcium channels for neuropathic pain. Biochem. Pharmacol. 70, 489–499.

Zieglgansberger, W., Berthele, A., Tolle, T.R., 2005. Understanding neuropathic pain. International Journal of Neuropsychiatric Medicine, CNS Spectrum 10 (4), 298–308.

Treating the discs

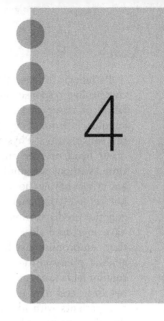

The discs act as flexible cushions between the spinal vertebra during mechanical shear and loading, cushioning the spine and giving it flexibility. Discs have an inner gel-like nucleus surrounded by an outer covering, the annulus fibrosus, wrapped in 13 concentric laminated bands around the nucleus, not unlike a jelly doughnut wrapped around its jam filling. The well-innervated disc annulus has no vascular supply and receives its nutrients by diffusion from the vertebral body vascular supply where it attaches to the end plates (White 1978). The disc is an osmotic system sensitive to load, pressure and concentration of proteoglycans that lives from motion (Kraemer 1995).

Water flows out of the disc during compression while standing or sitting upright and flows into the disc during decompression from relaxed sitting and lying. The disc itself has no blood supply and its nutrition is by diffusion from the end plate vasculature. To be optimally healthy the disc must be hydrated and mobile but not subject to excessive static compressive or repetitive flexed rotational loading. Inflammation in the disc is a response to excessive or prolonged loading, dehydration and micro tears in the annulus.

The outer three annular layers of the healthy disc are innervated by small myelinated and unmyelinated nerve fibers from the dorsal root ganglia and sympathetic trunks from multiple spinal levels. A disc at one spinal level may receive innervation from three or more spinal levels which means that inter-neurons in the cord are also involved. The vertebral end plate is as well innervated as the disc annulus suggesting that the end plate is an important source of discogenic pain (Lotz 2006).

The muscles at the spine stabilize the segment and protect the disc and the joint during movement. If the muscles are not effective the joint moves too much, the annulus is overstressed and the rate of degeneration increases: "... degeneration occurs as the result of imbalance of both static and dynamic spinal stabilizers. The disc degeneration that occurs is characterized by increased local inflammation and increased apoptosis of intervertebral disc cells" (Wang 2006).

The disc nucleus is rich in phospholipase A_2, a strongly proinflammatory substance that is very toxic and damaging to nerves (Olmarker 1993, 1995, Ozaktay 1995, 1998). When the disc bulges or ruptures the fragments of the nucleus expand from hydration when they are outside annular containment. The disc fragments create inflammatory damage to the nerves, the disc annulus and the surrounding tissues which is compounded by the immune system inflammatory response to a foreign body in the epidural space.

Degeneration is an inevitable response to mechanical loading and shear during repetitive motion or constant static loading as the spine ages. Studies have shown increases in IL-1, IL-6, TNFα and PGE_2 in injured discs. TNFα stimulates nerve growth factor and causes pain sensitive nerves to infiltrate the outer layers of the disc annulus and become sensitized. The degenerative process in the discs is complex and characterized by inflammation, loss of water and elasticity, tearing, scarring and disorganization of annular fibers, infiltration of nerves into the degenerated annulus and end plate tissues and dehydration and fragmentation of the nucleus (Kang 1996).

© 2011, Elsevier Ltd.
DOI: 10.1016/B978-0-443-06976-5.00004-6

Pathologic degeneration may be a chronic ineffective healing response consisting of ongoing accumulation of tissue damage in the end plate and disc annulus, inflammation, neo-innervation and nociceptor sensitization. Physiologic degeneration on the other hand may be an adaptation to loading over time, without accumulation of peripheral damage and thus having no appreciable inflammatory or nociceptive component (Lotz 2006). Patients with genetic predisposition to increased inflammation have increased degenerative response to activities that compromise disc health (Solovieva 2004). This genetic predisposition, when combined with environmental factors can create enhanced inflammatory response and may explain the difference between two patients with identical spinal imaging showing disc degeneration when one patient has tremendous pain symptoms and one has no pain at all.

Medical treatment for disc related injuries and pain includes pain medication, steroids to reduce the inflammatory response, physical therapy, exercises to stabilize the spine and move the disc fragment away from the nerve root as recommended by McKenzie (2006) and ultimately surgery. Epidural steroid and "caine" class anesthetic injections are used to reduce the nerve pain and inflammation and to keep the patient comfortable while the disc heals. Cauda equina symptoms, such as loss of bowel or bladder function, and severe motor weakness are indications for open spinal surgery without delay.

Microsurgery has better outcomes than large open back surgeries. It produces less perineural scarring because there is less muscle trauma, less internal bruising and fewer layers of tissue that have the potential to adhere to each other. Failed back syndrome, iatrogenic spine, or post-discotomy syndrome (PDS) result from the inflammation, soft tissue scarring and perineural fibrosis that accompany surgery.

Ultimately, if the pain can be managed and the surgery is put off long enough the symptoms resolve on their own and fewer than 10% of patients presenting with discogenic and radicular pain require surgery. Only 0.25%, one quarter of one percent, of individuals with "back problems" requires some form of surgery (Kraemer 1995).

Most surgeries are performed to provide pain relief for patients in the acute phase of disc inflammation. FSM has been shown to be effective in reducing neuropathic pain (Chapter 3) and in reducing IL-1, IL-6, TNFα and COX and LOX mediated inflammation, all of which have been implicated in discogenic pain. If FSM can be used to reduce inflammation and pain along with exercise therapies in the 99.75% of back pain patients who do not require surgery, more patients can recover function and avoid surgery and its complications. There are numerous case reports in which FSM treatment has done exactly this. The responses are consistent, predictable, reproducible and very encouraging to both patients and clinicians treating this difficult patient population.

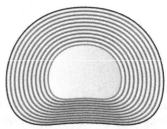

Figure 4.1 • A normal healthy disc is a flexible hydrated osmotic system that depends on the vertebral end plate vasculature for its nutrient supply. To be optimally healthy the disc must be hydrated and mobile but not subject to excessive static compressive or repetitive flexed rotational loading. Inflammation in the disc is a response to excessive or prolonged loading, dehydration and micro tears in the annulus (adapted with permission from White & Panjabi 1978).

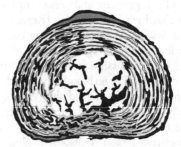

Figure 4.2 • The degenerated disc is mechanically different from the healthy disc. The disc nucleus is dehydrated and fibrosed and the protein polysaccharide content is altered from normal. The annulus is hardened and scarred from previous repairs of repeated microtrauma and may have one or more tears that allow the nucleus to protrude or extrude outside annular containment. The vertebral end plate is hardened and calcified impairing circulation to the disc. All of these factors change the load bearing characteristics of the disc and contribute to accelerated degeneration. Degeneration progresses along a continuum and depending on general health, hydration, physical activities and mechanical stresses and may accelerate, slow or in some cases even reverse (adapted with permission from White & Panjabi 1978).

Diagnosing the disc

Treating the disc with FSM is usually successful but the practitioner must know that the disc is what needs treating, which is not always as obvious as it sounds. The key to diagnosing discogenic pain is in the history, especially the mechanism of injury, the pain patterns and physical examination.

The mechanism of injury will involve flexion or combined flexion and rotation or some activity that exposes the patient to axial loading, lifting or flexion and rotation on a regular basis. In general, spinal flexion or combined flexion and rotation make the pain worse and extension may make the pain better as long as the patient does not have co-existing facet joint degeneration. Some patients know exactly what activity created the injury and some patients have no idea. Some patients have a history of activities that challenge the disc and then experience one event that makes the disc symptomatic. The challenge in taking the history is to identify which activities create spinal loading, flexion and rotation and might have caused the injury by asking questions about specific activities.

The patient may complain of low back, neck, shoulder, or thoracic spine pain or dermatomal nerve pain depending on what level has been injured and how badly it has been damaged. Some patients will have pain only in the area of the inflamed nerve root and their complaint will be "leg pain in the lateral calf" and not an L5 disc injury. Treating the leg or the muscle will not be satisfactory since the disc is ultimate the cause of the leg pain.

Cervical discogenic pain may present as neck, shoulder and arm pain or midscapular pain. The classic diagram (Fig. 4.3) published by Cloward describes the midscapular referred pain areas for the cervical discs. The patient with a cervical disc injury may present only with midscapular pain and shoulder pain (Cloward 1959). Treating the shoulder or the midscapular area will be unsatisfactory and only treatment aimed at the cervical disc will relieve the symptoms.

History questions

- What sorts of things were you doing in the days or weeks just before the pain started?
  - Look for activities that require flexion or combined flexion and rotation such as golf or tennis, yard work, laying floor coverings, painting, or moving.

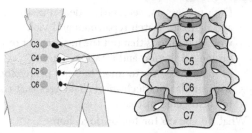

Figure 4.3 • The cervical disc annulus refers pain in between the shoulder blades stepwise down the spine according to the levels injured. The presence of mid-scapular pain helps diagnose the presence of an injured disc as the cause of neuropathic pain. It should be kept in mind that there are nine muscles, seven thoraco-costal joints and seven cervical facet joints that also refer to the midscapular area (adapted with permission from Cloward 1959).

- Were you lifting, leaning forward while using a keyboard, sitting, driving or bending over for long periods?
- Did you have any sort of trauma such as a fall or traffic accident?
  - Side impact accident force vectors put the discs at special risk especially if the spine is in rotation at the traumatized segment at the time of impact.
- Were you in one flexed or rotated position without moving for a prolonged period of time?
  - One patient fell asleep for 6 hours sitting up with his head tilted over to one side compressing the disc annulus and causing a small disc bulge that was read as "normal" on an MRI. The ensuing severe neck, shoulder and arm pain was clearly disc and nerve related but he waited 2 years for a diagnosis because his physicians didn't connect the mechanism of injury with the vulnerability of the discs to compression, rotation, connective tissue creep and shear. In 2 years no one had done a sensory examination.
- What do you do for a living?
  - Truck drivers, heavy equipment operators or workers who use equipment that vibrates while they are sitting have accelerated rates of degeneration in the discs and facets. The precipitating injury that is the "final straw" may seem minor but it will always involve axial compression, flexion or flexion and rotation. The most commonly degenerated discs are at L5–S1 but any lumbar disc can be at risk.

○ Data processors, secretaries, dental assistants and dentists, watch repairmen and violinists work in positions that put the neck into chronic prolonged flexion and rotation. These professions come to mind but any profession with similar biomechanical challenges is at risk for discogenic disease.

• What do you do for fun or do at home?

○ People who work in the yard or garden and who pull weeds by hand, who lay stones, or who dig holes or trenches with picks or shovels subject the spine to intense compressive forces with the neck and low back in a flexed position. People who work on cars often find themselves lifting heavy loads in awkward positions or working in one flexed position for prolonged periods of time. Some sports such as golf or tennis exert ballistic rotational forces on the discs that create chronic micro-injuries and eventually tissue failure.

How much does it hurt?

The pain level in acute discs is usually moderate to severe 5–8/10 on a 0 to 10 visual analog scale (VAS) tends to be worse when the muscles spasm to protect the area and worse with provocative activities. Chronic discogenic pain may be rated somewhat lower at a 3–4/10 VAS with pain excursions into the 5–8/10 level with provocative activities.

Where does it hurt?

The discs themselves have fairly well defined pain patterns creating pain at and near the spine. Cervical discs refer in between the shoulder blades as discussed above. If the disc injury creates minimal muscle spasm and just irritates the nerve the only symptom may be mild neuropathic pain in the dermatome adjacent to the injured disc. The L5–S1 disc is said to refer to the coccyx and is often mistaken for coccydynia. The L4–5 disc refers pain to the ischial tuberosities.

Nerve pain patterns

Sometimes isolated nerve pain is the only symptom that a disc has been injured. If the mechanism of injury or the patient's activities do not account for the pain, it suggests that an evaluation of the nerve and the discs would be worthwhile.

• **C3:** refers pain to the slope of the neck along the trapezius muscle and the patient may say they cannot tolerate a necklace or any clothing touching the neck

• **C4:** refers pain to the point of the shoulder and can mimic shoulder joint injury

• **C5:** refers pain into the upper arm

• **C6:** refers pain to the thumb and the lateral elbow

• **C7:** nerve root refers to the medial elbow

• **Thoracic nerve roots:** refer pain onto the chest or abdomen depending on the level affected

• **L1:** Lower abdomen

• **L2:** Groin, hip or upper thigh

• **L3:** Medial thigh and knee

• **L4:** Medial calf and ankle

• **L5:** Lateral calf, great toe and area between the first and second toe

• **S1:** Heel and lateral edge of the foot

• **S2:** Posterior leg

• **Pudendal** nerve: refers pain to the pelvis, genitals and groin through S2, S3, S4.

Muscle pain patterns

Muscle in the shoulder girdle is innervated by the C5 or C6 nerve roots. The nerve irritation creates taut muscles and the taut muscles may develop myofascial trigger points which have their own pain patterns referring into the arms and hands. The practitioner is referred to The Trigger Point Manual for complete listing of trigger point referral areas (Travell 1983).

Every muscle in the hip and low back is innervated by branches of the L3 nerve root. Disc related nerve irritation causes the muscles to become taut and eventually to develop myofascial trigger points. The trigger point referred pain patterns overlap the referred pain patterns from the discs and nerves and can complicate the diagnostic challenge. In some cases the trigger points are the only symptom and the perpetuating factor is the disc injury and inflammation (Travell 1992). Treating the muscle gives temporary relief and only treatment aimed at the disc will provide lasting improvement.

What makes it better – What makes it worse?

Flexion / combined flexion and rotation

The inability to tolerate flexion postures is diagnostic of disc injuries. The patient may complain

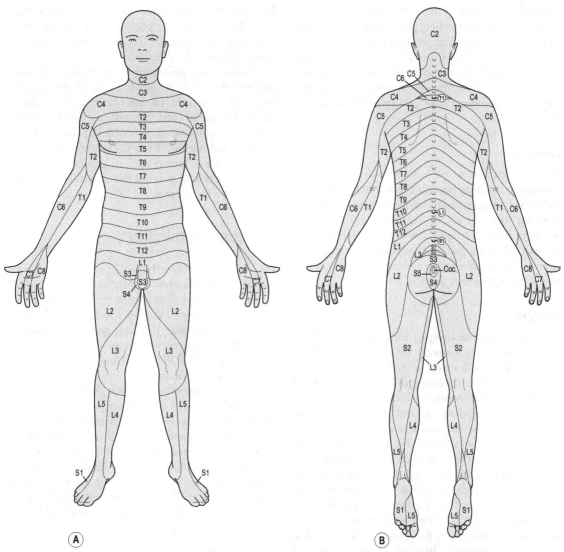

Figure 4.4 • This dermatome chart is only one of several versions of dermatomal sensory distribution commonly used. There are individual differences among patients and the sensory diagram is an approximation of nerve distribution in any given patient. Record the findings from the sensory examination on the dermatome diagram noting hyperesthesia, normal findings and reduced or absent sensation.

specifically that the pain is worse when driving a car because the seats put the lumbar spine into flexion and the legs are extended while using the pedals. This position creates flexion pressure on the discs, and stretches the sciatic nerve causing pain in the foot, leg or hip.

Patients with lumbar discogenic pain cannot lay supine with the knees flexed and must have the legs straight when supine so the lumbar spine is in extension. The patient can usually lay prone

comfortably as long as the facet joints are not also pain.

Cervical discs create neck pain and pain between the shoulder blades and in the cervical dermatomes that is worse with forward head postures created while using a keyboard, eating or reading. The pain will be worse when lifting or using the arms outstretched because the anterior cervical muscles contract to stabilize the spine during lifting, causing disc compression.

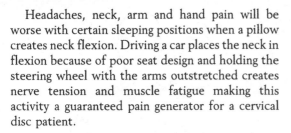

Headaches, neck, arm and hand pain will be worse with certain sleeping positions when a pillow creates neck flexion. Driving a car places the neck in flexion because of poor seat design and holding the steering wheel with the arms outstretched creates nerve tension and muscle fatigue making this activity a guaranteed pain generator for a cervical disc patient.

Valsalva

The pain may be worse with a bowel movement, sneezing or coughing because these activities increase abdominal pressure and increase pressure on the disc, exposing the nerves to increased inflammatory products from the disc. If neck, arm or hand pain or low back or leg pain or trunk and abdominal pain increases with coughing, sneezing or bowel movements it suggests that the disc is involved.

Imaging

The most common imaging for a disc is a CT or MRI; x-rays are not useful for disc injuries. Both CT and MRI will reveal a badly herniated disc. The challenge is in discerning the damaged inflamed disc that is a pain generator but appears as a "disc bulge" that is read as "normal" because it is not herniated outside the annulus and is consistent with the degeneration expected for the patient's age. A small piece of the nucleus may herniate but still be contained by the annulus. The inflammation will make the annulus appear very dark and the small piece of nucleus appears as a small white speck just inside it. The very well innervated annulus will become a strong pain generator but the disc will appear "normal". Imaging has limitations of resolution and cannot detect the microscopic internal changes in the disc that make it a pain generator. There is no way to tell from the imaging alone whether a disc is a pain generator. The imaging must be correlated with the clinical picture and physical examination.

Evaluating disc injuries

Most practitioners reading this text have been trained to perform a physical examination to evaluate the spine for discogenic injuries and pain. This brief description is meant to be a reminder rather than a comprehensive instruction. It is included to reinforce the notion that FSM treatment must match the diagnosis. The patient may present with a diagnosis of "disc injury and sciatica" but it is best if the practitioner confirms the diagnosis.

Evaluation of a disc injury through physical examination is done directly by physically challenging the disc, and indirectly by interrogating the sensory nerves, the spinal cord, the reflexes and the motor nerves which may be compromised by the inflammatory material released from the injured disc.

The reader is encouraged to pursue more complete instruction in physical examination techniques and orthopedic assessment.

Physical examination

The disc can be directly challenged by maneuvers that physically compress it or stress it in the direction of lesion. Cervical discs can be evaluated by gently pressing on the top of the head and loading the discs in axial compression. If a disc annulus is compromised the maneuver will cause pain between the scapulae (Cloward 1959) and may increase pain in the affected dermatome.

A Valsalva maneuver, in which the patient inhales, holds the breath and bears down, will compress the injured disc and move nerve towards the inflamed area causing local and occasionally dermatomal pain.

Nerve tension tests gently stretch the nerves and are painful when the nerve is inflamed due to disc injuries. They are non specific but can be revealing when combined with the history and other findings. Straight leg raise (SLR) is a nerve tension test for the L4, L5 and S1 nerves.

Dermatomal sensory exam

If the disc is injured the nerves and occasionally the spinal cord will become inflamed. Sensation in the nerve roots may be normal, numb or hypersensitive. In patient terms, the sensation created with a pin or pinwheel will be prickly and sharp (normal), dull (reduced) or very sensitive and unpleasant and "icky" (hyperesthesia). Nerves usually become hypersensitive long before they lose function and become numb.

A dermatomal sensory examination is performed by gently stroking a pinwheel, a pin or some sharp object such as a paper clip across the skin of the dermatome. All dermatomes, C2 through S3, should be tested to determine the sensory status beyond the area of pain complaint to evaluate for multiple levels of disc injury, more widespread central sensitization or spinal cord involvement.

Reflexes

Reflex testing is done with a brisk strike of a reflex hammer to create a brisk tendon stretch to evaluate the reflex arc associated with nerve root being interrogated. If the nerve root is not seriously compromised the reflex will be brisk, normal and rated +2/4. A normal deep tendon reflex does not mean that the disc is uninjured it only suggests that the disc is not likely to require surgery.

If the nerve is more seriously compromised the reflex will be reduced or absent at the level of the injured disc. Reflexes that are hyperactive below the level of the injured disc are as revealing as reduced reflexes. A deep tendon reflex has normal brisk amplitude because descending inhibitory impulses from the brain reach the segment in time to dampen the reflex arc. If the spinal cord is inflamed above the level of the reflex being tested the inflammation slows conduction in the cord and prevents the inhibitory impulses from reaching the segment in time and the reflex below the injured level will be hyperactive. A hyperactive patellar reflex indicates inflammation in the spinal cord at some level above L3 but is not specific as to what level. The best indicator of a cervical disc injury is a hyperactive patellar reflex. Analysis of the complete physical examination will usually reveal the precise level involved.

Muscle testing

Muscle testing is done by isolating the involved muscle and gently loading it to determine strength. If the muscle "locks and holds" when loaded it has full strength (+5/5). If it contracts but doesn't "hold" against testing pressure it is somewhat weak (+4/5). If it is unable to hold against any pressure it is weak (+3/5). And if it is unable to lift against gravity it is significantly weak (+2/5). The reader is referred to Hoppenfeld (1976) or a similar physical examination text for a more complete description of muscle testing and evaluation.

Loss of motor function (+3/5) suggests serious neural compromise and a surgical consult is advised even if the patient is going to be treated conservatively.

Myofascial involvement

The biomechanical abnormalities of the spinal segment associated with disc degeneration can contribute to the formation of myofascial trigger points in the muscles and fascia. Trigger points cause the muscles to be short and taut and contribute to the compression and loading of the discs and facets that accelerates the degenerative process.

Myofascial trigger points sensitize pain nerves that feed back into the spine. This neural input from the muscles compounds the nociceptive sensitization of the nerves to the disc from the dorsal rami and amplifies the pain response. Palpation of the muscles in the lumbar spine will almost always reveal trigger points in the psoas, quadratus lumborum and multifidi, most prominently at the level of the involved disc.

In the cervical spine, the scalenes, longus coli, levator scapulae, sternocleidomastoid (SCM) and trapezius will usually have trigger points in the area directly adjacent to the involved disc. Palpate the deep scalenes between the thyroid cartilage and the SCM and feel a taut band just along the border of the anterior disc line. This taut band is an indicator that the disc at that level is inflamed. When the disc is treated the band should soften and disappear as treatment progresses.

When discs in the thoracic spine are inflamed the thoracic paraspinals and trapezius directly adjacent to the disc will be taut and may contain trigger points; digestion may be affected. The rectus abdominus may be taut and have trigger points at the levels whose nerves are affected by the injured disc.

The practitioner treating a disc patient will of necessity end up treating the disc, the nerve and the muscles associated with that disc.

More than one diagnosis

Patients who have both facet and disc generated pain will have pain with both flexion and extension and may have trouble finding a relief position. Specifically, it is common in patients who have had whiplash injuries to have a C5–6 disc injury from the flexion component that creates neck and shoulder pain and a C2–3 facet joint injury from the extension component that creates upper cervical pain and a periorbital headache. As the patient flattens the cervical curve to relieve the upper facets the disc annulus compresses and the patient begins to experience discogenic midscapular and nerve pain. The patient will arch the neck to relieve the disc pain until the facet

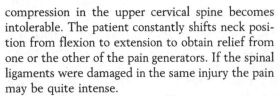

compression in the upper cervical spine becomes intolerable. The patient constantly shifts neck position from flexion to extension to obtain relief from one or the other of the pain generators. If the spinal ligaments were damaged in the same injury the pain may be quite intense.

Patients with chronic low back pain may have pain generators in the disc annulus, the facet joints, the muscles and the nerves. The same injuries that traumatize and damage the discs can also damage the muscles and facet joints. The psoas attaches to the anterior vertebral bodies and the discs and the lesser trochanter in the femur and acts as a trunk and hip flexor. Lumbar flexion may be painful because of a disc injury or it may be painful because trigger points in the psoas are activated when the muscle contracts to flex the trunk but the presence of trigger points in the psoas does not rule out the disc as a pain generator in lumbar flexion. The facet joints may cause pain when compressed during lumbar extension or the trigger points in the psoas may be activated when stretched during extension. The patient may have the disc, the muscle and the facet joint all contributing as pain generators.

As always the patient is entitled to more than one diagnosis. FSM practitioners have tools to treat each of these conditions and the only challenge is figuring out which to treat first in any given patient or whether to treat them all simultaneously (see Chapters 5, 6, 7, 11).

Treating spinal discs

Hydration

- The patient must be hydrated to benefit from microcurrent treatment.
- Hydrated means 1 to 2 quarts of water consumed in the 2 to 4 hours preceding treatment.
- Athletes and patients with more muscle mass seem to need more water than the average patient.
- The elderly tend to be chronically dehydrated and may need to hydrate for several days prior to treatment in addition to the water consumed on the day of treatment.
- *DO NOT* accept the statement, "I drink lots of water"
- *ASK* "How much water, and in what form, did you drink today before you came in?"
- Coffee, caffeinated tea, carbonated cola beverages do not count as water.
- Water may be flavored with juice or decaffeinated tea.

Channel A: condition frequencies

The frequencies listed are thought to remove or neutralize the condition for which they are listed except for 81 and 49 / which are thought to increase secretions and vitality respectively. They are listed alphabetically not in order of use or importance.

- Calcium ions   91
- Chronic inflammation   284
- Hemorrhage or bleeding   18
- Inflammation   40
- Scarring   13
- Sclerosis   3
- Secretions (Increase)   81
- Torn or broken   124
- Vitality (Restore)   49
- The basics
  ○ remove trauma   294
  ○ restore function   321
  ○ remove histamine   9

Channel B: tissue frequencies

- Disc as a whole: ___ / 630
  ○ This frequency is thought to address the entire disc structure.
- Disc Annulus: ___ / 710
  ○ The well innervated disc annulus is the most pain sensitive and most easily injured portion of the disc. It consists of coiled layers of sturdy connective tissue wrapped around the gel like nucleus. This tissue frequency responds best to treatment.
- Disc Nucleus: ___ / 330
  ○ The gel like disc nucleus fills the center of the disc and absorbs water to become a cushion for the vertebral bodies in the spine. It is very high in PLA_2 and very inflammatory.
- Dermatomal or Peripheral Nerve: ___ / 396
  ○ Any nerve outside the spinal cord
- Spinal cord: ___ / 10
  ○ Conducts impulses between the nerves and the brain

A/B pair for Inflammation
40 / 116
40Hz reduces inflammation, 116 is the frequency for the immune system. 40 / 116 reduced inflammation in the mouse model by 62% in a 4-minute

time-dependent response regardless of which tissue had been affected by the arachidonic acid.

A/B pair for Scar Tissue

- 58 / 00
- 58 / 01
- 58 / 02
- 58 / 32

These frequencies were discovered in a list of frequencies published by Albert Abrams in Electro-medical Digest in 1931. 58 / 00 was the frequency combination to remove "abnormal cellular stroma", probably meant to address the tendency of the cell to form scar tissue. 58 / 01 was used for scar in bony tissue. 58 / 02 was used for scar in soft tissue and 58 / 32 was used for scar tissue adhesions. These are A/B pairs in which channel A is not a condition and channel B is not a tissue but both frequencies form a frequency pattern that appears to eliminate or lengthen scar tissue.

In treating chronic complaints the 58/'s are used in order as listed above for approximately one to two minutes each at the beginning of the treatment to soften the tissues. If there is no bone involved in the complaint it is customary to leave out 58 / 01. For those practitioners who can feel the softening produced by the frequency, it is often helpful to run the frequency until the softening stops and the tissue becomes relatively more firm. There may be some patients in whom one or more of these frequencies will produce softening for up to 3 to 4 minutes.

The 58/'s will increase range of motion but do not change pain.

Caution: 58 / 00, 01, 02, 32

- Do not use these frequencies on injuries newer than 5 to 6 weeks old.
- Newly injured tissue must form scar tissue in order to repair itself.
- Removing the scar tissue seems to undo the healing by weeks in a new injury.
- The 58/'s can be used very briefly (15 seconds) to modify scar tissue as it is forming after the first four weeks.
- Never use this combination before the injury is 4 weeks old

This precaution is the result of trial and uncomfortable error. A patient was being treated for facet and soft tissue injuries caused by an auto accident that had occurred 3 weeks previously. She was pain free after four treatments in 21 days and was treated on a Tuesday. She returned on Thursday complaining that whatever had been done on Tuesday had "undone" 2 weeks worth of healing and she felt as much pain as she had 2 weeks previously. Review of the Tuesday treatment revealed that the 58/'s had been used in addition to the protocols that had been reducing the pain for the preceding 3 weeks. She was so pain free that it seemed as if the injury was much older and the date of injury was not checked before treatment. The presumption was made that the 58/'s had removed repair tissue necessary to keep the joint and soft tissues pain free and stable. Two more errors in the first year of treating with FSM in similar situations helped to determine that the 58/'s should not be used within 5 to 6 weeks of a new injury. They can be used briefly 4 weeks after the date of injury – for 5 to 10 seconds each – to thin out scar tissue as it is forming, especially in athletes who seem to heal faster.

This reaction is predictable and reproducible. Take this precaution seriously. The wise practitioner will only make this mistake once. It is better not to make it at all.

Treating chronic discs

Channel A Condition / Channel B Tissue

40 / 396, 10

- Reduce Inflammation / in the nerve and the spinal cord
- Treatment time: Reducing nerve pain usually takes 5 to 20 minutes. Treat the cord to reduce inflammation and minimize pain amplification for 2 to 4 minutes or more if time allows, depending on pain chronicity. Treating the disc is important for its repair but that may be a long term project taking a matter of weeks or months. Reducing nerve pain and spinal cord sensitization is important to keep the patient comfortable during the disc healing process. A disc at one spinal level may receive innervation from three or more spinal levels which means that inter-neurons in the cord are also involved. When treating the nerve always treat the cord to reduce inflammation and minimize the opportunity for central pain amplification.

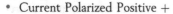

- Current Polarized Positive +
- Treatment Application: Position the positive leads over the spinal outflow of the nerve and the negative leads at the distal end of the nerve affected by the disc being treated

58 / 00, 02, 32

- **A/B pairs to remove scarring.** Use the 58/'s to remove the scar tissue from the disc annulus and the tissue in the surrounding area.
- **Treatment time:** 1–2 minutes or as needed. When used to treat chronic disc complaints the 58/'s are used in order as listed above for approximately 1 to 2 minutes each at the beginning of the treatment to soften or remove scar tissue. For those practitioners who can feel the softening produced by the frequency, it is often helpful to run the frequency until the softening is reduced and the tissue becomes relatively more firm. There may be some patients in whom one or more of these frequencies will produce softening for up to 3 to 4 minutes.
- **Current Polarized (+) or alternating (±) depending on patient response**

NOTE: Do not use 58/ in an acute exacerbation of a chronic disc problems. The disc needs to form scar tissue to repair the recent injury. The 58/'s may be used after the injury is 6 weeks old to soften the repair tissue and make the disc annulus more flexible and help prevent future re-injury.

40 / 630, 330, 710, 396

- Inflammation / disc as a whole, the nucleus, the annulus, and the nerve.
- The disc nucleus and annulus and nerve are most likely to be inflamed.
- Treatment time: Use these combinations for 2 to 4 minutes each.
- Current polarized (+) or alternating (±) depending on patient response.

284 / 630, 330, 710, 396

- Chronic inflammation / disc as a whole, the nucleus, annulus, and the nerve.
- Treatment time: Use these combinations for 1 to 2 minutes each or if you are sensitive to the feel of

tissue softening and time allows use the frequency as long as the softening happens.
- Current polarized (+) or alternating (±) depending on patient response.

91, 13 / 710, 396

- Calcium ions – hardening, scar tissue / disc annulus, and the nerve
- The frequency 91 Hz was originally thought to remove calcium from "stones" in the kidney or bile duct as indicated by its description on Van Gelder's list of frequencies. In July 2003, it was used for the first time to treat "hardening in the fascia" in the legs of a professional football player because his muscles and fascia felt like "stones" as they were being treated for scar tissue and hardening. 91 Hz produced remarkable softening in the fascia. Its usefulness in treating nerve pain was a late accidental discovery and its effectiveness was a pleasant surprise. It appears to soften virtually any chronically inflamed tissue.
- Calcium ions flow into nerve, fascia and other membranes during nerve depolarization and tissue inflammation (Winquist 2005). Using 91/ on any tissue removes something, presumed to be calcium, that perpetuates pain and hardens chronically inflamed tissue although there are no biopsy findings to confirm this. Clinically these frequency combinations produce profound softening of the tissue and reductions in pain and the exact mechanism of these changes are yet to be discovered.
- Treatment time: Use these combinations for 2 to 5 minutes each or if you are sensitive to the feel of tissue softening and time allows, use the frequency as long as the tissue softening happens.
- Current Polarized (+) or alternating (±) depending on patient response.

NOTE: Do not use 13 / 710 in acute exacerbations of chronic disc problems. The disc annulus needs scar tissue in order to repair. Do not use 13 / for 6 weeks following the acute episode.

81, 49 / 142, 710

- Increase secretions and vitality / in the fascia and the disc annulus

- 81 Hz is used for increasing secretions. / 142 Hz is used for the fascia. / 710 is for the disc annulus. The fascia secretes the ground substance necessary for repair of the fascia, ligaments and tendons and possibly the annulus (Myers 2001). Only use 81 / 710 when the discogenic pain is down to a 1–2/10. In the event that 81 Hz is actually increasing secretions, the secretions of the disc annulus are inflammatory when the disc is painful and increasing secretions may increase pain.
- Treatment time: Use for 1–2 minutes or if you are sensitive to the feel of tissue softening and time allows, use the frequency as long as the tissue softening happens.
- Current Polarized (+) or alternating (±) depending on patient response

49 / 630, 330, 710
- Restore vitality / in the disc as a whole, the nucleus and the disc annulus
- Treatment time: Treat for 1 minute each
- Current Polarized (+) or alternating (±) depending on patient response

If response is slow – narcotics

Experience has shown that patients who are on high levels of narcotics or who have had multiple injections with anesthetics respond slowly to treatment. This effect is reversed by the frequencies to "remove" narcotics and anesthetics. It is not thought that these frequencies actually remove the narcotic or anesthetic since they do not increase pain. It is much more likely that they somehow influence the membrane in such a way as to make it more receptive to treatment.

Use 43, 46, 19 / 396 first if the patient is on narcotics. The current application and lead placement are the same as for the disc treatment.

Treat the muscles

When treating the chronic disc remember to treat the muscles and trigger points in the muscles. The taut muscles act as confounding pain generators and compress the disc increasing the degenerative forces on both the disc and the facet joint.

Treat the psoas and lumbar paraspinal muscles in the low back.

Treat the scalenes and the cervical paraspinals in the neck.

Treat the thoracic paraspinals and the rectus abdominus in the trunk.

See Chapter 7 on treating muscles and myofascial pain for details of myofascial treatment.

58 / 00, 02, 32
- A/B pairs to remove scar tissue.
- If you have already used the 58/'s to treat the adhesions and scarring around the disc you may repeat them while focusing manual therapy on the muscles.

NOTE: Do not use 58/ in an acute exacerbation of a chronic disc problem. The disc needs to form scar tissue to repair the recent injury. The 58/s may be used after the injury is 6 weeks old to soften the repair tissue and make the disc annulus more flexible and help prevent future re-injury.

91, 13 / 62, 142, 396
- Remove calcium influx, scarring / from muscle belly, fascia and nerve.
- Use 91, 13 / 62, 142, 396 to treat the muscle belly and the fascia and visualize gently peeling the nerve away from the fascia. Use gentle movements to mobilize the fascia and the nerves.
- Treatment time: Use for 1–2 minutes or if you are sensitive to the feel of tissue softening and time allows, use the frequency as long as the softening happens.

40 / 116
- A/B pair to reduce inflammation.
- 40 / 116 seems to reduce inflammation in whatever tissue is involved. Use it in this case to reduce any inflammation not treated by 40 / and the disc tissues.
- Treatment time: Use for 4 minutes if time allows or use the frequency as long as the softening happens.

81, 49 / 142
- Increase secretions and vitality / in the fascia. The lead placement, current levels, polarity do not change when you treat the muscles. Focus the fingers on the soft tissues around the joint and on the muscles involved in the portion of the spine being treated.

Stenosis precaution

If there is dense scar tissue or bony stenosis of the nerve root or spinal cord or if a disc fragment is compressing the nerve root or cord at the involved level the patient's pain may increase when any current, especially polarized positive current is applied. If the patient is positioned comfortably, it is the only time the pain will increase during polarized positive treatment for nerve inflammation. Pain may increase in the dermatome or at the spine or both. Assess patient position to determine whether it is contributing to the pain increase.

Stop treating immediately if pain goes up during treatment. Move the patient to a seated position if possible. Move the contacts slightly up the spine superior to the nerve root being treated, reduce current levels and change the current from polarized positive to alternating. If this is going to reduce the reaction it will do so in five to ten minutes. If the pain continues to increase, stop treating with current. The pain should go back down in a few hours although it may take up to 24 hours to reduce to base line.

This reaction is diagnostic. If physical examination findings of reduced sensation and deep tendon reflexes at the involved level or hyperactive deep tendon reflexes below the involved level are present this reaction suggests the need for imaging to confirm the presence of compression and surgical referral if appropriate.

Treatment application for chronic disc pain

Current level: 100–300μamps

- Use lower current levels for very small or debilitated patients. Use higher current levels for larger or very muscular patients. In general higher current levels reduce pain more quickly. Do not use more than 500μamps as animal studies suggest that current levels above 500μamps reduce ATP formation while current levels below 500μamps increase ATP.

Current polarization

- **Alternating or Biphasic Current (±):** Current is used in alternating mode for treatment of most tissues except nerves. "Alternating DC current" is actually DC (direct) current that alternates its polarity from positive to negative during the machine duty cycle. Some patients respond better to alternating current than they do polarized positive current. Trying both applications is the best way to determine which will be optimal.

- **Polarized Positive Current (+):** Current is polarized positive for all nerve treatments and may be optimal in treating discs and muscle in some patients. In polarized positive current the DC wave form alternates from positive to "more positive" in a square wave pattern above the zero line on an oscilloscope. Some patients simply respond better to polarize positive current and some respond better to alternating or biphasic current. There is no explanation for this observed difference in response. Trying both is the best way to determine which will be optimal.

Waveslope: moderate to sharp

- The waveslope refers to the rate of increase of current in the wave as it rises zero up to the treatment current level for every frequency pulse. A sharp waveslope has a very steep leading edge on the square wave indicating a very sharp increase in current. A gentle waveslope has a very gradual leading edge on the waveform indicating a gradual increase in current.
- Use a moderate to sharp waveslope for chronic pain.
- Use a gentle waveslope for acute pain or new injuries. A sharp waveslope is irritating in new injuries.

Lead placement

FSM typically uses graphite gloves to conduct the current but adhesive electrode pads may also be used. The graphite gloves need to be kept moist so they conduct the current comfortably. The graphite gloves can be placed in a small warm wet towel or fabric sleeve or alligator clips can connect the leads to the wet contact.

Care should be taken to see that the wet fabric contacts do not touch each other. Current will follow the path of least resistance and the wet contacts are presumed to be less resistant than the patient therefore the current will flow in the wet contacts and avoid the tissue that needs treating.

To treat the disc only

- Place the **positive leads** in wet fabric to ensure a broad contact on the posterior spine at the involved spinal segment where the discs are painful in the cervical, thoracic or lumbar spine.
- Place the **negative leads** in wet fabric placed on the body anterior to the spinal contact to treat only the disc (Figs 4.5 to 4.8).

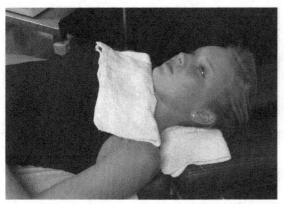

Figure 4.5 • Graphite gloves are placed in warm wet fabric contacts (face cloths). The graphite glove with the two positive leads in it is placed behind the neck and the graphite glove with the two negative leads in it is placed on the chest to allow current and frequencies to flow through the injured discs. This placement is used if there is no significant dermatomal nerve pain.

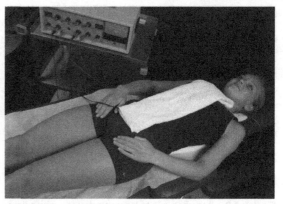

Figure 4.7 • Place the graphite glove with the negative leads attached inside a warm wet fabric contact (hand towel) and lay it down the center of the trunk so that all thoracic nerve roots and the discs can be treated.

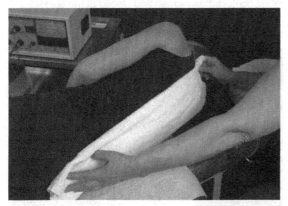

Figure 4.6 • Thoracic discs irritate thoracic nerves whose dermatomes are on the trunk. Place the graphite glove with the positive leads attached inside a warm wet fabric contact (hand towel) and lay it lengthwise down the spine.

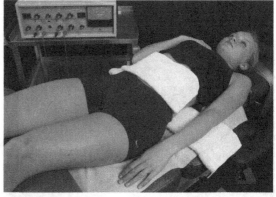

Figure 4.8 • Place the graphite gloves in separate warm wet fabric contacts (hand towel). If there is no dermatomal nerve pain the lumbar discs can be treated by placing the positive leads glove fabric contact behind the back and the negative leads contact on the abdomen. If two machines are being used to treat the disc and the nerve and muscle simultaneously place the positive leads from both machines in the contact behind the back. Place the negative leads glove from the machine running the disc protocol on the abdomen and place the negative leads glove from the machine running the nerve and muscle protocol at the distal end of the affected nerve.

OR

- Place the **positive leads** contact at the spine to treat the cervical or lumbar discs.
- Wrap the **negative leads** around the limb at the end of the dermatomal nerve if nerve pain is to be treated (Figs 4.9 & 4.10).

OR

- Place the **positive leads** contact lengthwise down the length of the spine so it contacts all cervical, thoracic and lumbar discs and nerve outflows from the spine (see Fig. 4.6).

- Place the **negative leads** contact either on the body anterior to the spinal contact or wrapped around the distal end of the affected nerve root.
- For cervical nerves place the negative leads at the end of the nerve as shown in Figure 4.9.

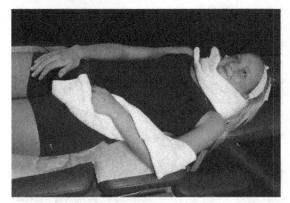

Figure 4.9 • If the nerve is to be treated at the same time as the disc, wrap the positive leads glove in a warm wet fabric contact (hand towel) and wrap the contact around the neck so the current flows through the nerve from proximal to distal. Wrap the negative leads glove in a warm wet fabric contact (hand towel) and wrap the contact around the nerve root to be treated. The C5, C6, C7, C8, T1 and T2 nerve roots are being treating in this photograph. To treat the C3 or C4 nerve roots the negative contact would be placed up near the shoulder at those dermatomes.

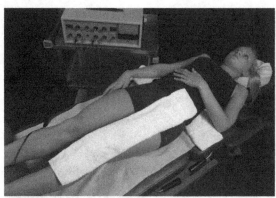

Figure 4.11 • If the nerve is to be treated at the same time as the disc the contact with the negative leads glove wrapped in it needs to be placed at the end of the nerve being treated in this case L3, L2, and L1. If all five nerve roots require treatment the towels can be connected to make one longer contact which is wrapped around the foot and extending up the leg to L1. The graphite glove with the positive leads is wrapped in the warm wet fabric contact (hand towel) and placed at the spine.

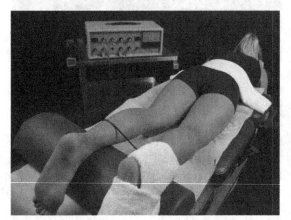
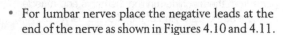

Figure 4.10 • If the nerve is to be treated at the same time as the disc the contact with the negative leads glove wrapped in it needs to be placed at the end of the nerve being treated in this case L4, L5 and S1. The graphite glove with the positive leads is wrapped in the warm wet fabric contact (hand towel) and placed at the spine.

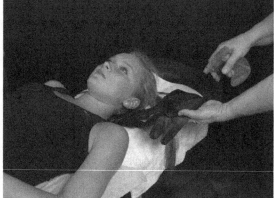

Figure 4.12 • The graphite glove can be placed directly on the skin after being wet thoroughly by spraying with water. The glove must be wet or the current will sting and prickle. There is not enough current to create a burn but it can be very uncomfortable.

- For lumbar nerves place the negative leads at the end of the nerve as shown in Figures 4.10 and 4.11.

OR

- **Graphite gloves** alone may be used
- If only the disc is to be treated and the nerve does not require treatment, the **positive leads** graphite glove can be placed directly on the skin under the spinal area to be treated after being wet thoroughly by spraying with water.
- **Note:** The glove must be wet or the current will sting and prickle. There is not enough current to create a burn but it can be very uncomfortable.
- The **negative leads** graphite glove can be placed directly on the skin on the body surface anterior to

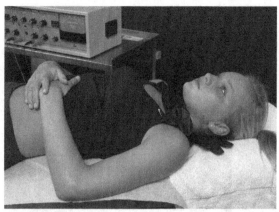

Figure 4.13 • The graphite glove can be placed directly on the skin if that is most convenient. Once the glove is moistened with water it usually stays moist for the duration of the treatment. The galvanic skin response to current flow usually creates slight sweating under the contact. This placement is for a cervical disc injury that has no neuropathic pain component. Place the positive leads contact at the back of the neck and the negative leads contact on the chest or on the front of the neck. This placement puts the contacts in the correct position for polarizing the current should that become necessary.

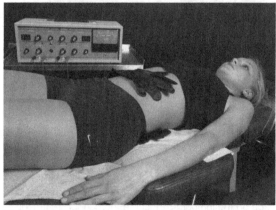

Figure 4.14 • The graphite glove can be placed directly on the skin if that is most convenient and there is no dermatomal neuropathic pain component. Once the glove is moistened with water it usually stays moist for the duration of the treatment. The galvanic skin response to current flow usually creates slight sweating under the contact. This placement is for a lumbar disc injury that has no neuropathic pain component. Place the positive leads contact at the low back and the negative leads contact on the abdomen. This placement puts the contacts in the correct position for polarizing the current should that become necessary.

the spinal area to be treated after being wet thoroughly by spraying with water.

OR

• **Adhesive Electrode Pads** may be used for convenience although the gloves seem to be more effective for reasons not understood. The adhesive electrode pads are especially useful for home treatment because they allow the patient to be active while being treated.

When applying treatment with adhesive electrode pads, the current and the frequencies must pass through the area to be treated in an interferential pattern, forming an "X" in three dimensions. The positive electrodes are placed at the spine at the level of the disc to be treated. The negative electrodes may be placed directly anterior or anterior and slightly inferior to the spinal contacts if the disc alone is being treated or if the nerve is to be treated the negative electrodes may be placed at the ends of the nerve root affected by the injured disc.

A diagram for the placement would look like this:

Positive Electrode Channel A	Positive Electrode Channel B
Area to be Treated	
Negative Electrode Channel B	Negative Electrode Channel A

Disc with no nerve involvement

• Place the **positive electrode from channel A** on the skin just lateral to the spinal segment at the level of the disc.
• Place the **negative electrode from channel A** so the current flows down an imaginary line diagonally through the body from the channel A positive electrode to the abdomen just anterior to the involved disc.
• For example to treat a lumbar disc with no nerve involvement place the positive lead from channel A on the right side of the low back. Place the negative leads from channel A on the left side of the abdomen at or below the same level as the disc being treated.
• Place the positive lead from Channel B on the left side of the low back and the negative leads from channel B on the right side of the abdomen.

Disc with nerve involvement

For example for a C6 disc with left hand pain from the C6 or C7 dermatome place the positive lead from channel A at the C6 disc level on the right side of the

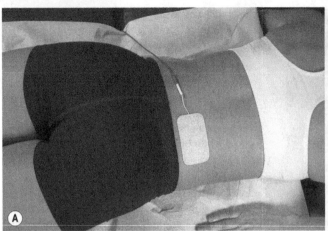
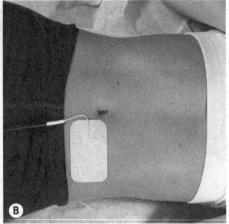

Figure 4.15 • A – Photo pad placement lumbar spine – channel A positive lead – Posterior. B – Photo pad placement lumbar spine – channel A negative lead – Anterior. To treat a lumbar disc with no nerve involvement, place the positive lead from channel A on the right side of the low back. Place the negative lead from channel A on the left side of the abdomen at or below the same level as the disc being treated. Place the positive lead from Channel B on the left side of the low back and the negative leads from channel B on the right side of the abdomen.

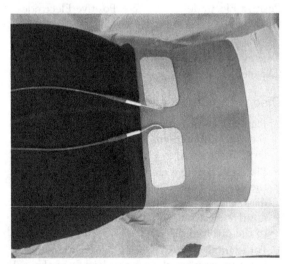

Figure 4.16 • Pads from Channel A and Channel B placed on the back for lumbar spine treatment.

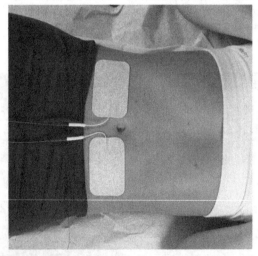

Figure 4.17 • Pads from both Channel A and Channel B in place on the lumbar spine and abdomen for treatment of lumbar disc without nerve involvement.

neck so it wraps around the neural foramen and place the negative lead from channel A on the dorsal surface of the hand at the distal end of the C6 and C7 dermatome. Create an interferential pattern by placing the positive leads from channel B on the left side of the neck and the negative leads from channel B on the palmar surface of the left hand at the distal end of the C6 and C7 dermatome.

Patient position

Patient supine

- **Treating the lumbar spine:** Position the patient so the knees and hips are straight and the low back naturally arched into extension unless the patient has accompanying facet disease. Extension is the comfort position for the lumbar discs. If there is

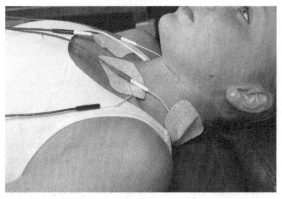

Figure 4.18 • Place the positive leads from channel A on the right side of the neck and the negative lead from channel A on the left upper chest just below the clavicle. Place the positive leads from channel B on the left side of the neck and the negative leads from channel B on the right upper chest just below the clavicle. The current and frequencies form an interferential pattern, crossing in three dimensions through the area to be treated.

accompanying facet joint pain find whatever neutral comfortable position is possible. The patient may be treated side lying.

• **Treating the cervical spine:** Position the patient with the chin in neutral so the neck is naturally

curved into slight extension. Extension is the comfort position for cervical discs. If there is coexisting facet generated pain the patient may have trouble finding a comfortable position. Placing a small one inch diameter roll under the C5–6 disc area to keep it in extension will allow the patient to flex and flatten the upper cervical spine and relieve the facet generated pain.

Patient prone

If the lumbar disc patient can lay prone it is the easiest position in which to treat the lumbar discs, nerves and muscles. The prone position puts the disc into extension, reduces radicular pain and the patient will prefer it as long as there is no coexisting facet joint disease. If there is accompanying facet joint pain find whatever neutral comfortable position is possible. The patient may be treated side lying.

If the cervical disc patient can be treated prone make sure the adjustable head rest is in neutral to allow a normal cervical curve. Do not put the neck in extension or the facet joints may become compressed and uncomfortable. Do not treat a cervical disc patient prone with the head turned to the side as it puts the disc in a rotational shear position. It is not possible to successfully treat a patient to reduce pain while their position is increasing pain.

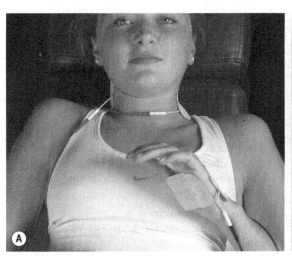
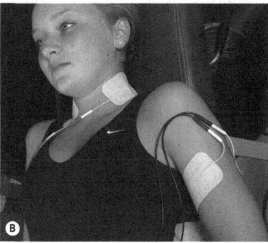

Figure 4.19 • A – Photo – pad placement cervical spine Channel A and Channel B – Cervical Disc and C6, C7 and C8 Nerve. B – Photo – pad placement cervical spine Channel A and Channel B – Cervical Disc and C4 and C5 Nerve. Place the positive lead from channel A on the right side of the posterolateral cervical spine over the neural foramen. Place the negative lead from channel A on the arm or hand at the level of the affected nerve, in this case C6, C7, and C8 on the hand. Place the positive lead from channel B on the left side of the cervical spine over the neural foramen and the negative lead from channel B on the other side of the hand. Placement for C4 nerve root is shown in B.

- **Treatment interval:** Chronic disc patients can and should be treated twice to three times a week for 4 to 6 weeks with at least one day separating the treatments. If the patient can afford a home microcurrent unit, it can be used daily as often as needed to eliminate nerve pain and to help speed repair of the disc.
- **Manual technique:** There is no manual therapy required while treating the disc which can be treated unattended. Manual therapy is helpful when treating the myofascial component of discogenic pain and when teasing apart the adhesions between the nerve and the fascia caused by the discogenic inflammation.
- For those trained in manual therapies using the hands while using FSM requires some adjustment of technique. The key is to let the frequency do the work and to use the hands with very gentle pressure and complete relaxation. The hands should be almost limp with just enough tone in the distal finger muscles to allow the fingers to gently assess the state of the tissue. The therapist should use the shoulder muscles and serratus to advance the arm and increase the pressure of the hand on the tissue being treated while keeping the hand relaxed. The hands are sensing change and softening in the muscles not forcing it. Let the frequency do the work. The patient's muscles will allow deeper palpation if the practitioners hands are relaxed and will defensively tighten if the contact is too firm or

Box 4.1

Summary for chronic discogenic pain

Treat the nerve
- 40 / 396, 10 (Polarize +)

Treat the disc (± or +)
- 58 / 00, 02, 32
- 40 / 630, 330, 710, 396
- 284 / 630, 330, 710, 396
- 91, 13 / 710, 396
- 81, 49 / 142, 710
- 49 / 630, 330, 710

If response is slow
- Use 43, 46, 19 / 396
- Use these frequencies first if the patient is on narcotics

Treat the muscle
- 58 / 00, 02, 32
- 91, 13 / 62, 142
- 40 / 116
- 81, 49 / 142

painful. Let the frequency do the work. If possible, move the fingers to the tissue being treated when the frequency for that tissue is running.

Treating acute discs

Use the acute disc protocol for the six weeks after an acute disc injury or an acute exacerbation of a chronic disc injury. When a patient presents within 12 hours of a fall, auto accident or any trauma in which the disc has been injured pain can be much reduced and recovery much accelerated by using FSM for the acute injury.

Caution: If the patient has lost reflexes, motor strength or sensation it is wise to request a surgical consult. 99% of acute disc injuries do not require surgical intervention but neuromuscular function should be monitored.
The patient can and should be treated while awaiting consult and imaging.

Caution: Do not use any frequencies to reduce hardening or scar tissue in an acute disc patient.

18 / 62
- Stop bleeding / arteries.
- 18Hz has been used clinically to stop bleeding in the menses and to prevent bruising. Use this only in the first 48 hours after the injury. It is used here because it is assumed that whatever trauma injured the disc may also have injured the vessels elsewhere.
- Treatment time: Use for 2 to 4 minutes or if you are sensitive to the feel of tissue softening and time allows, use the frequency as long as the softening happens.

40 / 396, 10 – Polarized +
- Reduce inflammation / in the nerves and the spinal cord.
- Treatment time: Treat the nerve to reduce inflammation using polarized positive current with the positive leads placed at the spine and the negative leads placed at the end of the inflamed nerve root. It may take 20 minutes to reduce nerve pain. Treat the nerve pain first since that is usually the most severe and bothersome pain and use the

frequencies to treat the disc after the nerve pain is less intense. The disc and the nerve can be treated simultaneously with two different machines – one focusing on the disc and one focusing on the nerve pain.

40 / 116

- **A/B pair for reducing inflammation.** 40Hz on channel A to reduce inflammation and 116 Hz on channel B thought to address the immune system were found to reduce LOX inflammation in the mouse model by 62% and COX inflammation by 30% in 4 minutes regardless of the tissue involved or the source of the inflammation. Reducing inflammation in human takes longer but does appear to be time dependent.

40 / 330, 630, 710 (± alternating or polarized +)

- Inflammation / disc nucleus, disc as a whole, disc annulus.
- Treatment time: Use these combinations for 4 to 10 minutes each. Research has shown 40Hz to have a time dependent response in a mouse model of inflammation. 50% of the reduction in inflammation was present at 2 minutes. The full response was present at 4 minutes. The nucleus and annulus are most likely to be inflamed. This part of the protocol will reduce the discogenic pain.

124 / 330, 630, 710

- **Remove the pattern of being "torn or broken" / disc nucleus, disc as a whole, disc annulus.** 124Hz is thought to remove the "fact of being torn or broken" from the injured tissue. This is a conceptual shift to the medically trained mind. In an energetic model, conditions have a physical consequence in the tissue – the physical structure of the disc is "torn or broken" – and at the same time there is an energetic or vibrational pattern that impresses itself on the semiconductor field that is the injured tissue. It is as if the pattern of being "torn or broken" has impressed itself on the disc's field, interfering with the normal healing processes and preventing tissue repair. The fact of being torn or broken is not just a disruption in tissue integrity; it is also a pattern in the field that may perpetuate the injury and prevent repair.
- In an energetic model it is thought that removing this pattern of being "torn or broken" allows the normal repair processes to become effective. This frequency rarely if ever changes symptoms but it seems to enhance tissue repair of "torn or broken" tissues.

- **Treatment time:** Use these combinations for 1 to 2 minutes each.

294, 321, 9, 124 / 330, 630, 710

- Trauma, Paralysis, Allergy Reaction, torn or broken / disc nucleus, disc as a whole, disc annulus.
- These four frequencies – "the basics" – do not tend to change symptoms but they appear to be important in restoring normal function to injured tissue. If you think of a time when you have suffered a physical injury you may notice that it is possible to distinguish between the symptoms from the injury and the effect of the "fact" of the trauma, the shock of it to your system. 294 / is thought to address the "fact of the trauma" or the shock to the system created by the trauma.
- When a tissue is traumatized it sometimes behaves as if it has "lost" a line of instructions not unlike a computer when it freezes for the same reason. 321 / is thought to "reboot" the tissue and is described as being used to neutralize "paralysis" moving it past the lost instruction and on to the next step to facilitate return to function.
- When any tissue is traumatized the first response is the secretion of histamine to initiate the inflammatory response. When treating to arrest the immediate effects of a new injury removing the histamine from the injured area seems to stop the inflammatory progression.
- These frequencies don't necessarily change symptoms but they seem to help speed recovery.
- Treatment time: Use for 1 to 2 minutes or if you are sensitive to the feel of tissue softening and time allows, use the frequency as long as the softening happens. Use these frequencies only on the first two to three treatments.

81, 49 / 142, 710

- 81Hz is used for increasing secretions. / 142 is used for the fascia. / 710 is for the disc annulus. The fascia secretes the ground substance necessary for repair of the fascia, ligaments and tendons and possibly the annulus (Meyers 2001).
- Use 81 / 710 ONLY when the discogenic pain is down to a 1–2/10. In the event that 81Hz is actually increasing secretions, the secretions of the disc annulus are inflammatory when the disc is painful and increasing them may increase pain.
- **Treatment time:** Use for 1–2 minutes or if you are sensitive to the feel of tissue softening and time allows, use the frequency as long as the tissue softening happens.

81, 49 / 396

- **Treatment time:** If there has been any motor weakness run 81 / 396 for 2 to 4 minutes once the pain is down or gone. Do not use 81 / 396 if the nerve pain is still present. If 81 / is indeed increasing secretions and the nerve is still inflamed then the secretions that will increase are inflammatory and the pain will go up. If the pain is down to the 0–2/10 range 81 / 396 can be used safely and has been known to increase muscle function. Use 49 / 396 for approximately one minute.

Stenosis precaution

If there is dense scar tissue or bony stenosis of the nerve root or spinal cord or if a disc fragment is compressing the nerve root or cord at the involved level, the patient's pain may increase when polarized positive current is applied. It is the only time the pain will increase during polarized positive treatment for nerve inflammation. It may increase in the dermatome or at the spine or both.

Stop treating immediately if pain goes up during treatment. Move the patient to a seated position if possible. Move the contacts slightly up the spine superior to the nerve root being treated, reduce current levels and change the current from polarized positive to alternating. If this is going to reduce the reaction it will do so in five to ten minutes. If the pain continues to increase, stop treating with current. The pain should go back down in a few hours although it may take up to 24 hours to reduce to base line.

This reaction is diagnostic. If physical examination findings of reduced sensation and deep tendon reflexes at the involved level or hyperactive deep tendon reflexes below the involved level are present this reaction suggests the need to perform an MRI to confirm the presence of compression.

Treatment application for acute disc pain

Treatment application and manual technique for acute disc pain is the same as for chronic disc pain with the exception of the waveslope and treatment interval. The patient may be more antalgic than the chronic disc patient so movement and patient positioning become even more critical.

Waveslope: gentle

The waveslope refers to the rate of increase of current in the wave as it rises in alternating mode from zero up to the treatment current level every

2.5 seconds on the Precision Microcurrent. Other microcurrent instruments may have slightly different duty cycles and the wave form may change more or less frequently. A sharp waveslope has a very steep leading edge on the wave shape indicating a very sharp increase in current. A gentle waveslope has a very gradual leading edge on the waveform indicating a gradual increase in current.

If the device being used allows the option, use a gentle waveslope for acute pain or new injuries as a sharp waveslope is irritating.

Patient position

The patient is even more sensitive to position in the acute disc injury than in chronic disc pain. Be sure the injured area is in extension unless there is accompanying facet joint generated pain. If there is accompanying facet joint pain find whatever neutral comfortable position is possible. The patient may be treated side lying or in any position that can be negotiated comfortably.

Muscle spasm and splinting caused by disc inflammation can make movement difficult. If the patient has trouble getting onto a treatment table, the best way to reduce the splinting is to use 40 / 396, 710 for about 10 minutes.

Treatment interval

Patients with acute disc injuries can and should be treated twice to three times a week for 4 to 6 weeks if time and finances allow it. The disc should heal in that time if no exacerbation has occurred. If the

Box 4.2

Summary for acute discs

Stop the bleeding
- 18 / 62

Treat the nerve
- 40 / 396, 10 (polarize +)

Treat the disc
- 40 / 116, 630, 330, 710, 396
- 294, 321, 9, 124 / 330, 630, 710
- 81, 49 / 142, 710 (After pain is reduced)
- 49 / 630, 330, 710

Treat the nerve
- 40, 81, 49 / 396 polarized + to reverse muscle weakness

If response is slow
- Use 43, 46, 19 / 396
- Use first if the patient is on narcotics

patient can afford a home microcurrent unit it can be used daily as often as needed to eliminate nerve and disc pain. Acute disc injuries usually recover fairly rapidly but each patient will respond differently depending on general health, emotional state, previous disc injuries and physical conditioning.

Adjunctive therapies

FSM treatment alleviates the pain and accelerates the healing process. Using proper posture, exercises and supplements will enhance the recovery and support the "stable state" required to maintain the benefits of treatment. The following recommendations are intended to provide guidance for FSM practitioners in very basic disc rehabilitation processes and are not intended as a comprehensive guide to disc rehabilitation. The practitioner is advised to consult with a rehabilitation specialist or training course for more complete instruction.

Posture recommendations

The patient should avoid flexion in the affected area of the spine in any form at all costs during the initial phases of disc healing. The patient should be advised to keep the lumbar spine in extension by keeping in mind the admonition to "stick your tail out" when sitting, standing or lifting and to use this lumbar extension as a way to keep the cervical spine in neutral with the ears over the shoulders. As the disc stabilizes and heals more completely the patient can begin to strengthen the core muscles and assume a more neutral posture.

The patient should be instructed to avoid activities or movements that create spinal flexion and combined flexion and rotation such as lifting, twisting, bending forward and improper sitting postures. Sitting posture that protects the cervical spine discs involves lumbar extension and erect spinal posture to bring the head and ears directly over the shoulders. The patient should sit up on the ischial tuberosities and rock the pelvis forward creating lumbar extension. This protects both the lumbar and cervical discs. Forward head posture causes strain on the neck muscles and the discs and increases compressive load on the discs and facet joints. Sitting in a car generally places the lumbar spine in flexion because the seat base is usually too long and the legs are outstretched. The patient should place a rolled up towel or a small pillow behind the low back to maintain the lumbar curve. This will protect both the lumbar and cervical discs.

The patient should be instructed to avoid prolonged static posture since it contributed to dehydration of the disc. The discs are hydroscopic structures and absorb and release water much like a sponge when compressed and then released. Gentle frequent small range movements as tolerated in segmental flexion and extension will help keep the discs hydrated.

The patient should consult with a therapist who can instruct them in proper posture and exercises to strengthen the muscles around the discs and mobilize the spine in a pain free range to increase circulation around the disc and increase the osmotic action required to rehydrate the discs. Extension exercises have been used to reposition the disc nucleus more centrally in the center of the annulus (McKenzie 2006). Patients with acute discs may benefit from a firm curved back brace to support the spine until exercises can strengthen the supporting muscles.

Both acute and chronic disc injuries will benefit from appropriate exercise prescribed and supervised by a physiotherapist or physical therapist, chiropractor, or physiatrist who specializes in exercise therapy. The following recommended exercises have been used clinically and found to be helpful but are by no means meant to replace expert advice.

Lumbar disc exercises

Have the patient lay prone and lift the straight leg and hip about a half inch off the bed. The glutes, the ipsilateral lumbar paraspinals and then the contralateral lumbar paraspinals should fire in that order. If the muscles do not fire in that order, reduce the load by reducing the height of the leg lift. It may be necessary to reduce the movement to the point of simply contemplating the lift. If the patient has coexisting facet joint disease, lying prone creates facet compression and this exercise is not advised.

Do five on each side morning and night – when in doubt do fewer reps more often, especially at first. Pelvic tilts need to be done with a towel rolled up to support the lumbar curve. Three sets of five morning and night are recommended.

Cervical disc exercises

Have the patient lay prone on the bed with the forehead resting on the back of the hands with the neck in neutral, chin slightly tucked. Lift the head just enough to engage the small intersegmental posterior cervical muscles by initiating the intention to lift the head. If the long spinal extensors or the trapezius engage the effort is too great and the patient should be instructed to reduce the effort. This is a very tiny movement; the forehead is never raised off the back of the hands. The bone may lift slightly but the skin doesn't lose contact with the back of the hands. After performing this central movement five times, the patient turns the head 10 degrees to the right and lifts the head the same way to engage the small inter-segmental cervical muscles that initiate rotation. After performing this right rotated movement the patient turns the head 10 degrees to the left and lifts five times. This is harder than it looks and if done properly the patient may feel muscle fatigue after less than five repetitions. Instruct the patient to stop when the muscles feel tired even if the fatigue occurs after only a few repetitions. The patient should be reassured that strength and stamina will build more quickly if the muscles do not become exhausted. Do five repetitions twice a day.

Chiropractors, osteopaths and physical therapists should exercise caution in side posture or rotary adjustments that may shear the disc. Manipulation and mobilization can be effective in reducing disco-genic pain and they have been known to make it worse. The patient should be positioned in such a way as to minimize combined flexion and rotation.

Nutritional support

Professional grade nutritional supplements can be helpful in reducing inflammation and relaxing muscles. Essential fatty acids (EPA/DHA) reduce inflammation at doses of one to eight grams per day as long as there is no contraindication to this dosage. Magnesium malate and magnesium glycinate are well absorbed and help relax muscle tissue. Glucosamine and chondroitin sulfate and MSM (methylsulfonylmethane) are said to be effective in reducing pain in degenerative joints. SAMe (s-adenosyl methionine) is becoming more widely used for reducing joint inflammation and pain. A complete listing of nutritional adjunctive therapies is beyond the scope of this text but the reader is encouraged to become knowledgeable in this area and to customize treatment to the patient's needs.

Acute disc case report

- Case report presentation, November 2003 FSM symposium
- Christopher J Bump, DC

History

DL is a 50-year-old female who originally presented for concerns about allergies and skin rashes in 2001.

The patient presented once again on April 19, 2002 for low back pain. Examination findings included reduced lumbar range of motion and pain. She had 25 degrees of flexion, 5 degrees extension, and lateral bending right and left both limited at 15 degrees. SLR, DTRs and sensory dermatome testing was essentially negative. Her para-spinal muscles, quadratous lumborum, and gluteus medius were splinted, with the right side more severe than the left. There was palpable tenderness at the L4–5 and L5–S1 vertebral levels. She was treated one time, utilizing SOT blocking, myofascial/trigger point therapy and Cox flexion–distraction technique. FSM was used additionally. Frequencies used were 294, 321, 9, 29, /142, 46 and also 94 / 200 (nervous tension). She was given stretches to do at home, and a natural anti-inflammatory. She did not return for a follow-up visit as her condition cleared after this initial intervention.

DL presented again on July 12, 2002 seeking advice for a diagnosis of disc herniation. The disc her-niation was a large centrally located disc extrusion causing severe spinal canal stenosis at the L4–5 level. Also, at the L5–S1 level there was a left side hernia-tion compressing the left neural foramina. She had sought the care of an orthopedic surgeon as she could not lift or feel her right foot. She had only mild achy-ness in her low back, but there was a burning pain radiating to her right calf. The orthopedic surgeon recommended immediate surgery but the patient wanted a second opinion.

Having treated HNP and disc conditions for 20 years I was quite apprehensive about attempting even a short course of intervention with such a severe disc condition as the L4–5 disc was actually extruded and her neurological symptoms were significant. The cause of the herniation was uncertain, however DL had recently begun a vigorous walking program and she suspected that was the provocation.

Examination

Height 5ft5 3/4ins, weight 194, BMI (Body Mass Index) 33. Blood pressure 142/118, and respiration was shallow and rapid at 20 breaths per minute. Lumbar range of motion was painful in extension at neutral position, and lateral bending right and left was painful in both directions at 20 degrees.

Kemp's test was positive to the right.

Heel-walk test was positive on the right – she could not lift the forefoot sufficiently to allow her to walk on her heels.

Straight Leg Raise was positive right at 70 degrees. Braggard's test was positive right. Both patellar and Achilles deep tendon reflexes were diminished, graded 2 on a scale of 1–5, bilaterally. Dermatome/sensory distribution was diminished in the L4, L5, and S1 dermatomes, bilaterally. Calf circumference right 16ins, left 16 1/2ins. There was noted fixation of the L4–5 and L5–S1 vertebral motor units, and associated muscle splinting.

Imaging

MRI findings from study performed by Radiological Associates on 7/10/2002 revealed the following:

1. Central and right Para central herniation with disc extrusion at L4–5 causing marked right central canal stenosis seen on axial sequence image #15.
2. Left sided L5–S1 herniation compressing the left L5–S1 neural foramina at its origin

Diagnosis

Multiple herniated nucleus pulposus with associated neuropathy, muscle atrophy and spasm.

Treatment

As mentioned above, I was apprehensive about accepting this case, as my experience with disc extrusions involved referral to a neurosurgeon. However, the patient was persistent about wanting to avoid surgery at all costs, and asked if I might try anything I could. Because I utilize non-osseous manipulative chiropractic techniques, that include Cox flexion–distraction and SOT, I agreed to do a short trial of treatment and to continue to treat as long as her condition improved. In other words, I agreed to treat her conditionally. My previous experience treating mild to moderate disc herniation has been favorable, but disc extrusions were always a referred out to surgical specialists.

DL was treated 22 times from July 12th 2002 through October 9, 2002. Her treatment schedule was intense in the first 4 weeks at three times per week. As she improved therapy was administered twice weekly, and then once per week.

Treatment was simple, and remained basically the same throughout the 12 weeks of her care. She was

blocked according to SOT Category III for right short leg, and her L3–4, L4–5, and L5–S1 vertebral motor units were distracted using Cox flexion-distraction technique.

Frequency-specific microcurrent was used in each session. As the patient was lying prone, a moistened conductive material was placed, with black-leads attached, under her abdomen, between her symphysis pubis and naval. Another moistened conductive material attached to the red leads, and placed over her lower lumbar spine. The initial settings used were set at 100µamps in a bi-phasic, or alternating, polarity. They were 294, 321, 9, 124, 40 / 330, 630, 710. The treatment was approximately 30 minutes long for the first session, with the frequencies being changed every 2 minutes.

The patient returned on July 15 with a significant reduction in pain going from an 8–9 on a visual analog scale down to a 6. She continued to make progress with her symptoms reducing in a progressive fashion over time. She experienced minor exacerbations with over-exertion, but recovered quickly from each event. Both the pain and tingling down her right leg into her great-toe improved and her heel-walk test strengthened. The frequencies stayed the same for the first two weeks. After the acute phase of treatment 294 and 321 were not used but 284 for chronic inflammation was added.

The majority of treatment was done with the following settings, all done at 100µamps: 284, 40, 3 / 330, 630, 710, 396. The frequencies were chosen for their ability to treat trauma 294, paralysis 321, histamine 9, acute inflammation 40, chronic inflammation 284, adhesions 3, and torn or broken tissue 124. These condition frequencies were directed at the disc, which has three different frequencies 330, 630 and 710.

The patient was referred to a neurologist early in treatment on July 19, 2002. He recommended a course of conservative treatment to begin with, based on her signs, symptoms, response to treatment already, and her unwillingness to undergo surgery.

After a follow-up visit with the neurologist on September 10, he recommended that she continue with the FSM and Chiropractic treatment and that surgery would not be necessary. Her foot drop continued to improve; she began an exercise/walking routine on the August 15, just 4 weeks after beginning treatment. By the end of August into early September she had symptoms only with significant exertion and they resolved within hours.

She remained essentially symptom free through September and was released from care on October 9, 2002. I made an attempt to have a follow-up MRI done but because of the patient's lack of symptoms, the neurologist, orthopedist and insurance company declined authorization.

As of June 2003, the patient remains symptom free and continues to enjoy a very active life-style.

Impression

This case is both unique and interesting demonstrating the versatility and potency of FSM. As mentioned above, given the severity of her disc injury I would have in the past referred her back to the orthopedic or neurologist. And had it not been for her insistence on avoiding surgery at all costs, I probably would not have attempted any therapeutic intervention. However, having used other conservative procedures with previous success in the treatment of mild and moderate herniated discs, I felt at least, I could do no harm. What was most impressive about this case was the severity of herniation, with disc extrusion, the complication of presenting symptoms and the rapid and enduring response to treatment.

And choosing which frequencies to use and which tissues to treat was fairly straightforward.

Conclusion

In conclusion I would like to emphasize once again what was most impressive for me regarding the use of FSM in this case. First was the speed with which DL responded to intervention. In the past, severe foot-drop would respond very slowly, taking months to correct, not weeks. This is especially so given the severity of DL's neurological deficit. Second, just agreeing to treat this condition was beyond what I normally would treat, but having FSM as a therapeutic tool allowed me to do so with a degree of curiosity, excitement and apprehension. Third, this case offers a clear, practical application for FSM that can be incorporated with other therapies. It is my professional opinion, based on 20 years of clinical experience, using both SOT and Cox flexion-distraction techniques that they alone would not have been enough to correct DL's condition. FSM was the variable added to the intervention that in my opinion resulted in such profound and dramatic response.

Bibliography

Cloward, R.B., 1959. Cervical discography: mechanisms of neck, shoulder and arm pain. Ann. Surg. 150, 1052–1064.

Hoppenfeld, S., 1976. Physical examination of the spine and extremities. Appleton-Century Crofts. Division of Prentice Hall, New York.

Kang, J.D., Georgescu, H.I., Intyre-Larkin, L., et al., 1996. Herniated lumbar intervertebral discs spontaneously produce matrix metalloproteinases, nitric oxide, interleukin E2. Spine 21, 271–277.

Kraemer, J., 1995. Natural course and prognosis of intervertebral disc diseases. Spine 20, 635–639.

Lotz, J.C., Ulrich, J.A., 2006. Innervation, inflammation and hypermobility may characterize pathologic disc degeneration: review of animal model data. J. Bone Joint Surg. 88 (Suppl. 2), 76–82.

McKenzie, R., 2006. Treat your own back. Spinal Publications, New Zealand.

Meyers, T., 2001. Anatomy trains. Churchill Livingstone, Edinburgh, pp. 9–49.

Olmarker, K., Rydevik, B., Nordberg, C., 1993. Autologous nucleus pulposus induces neurophysiologic and histologic changes in porcine cauda equina nerve roots. Spine 18, 1425–1432.

Olmarker, K., Blomquist, J., Stromberg, J., et al., 1995. Inflammatogenic properties of nucleus pulposus. Spine 20, 665–669.

Ozaktay, A.C., Cavanaugh, J.M., Blagoev, D.C., 1995. Phospholipase A$_2$-induced electrophysiologic and histologic changes in rabbit dorsal lumbar spine tissues. Spine 20, 2659–2668.

Ozaktay, A.C., Kallakuri, S., Cavanaugh, J.M., 1998. Phospholipase A$_2$ sensitivity of the

dorsal root and dorsal root ganglion. Spine 23, 1297–1306.

Soloviuva, S., Kouhia, S., Leino-Arjas, P., et al., 2004. Interleukin polymorphisms and intervertebral disc degeneration. Epidemiology 15, 626–633.

Travell, J.G., Simons, D.G., 1983. Myofascial pain and dysfunction: the trigger point manual, vol. 1. Williams &Wilkins, Baltimore.

Travell, J.G., Simons, D.G., 1992. Myofascial pain and dysfunction: the trigger point manual, vol. 2. Williams &Wilkins, Baltimore.

Wang, Y.J., Shi, Q., Cheung, K.C., et al., 2006. Cervical intervertebral disc degeneration induced by unbalanced dynamic and static forces: a novel in vivo rat model. Spine 31, 1532–1538.

White, A.A., Panjabi, M.H., 1978. Clinical biomechanics of the spine. JB Lippincott Company, Philadelphia.

Treating facet joint generated pain

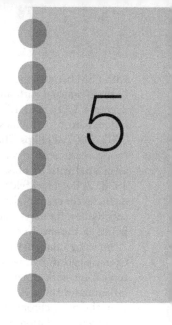

5

Facet joints are the posterior articulating joints in the spine. They carry most of the compressive load when the spine is in extension and guide motion during flexion, extension and rotation. High and low threshold mechanoreceptors and mechanically sensitive pain receptor nerves fire as the joint capsule is stretched and the cartilaginous joint surface compressed during joint movement. Proprioceptive nerve endings in the joint capsule fire during normal range of motion of the joint. Abundant free and encapsulated nerve endings and small nerve fibers capable of secreting substance P and calcitonin gene-related peptide (CGRP) enervate the capsule and joint surfaces. During trauma the joint approaches end range extension stretching the joint capsule and compressing the cartilage to the point of injury. Injury and inflammation of the facet joint and surrounding muscles excite and sensitize the nerves at the joint (Cavanaugh 1996). Excessive capsule stretch, seen in whiplash and hyperextension injuries, activates nociceptors in the joint capsule, leads to prolonged neural after-discharges and can cause damage to the capsule and to the axons in the capsule and is a probable cause of persistent neck and back pain. Facet joints have been implicated as a major source of low back and neck pain (Cavanaugh 2006).

Facet joints become painful as the joint tissues degenerate and become inflamed (Beaman 1993). The cartilage surface becomes irregular, frayed and calcified. The periosteum and subchondral bone becomes inflamed and calcified. Nerve fibers infiltrate the inflamed and degenerated tissues and secrete substance P in the eroded areas sending pain signals to the brain via the nerves and spinal cord. The nerves at the facet joint capsule transmit proprioceptive information in normal joints and pain information in inflamed or injured joints. Chen found more c-fiber receptors on the dorsolateral aspect of the facet joint where muscles and tendons were attached (Chen 2006). Inflammation leads to decreased firing thresholds and elevated baseline discharge rates of nerve endings in facet capsules (Cavanaugh 2006). Chronic inflammation leads to fibrosis between the nerves and soft tissues such as the capsule, the muscles and the fascia (Lewis 2004). These adhesions can make even normal motion painful as the nerves are stretched by the movement of the soft tissues to which they are adhered.

The reduced firing threshold, increased baseline neural discharge and perineural fibrosis in the injured and degenerated facet joint tissues feeds constant neural input into the spinal cord which feeds back to the muscles around the joint contributing to the formation of taut bands and myofascial trigger points in the paraspinal and postural muscles (Gerwin 2004). The myofascial trigger points compound the pain (Travell 1983, 1992) and the taut bands complicate joint function when the shortened sensitized muscle fibers contribute to joint compression and sensitized neural input and help perpetuate joint inflammation. This interaction between the nerve, joint and muscle forms a feed-back–feed-forward neuro-mechanical cycle that is very difficult to break once it becomes established and is the reason that chronic low back and neck pain is so pervasive and difficult to treat. To interrupt it effectively, all three aspects of dysfunction should be addressed at once. FSM makes this possible in most cases.

Identifying which pathologies in which tissues are creating the pain becomes important when treating

DOI: 10.1016/B978-0-443-06976-5.00005-8

with FSM because the frequency choices are specific to the tissue and pathology. FSM has been shown to decrease COX and LOX mediated inflammation, inflammatory cytokines and CGRP (McMakin 2005, 2007, Phillips 2000). FSM has been shown to decrease scar tissue and to reduce the pain associated with myofascial trigger points (McMakin 1998, 2004, Huckfeldt et al 2003). FSM has frequencies for calcium deposits and calcium influx into soft tissues, for nerve pain and for myofascial trigger points in the involved muscles.

By using adjunctive modalities such as appropriate exercise and stretching, posture re-education, oral or topical anti-inflammatory medications and oral anti-inflammatory nutrients such as fish oils (EPA/DHA) even the most chronic facet joint pain can improve. Complete resolution of acute or chronic facet pain may require more invasive interventions such as steroid and lidocaine injections into the joint under fluoroscopy to "get on top of" the inflammation so the more conservative modalities can be effective. Studies show that facet injections as a sole treatment modality aren't effective for long term facet joint pain relief but clinical experience has shown that when combined with other therapies such as FSM, appropriate exercise, nutritional supplementation and postural reeducation they can be a very successful adjunct.

Diagnosing facet joint pain

When the patient complains of neck, thoracic or lumbar spine pain, or "backache" the facet joints

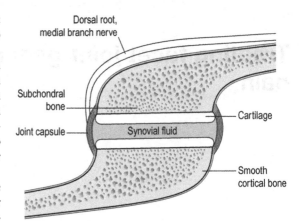

Figure 5.1 • A healthy facet joint has intact cortical bone, periosteum and cancellous bone. The joint capsule and ligaments are not thickened; the cartilage is hydrated and smooth and the synovial fluid is uniformly lubricating.

should be considered and examined for involvement. In general, the pain from the inflamed joint will be at the spine and radiating in a scleratomal pattern into the area just adjacent to the joint. Facet joint referred pain rarely goes below the knee in the lumbar spine and is most commonly seen in the upper back and shoulder in cervical spine facets.

The pain level may be rated from mild, 3–4/10 on a 0 to 10 visual analog scale (VAS) to severe, 7–8/10 VAS depending on the severity of recent injury, previous facet joint damage, degeneration, inflammation and scarring.

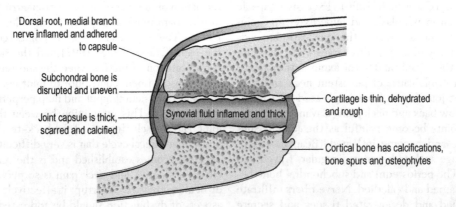

Figure 5.2 • Inflammation and chronic inflammation of the facet joint causes thickening of the joint capsule and ligaments and calcium deposits at the periosteum, the ligaments and the joint capsule. The cartilage is thinned and uneven and the synovial fluid is thick.

The pain will be worse with extension and sitting which compress the posterior joints and better with flexion which gaps the joints and relieves the pressure. The patient will state that they cannot lay prone at all and if laying supine must have the knees and hips flexed at 90 degrees. The pain will be worse with rotary motions that compress the joint on one side and move soft tissues that are adhered to nerves and the joint capsule. Movements that use trigger point laden muscles will create both local and referred pain from the myofascial trigger points. Inflammation in the facet joints can trigger neural pain and create dermatomal nerve pain although this is less common. The same injuries that traumatize and damage the facet joints can also damage the discs and the patient may have pain with flexion or rotation caused by disc inflammation (see Chapter 4).

The saying "The patient is entitled to more than one diagnosis" is especially true of patients with facet generated pain. The patient may have overlapping facet joint, neuropathic, discogenic and myofascial trigger point pain.

History of causation consistent with facet Injury

Any trauma that creates sudden spinal extension or compression can injure a facet joint. The most common traumatic mechanisms are automobile accidents and falls.

Prolonged static posture in extension while sitting or chronic poor muscle balance can lead to chronic segmental joint extension; compressing the facet joint and leading to local joint damage – most commonly seen in the lumbar or cervical spine.

The psoas muscle is the ultimate culprit in most chronic low back facet generated pain. The psoas and iliacus form the iliopsoas and attach to the anterior vertebral bodies and discs of the lumbar spine and the lesser trochanter of the femur. The psoas is a trunk flexor. When the psoas is tight it should pull the trunk into flexion but the posterior lumbar and thoracic paraspinal muscles tighten to keep the torso upright. These opposing mechanical forces compress both the facet joints and the discs but the facet joints seem to take the brunt of the insult.

A similar muscular imbalance exists in the cervical spine with the scalenes as neck flexors and the posterior neck muscles opposing to keep the neck upright. The lower cervical discs and the upper cervical facet joints are compromised in this case. Chronic forward head posture while seated reading or typing at a computer is responsible for muscle pain and fatigue and facet joint compression and degeneration.

Physical examination

Most practitioners reading this text have been trained to perform a physical examination to evaluate spine and facet joint pain. This brief

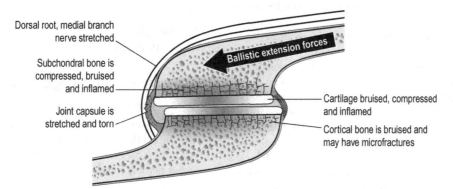

Figure 5.3 • During trauma ballistic extension forces stretch the facet joint capsule beyond its normal limits, compress and bruise the cartilage and subcortical bone, may cause micro-fractures in the cortical bone and traction injuries to the dorsal root medial branch. The damage causes inflammation; post-traumatic fibrosis impairs circulation and often leads to chronic inflammation and progressive joint degeneration. The capsule and ligaments are further stretched during the rebound flexion in a whiplash injury.

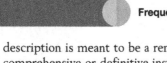

description is meant to be a reminder rather than a comprehensive or definitive instruction. The reader who desires more complete instruction is referred to Hoppenfeld (1976) or Souza (2009) or a similar resource.

This examination procedure may seem incredibly simply but it has been completely foolproof in the authors, experience when combined with a probable history and mechanism of injury. To examine the lumbar and thoracic spine facet joints, lay the patient prone and briefly and gently apply pressure to the suspect facet joints with the thumb placed perpendicular to the spine and parallel to the direction of the facet joint. If the patient says "ouch" then that facet joint is a pain generator. As the joint is compressed and patient reports pain, the paraspinal muscles will usually splint. If the examination is too forceful it will increase the patient's pain and in the worst case may contribute to further facet joint damage.

To examine the cervical spine facet joints have the patient lay supine or seated and gently and briefly use the finger pads to compress the joints. If the patient is supine gently lift up into the joints with the finger pads following the joint line and feel for the muscle splinting and guarding that accompanies the patient's report of pain. The joint capsule and surrounding muscles will feel like a tight firm ball just lateral to the midline. If the patient is seated support the head with one hand and gently and briefly use the pads of the fingers to compress the joints. If the patient says "ouch" then that joint is a pain generator. The postural muscles will be activated while the patient is seated and may camouflage the local muscle splinting that occurs when the joint is compressed.

If it is necessary for forensic or medical legal purposes to confirm that the joint identified by the physical examination is indeed a pain generator, the practitioner may order a facet block to be done to the joint in question. Facet blocks should be done, with some pain medication or light sedation, under fluoroscopy by physicians trained and certified by ISIS (International Spinal Injection Society) or some similar body. The block may be done with local anesthetic for diagnosis only but it is more common to do a block that is both diagnostic and therapeutic which combines an anti inflammatory steroid with a local anesthetic. If the block reduces or eliminates the joint pain it confirms that the joint was a pain generator.

Treating chronic facet joint pain

Hydration

- The patient must be hydrated to benefit from microcurrent treatment.
- Hydrated means 1 to 2 quarts of water consumed in the 2 to 4 hours preceding treatment
- Athletes and patients with more muscle mass seem to need more water than the average patient.
- The elderly tend to be chronically dehydrated and may need to hydrate for several days prior to treatment in addition to the water consumed on the day of treatment
- *DO NOT* accept the statement, "I drink lots of water"
- *ASK* "How much water, and in what form, did you drink today before you came in?"
- Coffee, caffeinated tea, carbonated cola beverages do not count as water.
- Water may be flavored with juice or decaffeinated tea.

Channel A: condition frequencies

The frequencies listed alphabetically are thought to remove or neutralize the condition for which they are listed except for 81, 49 / which are thought to increase secretions and vitality respectively

- Calcium ions, hardening   91 /
- Chronic inflammation   284 /
- Hemorrhage or bleeding   18 /
- Inflammation   40 /
- Scarring   13 /
- Sclerosis   3 /
- Secretions (Support)   81 /
- Vitality (Restore)   49 /

3 Channel B: facet joint tissue frequencies

- Bone: ___/ 59 and ___/ 39
  - Both frequencies are used when treating bone. It is presumed that one frequency is for cortical bone and one is for cancellous bone but it is not known what portion is addressed by which frequency.
- Periosteum: ___/ 783
  - The periosteum lines the outside of the bone, interweaves with tendinous and ligamentous attachments and is very well innervated and pain sensitive.

- Cartilage: ___ / 157
  - Cartilage lines the facet joint and becomes damaged, degenerated, calcified and inflamed when traumatized by acute or chronic compression of the joint surface.
- Joint Capsule: ___ / 480
  - The joint capsule attaches to the periosteum, surrounds the joint and becomes fibrosed, calcified, scarred and inflamed when over stretched by trauma.
- Tendons: ___ / 191
  - The tendons attach the muscles and fascia to the postero-lateral joint capsule and periosteum.
- Ligament: ___/100
  - The spinal ligaments connect adjacent joints by attaching bone to bone at the periosteum.
- Nerve: ___/ 396
  - The recurrent nerves innervating the joint capsule transmit proprioceptive information in the normal facet joint and pain information in the degenerated joint. They infiltrate the joint in response to chronic inflammation becoming fibrosed and scarred to the capsule and fascia as degeneration progresses. Dermatomal nerve roots may become painful as inflammatory peptides diffuse out from the inflamed facet joint tissues.
- Fascia: ___/142
  - The fascia is the thin connective tissue covering surrounding the muscles and all soft tissues. The fascia becomes inflamed, calcified and fibrosed during the degenerative process.
- Artery and Elastic Tissue in the Muscle Belly: __/ 62
  - 62 is the frequency used for the artery and the elastic tissue in the arterial walls. The muscle belly responds to this frequency either because it is full of small arteries or because the elastic tissue in the muscle belly is somehow related to the artery wall.

A/B pairs for scar tissue

- 58 / 00
- 58 / 01
- 58 / 02
- 58 / 32

These frequencies were discovered in a list of frequencies published by Albert Abram's in Electro-medical Digest in 1931. 58 / 00 was the frequency combination to remove "abnormal cellular stroma", whatever that might have been. 58 / 01 was used for scar in bony tissue. 58 / 02 was used for scar in soft tissue and 58 / 32 was used for scar tissue adhesions.

In treating chronic complaints the 58/'s are used in order as listed above for approximately 1 to 2 minutes each at the beginning of the treatment to soften the tissues. If there is no bone involved in the complaint it is customary to leave out 58 / 01. For those practitioners who can feel the softening produced by the frequency, it is often helpful to run the frequency until the softening is reduced and the tissue becomes relatively more firm. There may be some patients in whom one or more of these frequencies will produce softening for up to 3 to 4 minutes.

The 58/'s will increase range of motion but do not change pain.

Caution: 58 / 00, 01, 02, 32
- Do not use these frequencies on injuries newer than 5 to 6 weeks old.
- Newly injured tissue must form scar tissue in order to repair itself.
- Removing the scar tissue seems to undo the healing by weeks in a new injury.
- The 58/'s can be used very briefly (15 seconds) to modify scar tissue as it is forming after the first four weeks.
- Never use this combination before the injury is 4 weeks old

This precaution is the result of trial and uncomfortable error. A patient was being treated for facet and soft tissue injuries caused by an auto accident that had occurred 3 weeks previously. She was pain free after four treatments in 21 days and was treated on a Tuesday. She returned on Thursday complaining that whatever had been done on Tuesday had "undone" 2 weeks of healing and she felt as much pain as she had 2 weeks previously. Review of the Tuesday treatment revealed that the 58/'s had been used in addition to the protocols that had been reducing the pain for the preceding 3 weeks. She was so pain free that it seemed as if the injury was much older and the date of injury was not checked before treatment. The presumption was made that the 58/'s had removed repair tissue necessary to keep the joint and soft tissues pain free and stable. Two more errors in the first year of treating with FSM in similar situations helped to determine that the 58/'s should not be used within five to six weeks of a new injury. They can be used briefly four weeks after the date of injury – for 5 to 10 seconds each – to thin out scar tissue as it is forming, especially in athletes who seem to heal faster.

This reaction is predictable and reproducible. Take this precaution seriously. The wise practitioner will only make this mistake once; it is better not to make it at all.

Treatment protocol chronic facet pain

Channel A condition / Channel B tissue

58 / 00, 01, 02, 32
• A/B pair for Removing scar tissue and adhesions
• Treatment time: When used to treat chronic complaints the 58/'s are used in order as listed above for approximately 1 to 2 minutes each at the beginning of the treatment to soften the tissues and remove scar tissue. Facet joints have bone as a tissue so 58 / 01 is usually included in the protocol. For those practitioners who can feel the softening produced by the frequency, it is often helpful to run the frequency until the softening is reduced and the tissue becomes relatively more firm. There may be some patients in whom one or more of these frequencies will produce softening for up to 3 to 4 minutes.

40 / 396, 59, 39, 783, 157, 480, 191, 100
• Inflammation / Nerve, bone, periosteum, cartilage, capsule, tendon, ligament.
• Treatment time: Use these combinations for 2 to 4 minutes each. Research has shown 40Hz to have a time dependent response in a mouse model of inflammation. 50% of the reduction in inflammation was present at 2 minutes. The full response was present at 4 minutes. Treat the nerve first as it seems to relax the muscles and allow better palpation of the facet tissues. The periosteum is the most pain sensitive part of the bone and the nerve and the joint capsule are the most sensitive to inflammation and should

respond best to this frequency. This protocol should reduce the joint pain but will not change range of motion.

284 / 396, 59, 39, 783, 157, 480, 191, 100
• Chronic inflammation / Nerve, bone, periosteum, cartilage, capsule, tendon, ligament.
• Treatment time: Use these combinations for 1 to 2 minutes each or if you are sensitive to the feel of tissue softening and time allows use the frequency as long as the softening happens.

91, 13 / 142, 396, 480, 783, 157, 191
• Calcium ions, scar tissue / fascia, nerve, joint capsule, periosteum, cartilage, and tendons.
• 91 / 783, 480, 157, 396 seems to reduce joint pain most effectively and softens the joint capsule dramatically.
• 13 / 142, 396, 480 usually increase range of motion most effectively. Scarring between the capsule and the nerve appear to create sharp pain with palpation and respond well to treatment. See manual technique below.
• Treat all the tissues if time allows.
• Treatment time: Use these combinations for 1 to 2 minutes each or if you are sensitive to the feel of tissue softening and time allows, use the frequency as long as the softening happens.

81, 49 / 142
• 81Hz is used for increasing secretions. / 142Hz is used for the fascia. The fascia secretes the ground substance necessary for repair of the fascia, ligaments and tendons.

49 / 59, 39, 783, 157, 480
• 49 / treat one or two tissues that responded best to 40 / for 1 minute each. Treat all tissues with 49 / if time allows.

If response is slow: narcotics

Experience has shown that patients who are on high levels of narcotics or who have had multiple injections with anesthetics respond slowly to treatment. This effect is reversed by the frequencies to "remove" narcotics and anesthetics. It is not thought that these frequencies actually remove the narcotic or anesthetic since they do not increase pain. It is much more likely that they somehow influence the membrane in such a way as to make it more receptive to treatment.

Use **43, 46, 19 / 396 first** if the patient is on narcotics. The current application and lead placement are the same as for the joint treatment.

Stenosis precaution

If there is dense scar tissue or bony stenosis of the nerve root or spinal cord or if a disc fragment is compressing the nerve root or cord at the involved level the patient's pain may increase when polarized positive current is applied. If the patient is positioned comfortably, it is the only time the pain will increase during polarized positive treatment for nerve inflammation. It may increase in the dermatome or at the spine or both. Assess patient position to determine whether it is contributing to the pain increase.

Stop treating immediately if pain goes up during treatment. Move the patient to a seated position if possible. Move the contacts slightly up the spine superior to the nerve root being treated, reduce current levels and change the current from polarized positive to alternating. If this is going to reduce the reaction it will do so in 5 to 10 minutes. If the pain continues to increase, stop treating with current. The pain should go back down in a few hours although it may take up to 24 hours to reduce to base line.

This reaction is diagnostic. If physical examination findings of reduced sensation and deep tendon reflexes at the involved level or hyperactive deep tendon reflexes below the involved level are present this reaction suggests the need to x-ray or perform an MRI to confirm the presence of compression.

Treat the muscles

When treating the facet joint remember to treat the muscles and trigger points. The taut muscles act as confounding pain generators and at the same time compress the facet joint increasing the degenerative forces on both the facet joint and the disc (see Chapter 7).

Treat the psoas and lumbar paraspinals muscles in the low back.

Treat the scalenes and the cervical paraspinals in the neck.

Treat the thoracic paraspinals and the rectus abdominus in the trunk.

See the chapter on treating muscles and myofascial pain for details.

58/ 00, 02, 32

- If you have already used the 58/'s to treat the adhesions and scarring around the facet joint there is no need to repeat them but it doesn't hurt to repeat them with the focus on the myofascial tissue being treated.

91, 13 / 62 (396, 142)

- You have already used 91, 13 / to treat the fascia and the nerve so you need not repeat them just add / 62 to treat the muscle belly.
- Treatment time: Use for 1–2 minutes or if you are sensitive to the feel of tissue softening and time allows, use the frequency as long as the softening happens.

40 / 116

- 40 / 116 seems to reduce inflammation in whatever tissue is involved. Use it in this case to reduce any inflammation not treated by 40 / and the facet joint tissues.

81, 49 / 142

- The lead placement, current levels, polarity do not change when you treat the muscles. Focus the fingers on the soft tissues around the joint and on the muscles involved in the portion of the spine being treated.

Treatment application

- **Current level:** 100–300μamps. Use lower current levels for very small or debilitated patients. Use higher current levels for larger or very muscular patients. In general higher current levels reduce pain more quickly. Do not use more than 500μamps as animal studies suggest that current levels above 500μamps reduce ATP formation while current levels below 500μamps increase ATP.

- **± Polarization or Polarized Positive +:** Current is used in alternating mode. Alternating DC current is actually pulsed DC (direct) current that alternates its polarity from positive to negative. Some patients respond better to polarized positive current for reasons that are not understood. It is best to try both on each patient at each session.

- **Waveslope:** Moderate to sharp for chronic facet pain. Use a gentle wave slope for acute facet pain.
  - ○ The waveslope refers to the rate of increase of current flow on the leading edge of the square wave. A sharp waveslope has a very steep current up ramp; a gentle waveslope has a gradual current up ramp.

- **Contact placement for spinal facet joints**
  - ○ FSM typically uses graphite gloves to conduct the current. The graphite gloves need to be kept moist so they conduct the current comfortably. The graphite gloves can be placed in or leads attached with alligator clips can be attached to a small warm wet towel or fabric sleeve.

○ Care should be taken to see that the wet fabric contacts do not touch each other. Current will follow the path of least resistance and the wet contacts are presumed to be less resistant than the patient therefore the current will flow in the wet contacts and avoid the tissue that needs treating.

○ Place the **positive leads** in wet fabric to ensure a broad contact on the posterior spine at the involved spinal segment where the facet joints are painful in the cervical, thoracic or lumbar spine.

○ Place the **negative leads** in wet fabric placed on the body anterior to the spinal contact.

OR

• Wrap the **positive leads** contact around the spine or lay the contact over the spine to treat the facet joints.

• Wrap the **negative leads** around the adjacent limb at the end of the referred pain area if myofascial trigger points are being treated at the same time.

OR

• The **positive leads** graphite glove can be placed directly on the skin under the spinal area to be treated after being wet thoroughly with water.

• The **negative leads** graphite glove can be placed directly on the skin on the body surface anterior to the spinal area to be treated after being wet thoroughly with water.

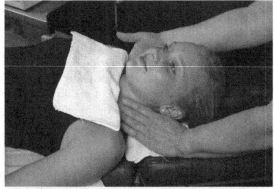

Figure 5.4 • To treat the cervical facet joints, place the positive leads glove in a warm wet fabric contact (hand towel) at the posterior cervical spine. Place the negative leads glove in a warm wet fabric contact (face cloth) at the anterior cervical spine or on the upper chest. Place the hands under the towels to palpate the tissue changes, mobilize the joints and work the muscles paying close attention to the periosteum at the joint line and the capsule over the joint while running 91 / 783, 480.

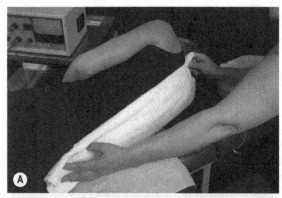
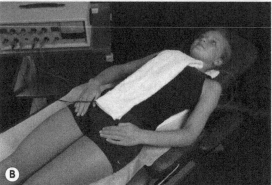

Figure 5.5 • To treat the thoracic facet joints wrap the positive leads glove in a warm wet fabric contact (hand towel) or attach the leads to the contact with alligator clips and place it lengthwise down the posterior spine with the patient supine with knee bent and back flat. Wrap the negative leads glove in a warm wet fabric contact (hand towel) and place it lengthwise down the trunk so the current flows through the tissue in three dimensions. The practitioner's hands can be placed under the contacts to work the soft tissues and mobilize the joints.

OR

• **Adhesive Electrode Pads** may be used for convenience although the gloves seem to be more effective for reasons not understood. The adhesive electrode pads are especially useful for home treatment because they allow the patient to be active while being treated.

When applying treatment with adhesive electrode pads, the current and the frequencies must pass through the area to be treated in an interferential pattern, forming an "X" in three dimensions. The positive electrodes are placed at the spine at the level of the facet to be treated. The negative electrodes may be placed directly anterior or anterior and

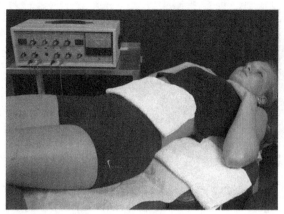

Figure 5.6 • Place the positive leads contact under the spine with the patient positioned supine with knees bent and back flat. Place the negative leads contact on the abdomen. Place the hands under the towels to palpate the tissue changes, mobilize the joints and work the muscles, especially the psoas and quadratus lumborum and lumbar paraspinals.

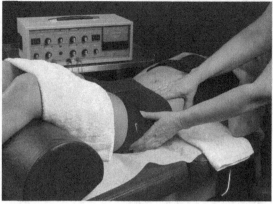

Figure 5.8 • Place the positive leads glove or attach the negative leads by alligator clips to the warm wet cloth contact (hand towel) and place it under the low back with the patient supine. Place the negative leads glove or attach the negative leads by alligator clips to a warm wet towel draped across the abdomen and upper thigh to treat the facet joints and the nerves and muscles of the low back, hip and thigh. Use the hands under the towels to palpate the changes, work the muscles, and mobilize the facet joints.

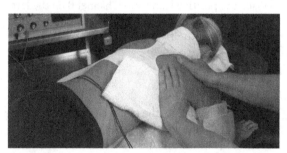

Figure 5.7 • Place the positive leads glove or attach the negative leads by alligator clips to the warm wet cloth contact (hand towel) and place it behind the neck with the patient supine. Place the negative leads glove or attach the negative leads by alligator clips to a warm wet towel draped across the scapula, under the axilla and wrapped around the upper arm to treat the facet joints and the nerves and muscles of the neck, upper back, and shoulder. Use the hands under the towels to palpate the changes, work the muscles, and mobilize the facet joints.

slightly inferior to the spinal contacts for the facet being treated.

A diagram for the placement would look like this:

Positive Electrode   Positive Electrode
Channel A   Channel B
          Area to be Treated
Negative Electrode   Negative Electrode
Channel B   Channel A

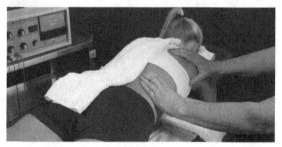

Figure 5.9 • To treat the thoracic facet joints, nerves and muscles with the patient prone wrap the positive leads glove in a warm wet fabric contact (hand towel) or attach the leads to the contact using alligator clips and place it lengthwise down the posterior spine. Wrap the negative leads glove in a warm wet fabric contact (hand towel) or attach the negative leads to the contact using alligator clips and place it lengthwise down the trunk under the prone patient so the current flows through the tissue in three dimensions. The practitioner's hands can be placed under the contacts to palpate the changes, work the soft tissues and mobilize the joints.

Facet joint pain with no referral

• Place the **positive electrode from channel A** on the skin just lateral to the spinal segment at the level of the facet joint.
• Place the **negative electrode from channel A** so the current flows down an imaginary line

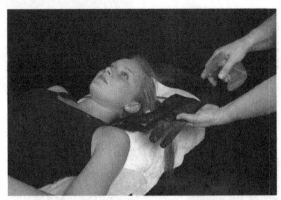

Figure 5.10 • The graphite glove can be placed directly on the skin after being wet thoroughly by spraying with water. The glove must be wet or the current will sting and prickle. There is not enough current to create a burn but it can be very uncomfortable.

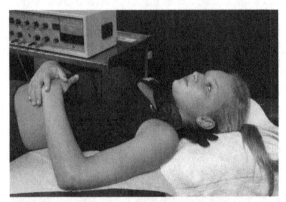

Figure 5.11 • The graphite glove can be placed directly on the skin if that is most convenient. Once the glove is moistened with water it usually stays moist for the duration of the treatment. The galvanic skin response to current flow usually creates slight sweating under the contact. This placement is for cervical facet joint pain. Place the positive leads contact at the back of the neck and the negative leads contact on the chest or on the front of the neck. This placement puts the contacts in the correct position for polarizing the current should that become necessary.

diagonally through the body from the channel A positive electrode to the abdomen just anterior to the involved facet joint.

• For example, to treat a lumbar facet, place the positive lead from channel A on the right side of the low back. Place the negative leads from channel A on the left side of the abdomen at or below the level of the facet being treated.

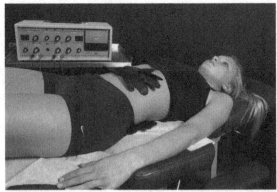

Figure 5.12 • The graphite glove can be placed directly on the skin if that is most convenient. Once the glove is moistened with water it usually stays moist for the duration of the treatment. The galvanic skin response to current flow usually creates slight sweating under the contact. This placement is for lumbar facet joint pain. Place the positive leads contact at the low back and the negative leads contact on the abdomen. This placement puts the contacts in the correct position for polarizing the current should that become necessary.

• Place the positive lead from Channel B on the left side of the low back and the negative leads from channel B on the right side of the abdomen.

Patient position

Patient supine

• In the lumbar spine, the knees and hips should be bent so that the low back is flat. This is the comfort position for the lumbar facet joints unless the patient has accompanying disc pain generators. If there is accompanying discogenic pain find whatever neutral comfortable position is possible. The patient may be treated side lying.

• In the cervical spine, the chin should be tucked so the neck is flat. This is the comfort position for cervical spine facets.

• If a patient continually moves the neck while lying supine they may have both facet and disc pain generators. The most common pattern seen after whiplash injuries is a C5–6 or C6–7 disc injury combined with an upper cervical facet joint injury usually at C2–3. The disc injury produces neck and shoulder pain and the C2–3 facet joint injury produces a headache and peri-orbital pain. As the patient flattens the cervical curve to relieve the upper facets the disc annulus compresses and the patient begins to experience discogenic

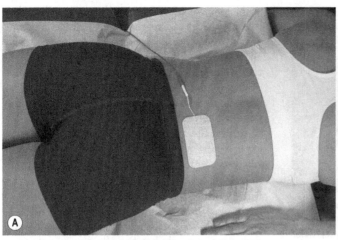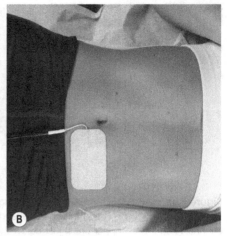

Figure 5.13 • To treat lumbar facet joint pain with adhesive electrode pads place the positive lead from channel A on the right side of the low back. Place the negative lead from channel A on the left side of the abdomen at or below the same level as the facet joint being treated. Then place the positive lead from channel B on the left side of the low back and the negative leads from channel B on the right side of the abdomen.

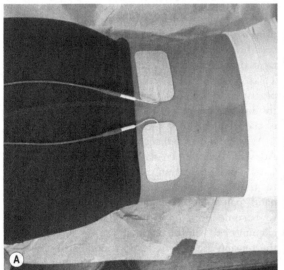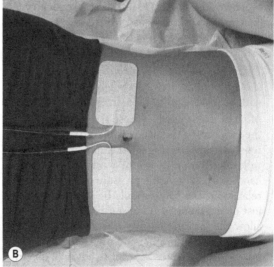

Figure 5.14 • Pads from both channel A and channel B in place on the lumbar spine and abdomen for treatment of lumbar facet joint pain. The current and frequencies form an interferential pattern, crossing in three dimensions through the area to be treated.

midscapular pain and neck and shoulder pain. The patient will arch the neck to relieve the disc pain until the facet compression in the upper cervical spine becomes intolerable. This is more pronounced while the patient is supine but can be seen while they are seated as well. Placing a small one inch diameter roll under the C5–6 disc area to keep it in extension will allow the patient to flex

and flatten the upper cervical spine and relieve the facet joint compression.

Patient prone

If the facet patient must lay prone for treatment access to the posterior lumbar or cervical muscles place a pillow or bolster under the abdomen to create lumbar flexion. Tip the head rest or face rest down to

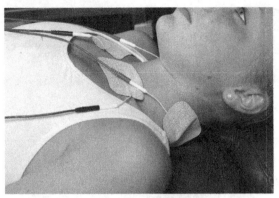

Figure 5.15 • Place the positive leads from channel A on the right side of the neck and the negative lead from channel A on the left upper chest just below the clavicle. Place the positive leads from channel B on the left side of the neck and the negative leads from channel B on the right upper chest just below the clavicle. The current and frequencies form an interferential pattern, crossing in three dimensions through the area to be treated.

create cervical flexion. Do not treat a cervical facet patient prone with the head turned to the side. It is not possible to treat a patient successfully to reduce pain while their position increases pain.

- *Treatment interval*: Facet joint patients can and should be treated twice a week for 4 to 6 weeks with at least one day separating the treatments.
- *Manual technique*: For those trained in manual therapies using the hands while using FSM requires some adjustment of technique. The key is to let the frequency do the work and to use the hands with very gentle pressure and complete relaxation. The hands should be almost limp with just enough tone in the distal finger muscles to allow the fingers to gently assess the state of the tissue. The therapist should use the shoulder muscles and serratus anterior to advance the arm and increase the pressure of the hand on the tissue being treated. The hands are sensing change and softening in the muscles not forcing it. The patient's muscles will relax and allow deeper palpation if the practitioner's hands are relaxed and will defensively tense if the contact is too firm or if the palpating fingers are too tense.
- When using 91, 13 / 480, 396 on the cervical spine place the pads of the fingers under the joint line and gently lift the facet joint on one side of the spine about 2mm. Release this side back to neutral and gently lift the joint on the other side about 2mm. This creates a small amount of segmental rotation

at the joint capsule. The nerve becomes adhered to the inflamed and hardened joint capsule and the goal is to gently tease the nerve off of the capsule to allow increased range of motion. The manual technique here is unlike anything most physical medicine practitioners do. It is a gentle slow segmental rocking movement intended to move the joint through its range while allowing the frequency to release the scar tissue and hardening. It is best experienced by relaxing the fingers and using them to sense and follow the frequency effect.

- *Let the frequency do the work*. If possible, move the fingers to the tissue being treated when the frequency for that tissue is running. When the frequencies are softening scar tissue or mineral deposits use gentle but firm finger pressure to assist the process.

What tissue is it? What is wrong with it?

As proficiency with FSM increases the practitioner using a manual microcurrent device can become more specific with the choice of frequencies for tissues to be treated and pathologies to be removed from them. This process usually occurs gradually as the skilled practitioner becomes more familiar with palpating the local anatomy and more sensitive to the effects of the frequencies on the structures being treated.

With an illustrated anatomy text such as Netter's Atlas of Illustrated Anatomy (Netter 1991) as a visual guide, palpation can become very specific as to tissue. Following the recommended "relaxed hand" palpation technique allows the sensing fingers to become quite sensitive. When the finger tips encounter a painful tissue it can be identified by the tension in the muscles surrounding the area, by the patient's verbal response or by the subtle sense that the tissue is simply "different" from the less painful tissue in the area. If the practitioner will attend to the subtle awareness that the tissue is simply "different" this distinction alone is sufficient to create a very skilled palpation sense. This level of skill is within the grasp of every practitioner given time, motivation, practice and patience.

When palpation identifies a taut or tender area the practitioner can pause and ask internally, "What tissue is it?" Make a guess as to what tissue it is-based on the texture and the visual landmarks provided by the illustrated anatomy text. Then ask internally, "What is wrong with this tissue?" For example, the fingers may palpate what feels like the surface of the periosteum where a tendon attaches that feels as if it is both inflamed and calcified.

This awareness actually forms a hypothesis. Test the hypothesis by treating with 40, 91 / 783, 191 (remove inflammation and calcified hardening from the periosteum and tendon). If the tissue softens and the local palpatory pain is reduced, then the hypothesis was very likely correct. If nothing changes then reconsider the anatomy and/or the pathology.

Perhaps the problem tissue is indeed the periosteum and the tendon but perhaps they are scarred down, tethering and stretching the nerve fibers rather than being inflamed and calcified. This assessment forms a new hypothesis which can be tested by running the frequencies 13, 3 / 783, 191, 396 (remove scar and sclerosis from the periosteum, tendon and the nerve).

Repeat this process as needed to complete the treatment and achieve maximum improvement in the tissue. This process may be overwhelming to the novice FSM practitioner because there are so many new tasks and details to master but it actually simplifies and optimizes treatment as soon as it can be accomplished.

Adjunctive instructions for the facet pain patient

The patient should be instructed to avoid activities or movements that create spinal extension such as improper sitting postures or leaning backwards. Sitting posture that protects the cervical spine facet joints involves lumbar extension and erect spinal posture to bring the head and ears directly over the shoulders. Forward head posture causes strain on the neck muscles and the discs and increases compressive load on the facet joints.

The patient should consult with a therapist who can instruct them in proper posture and exercises to strengthen the core abdominal muscles and the muscles around the facet joints and to mobilize the joints in a pain free range to increase circulation and facilitate tissue repair.

Chiropractors, osteopaths and physical therapists should avoid lumbar side posture or rotary adjustments which by their nature gap one joint and jam the joint on the opposite side unless the facet pain is strictly one sided. It is possible to adjust bilateral facets by positioning the patient supine on a drop table and performing a gentle drop table adjustment with a light thrust from the front. The same adjustment can be performed as a mobilization with the patient flexed to 90 degrees at the hips and knees.

Nutritional support

Professional grade nutritional supplements can be helpful in reducing inflammation and relaxing muscles. Essential fatty acids (EPA/DHA) reduce inflammation. Magnesium malate and magnesium glycinate are well absorbed and help relax muscle tissue. Glucosamine and chondroitin sulfate and MSM (methylsulfonylmethane) are said to be effective in reducing pain in degenerative joints. SAMe (s-adenosyl methionine) is becoming more widely used for reducing joint inflammation and pain. A complete listing of nutritional adjunctive therapies is beyond the scope of this text but the reader is encouraged to become knowledgeable in this area and to customize treatment to the patient's needs.

Narcotics

If patients are on high levels of narcotics or have had multiple injections with anesthetics it is sometimes necessary to run the frequencies to "remove" narcotics and anesthetics. It is not thought that these frequencies actually remove the narcotic or anesthetic. It is much more likely that they somehow influence the membrane in such a way as to make it more receptive to treatment.

 Box 5.1

Summary for treating chronic facet joint pain

Treat the joint (± or +)
- 58 / 00, 01, 02, 32
- 40 / 396, 59, 39, 783, 157, 480, 191, 100
- 284 / 396, 59, 39, 783, 157, 480, 191, 100
- 91, 13 / 142, 396, 480, 783, 157, 191
- 91 / 783, 480, 157, 396
- 13 / 142, 396, 480 (with motion)
- 81, 49 / 142
- 49 / 59, 39, 783, 157, 480

If response is slow
- Use 43, 46, 19 / 396
- Use these frequencies first if the patient is on narcotics

Treat the muscles (± or +)
- 58 / 00, 02, 32
- 91, 13 / 62 (396, 142)
- 40 / 116
- 81, 49 / 142

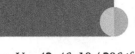

- Use **43, 46, 19 / 396** if the patient is on narcotics. The current application and lead placement are the same as for the facet or nerve treatment.

Treating acute facet joint pain

Hydration

- The patient must be hydrated to benefit from microcurrent treatment.
- Hydrated means 1 to 2 quarts of water consumed in the 2 to 4 hours preceding treatment
- Athletes and patients with more muscle mass seem to need more water than the average patient.
- The elderly tend to be chronically dehydrated and may need to hydrate for several days prior to treatment in addition to the water consumed on the day of treatment
- *DO NOT* accept the statement, "I drink lots of water"
- *ASK* "How much water, and in what form, did you drink today before you came in?"
- Coffee, caffeinated tea, carbonated cola beverages do not count as water.
- Water may be flavored with juice or decaffeinated tea.

Channel A: condition frequencies

The frequencies listed are thought to remove or neutralize the condition for which they are listed except for 81, 49 / which are thought to increase secretions and vitality respectively

- Bleeding or hemorrhage   18 /
- Torn or broken   124 /
- Inflammation   40 /
- Secretions (increase)   81 /
- Vitality (restore)   49 /
- The basics
- Remove trauma   294 /
- Restore function   321 /
- Remove histamine   9 /

Channel B: facet joint tissue frequencies

- Bone: ___ / 59 and ___ / 39
  - It is presumed that one is for cortical bone and one is for cancellous bone but it is not known which is for what tissue. When treating bone both frequencies are used.

- Periosteum: ___ / 783
  - The periosteum lines the bone and is very pain sensitive. Tendons, ligaments and the joint capsule attach to the periosteum by interweaving with the fibers that cover it.
- Cartilage: ___ / 157
  - Cartilage lines the facet joint and becomes damaged, degenerated, calcified and inflamed when traumatized by acute or chronic compression of the joint surface.
- Joint Capsule: ___ / 480
  - The joint capsule surrounds the joint and becomes scarred and inflamed when over stretched by trauma.
- Tendons:___ / 191
  - The tendons attach the muscles and fascia to the posterolateral joint capsule and periosteum.
- Ligament: ___ /100
  - The spinal ligaments connect bone to bone and connect the adjacent joints.
- Nerve: ___ / 396
  - This refers to the dermatomal nerves that may be irritated by the facet joint inflammation and the recurrent nerves that innervate the joint capsule and infiltrate the joint in response to chronic inflammation.
- Fascia: ___ /142
  - The fascia is the thin connective tissue covering surrounding the muscles and virtually all visceral tissue.
- Artery and Elastic Tissue in the Muscle Belly: ___ / 62
  - 62Hz is the frequency used for the artery and the elastic tissue in the arterial walls. The muscle belly responds to this frequency either because it is full of small arteries or because the elastic tissue in the muscle belly is somehow related to the artery wall.
- A/B Pair
  - 40 / 116
  - Reduce inflammation
  - Animal research in mice demonstrated a 62% reduction in swelling as a measure of LOX mediated inflammation when the frequency 40 / 116 (reduce inflammation in the immune system) was used. This was a 4-minute time-dependent response with half the effect being present at 2 minutes and the full effect present at 4 minutes.

Treatment protocol acute facet pain

Use in the first week following an injury to the facet joint

When a patient presents within 12 hours of a fall, auto accident or any trauma in which the joint has been hyperextended pain can be much reduced and recovery much accelerated by using FSM for the acute injury. The channel A condition frequencies are different than for the chronic conditions. It is important to remember that the body needs fibrosis to repair the newly injured tissue and no frequency thought to remove fibrosis should be used in the 6 weeks following the injury.

The 4-hour window

If a patient can be treated within 4 hours of the time of a new injury, as long as the tissue is intact, the healing is tremendously accelerated. Every effort should be made to encourage patients to be treated within this critical time period.

18 / 62

- 18Hz has been used clinically to stop bleeding post-operatively, in the menses and to prevent bruising. 62Hz is the frequency for the arteries. Use this only in the first 48 hours after an injury.
- Treatment time: Use for 4 to 10 minutes or if you are sensitive to the feel of tissue softening and time allows, use the frequency as long as the softening happens.

124 / 59, 39, 783, 157, 480, 191, 62, 100

- Something torn or broken / bone, periosteum, cartilage, capsule, tendon, artery or muscle belly, ligament.
- 124Hz is thought to remove the "fact of being torn or broken" from the injured tissue. This is a conceptual shift to the medically trained mind. In an energetic model, conditions have a physical consequence in the tissue – the periosteum or joint capsule is "torn or broken" – and at the same time there is also an energetic or vibrational pattern that impresses itself on the semiconductor field that is the injured tissue. It is as if the pattern of being "torn or broken" has impressed itself on the field representing the tissue, interferes with the normal healing processes and prevents tissue repair. In an energetic model it is thought that removing this pattern of being "torn or broken"

enables the normal repair processes to become effective. This frequency rarely if ever changes symptoms but it seems to enhance tissue repair of "torn or broken" tissues.

- Treatment time: Use for 1 minute with each tissue or if you are sensitive to the feel of tissue softening and time allows, use the frequency as long as the softening happens. Use this frequency only on the first two to three treatments.

294, 321, 9, 49 / 480, 157, 783

- Trauma, Paralysis, Allergy Reaction, vitality / joint capsule, cartilage, periosteum.
- These four frequencies – the basics – do not tend to change symptoms but they appear to be important in restoring normal function to injured tissue. If you think of a time when you have suffered a physical injury you may notice that it is possible to distinguish between the symptoms from the injury and the effect of the "fact" of the trauma, the shock of it to your system. 294 / is thought to address the "fact of the trauma" or the shock to the system created by the trauma.
- When a tissue is traumatized it sometimes behaves as if it has "lost" a line of instructions not unlike a computer when it freezes for the same reason. 321 / is thought to "reboot" the tissue and is described as being used to neutralize "paralysis" moving it past the lost instruction and on to the next step to facilitate return to function.
- When any tissue is traumatized the first response is the secretion of histamine to initiate the inflammatory response. When treating to arrest the immediate effects of a new injury removing the histamine from the injured area seems to stop the inflammatory progression.
- Any tissue that has been traumatized returns to full function more efficiently if "vitality", 49Hz, is restored. These frequencies don't necessarily change symptoms but they seem to help speed recovery.
- Treatment time: Use for 1 to 2 minutes or if you are sensitive to the feel of tissue softening and time allows, use the frequency as long as the softening happens. Use these frequencies only on the first two to three treatments. In the interests of time only three tissues have been included. If time allows and there is information that suggests a particular tissue has been particularly traumatized any tissue may be added to the channel B sequence.

40 / 59, 39, 783, 396, 157, 480, 191 142, 62, 100
- Inflammation / bone, periosteum, nerve, cartilage, capsule, tendon, fascia, artery, muscle belly, ligament.
- Treatment time: Use these combinations for 2 to 4 minutes each. The key to reducing acute facet joint pain is to reduce inflammation as rapidly and dramatically as possible. Research has shown 40Hz to have a consistent positive effect in reducing inflammation in both humans and animals. Animal research showed a 4-minute time-dependent response but human research showed up to 90 minutes was required to reduce cytokines when treating the spinal cord (see Chapters 1 & 8). If the practitioner is sensitive to the sensation of softening and time allows, use 40Hz for as long as the tissue is softening.

A/B Pair

40 / 116
- Reduce inflammation in any tissue.
- Animal research in mice demonstrated a 62% reduction in swelling as a measure of LOX mediated inflammation when the frequency 40 / 116 (reduce inflammation in the immune system) was used. This was a 4-minute time-dependent response with half the effect being present at 2 minutes and the full effect present at 4 minutes. 40 / 116 reduced inflammation generally regardless of the tissue that had been inflamed by the chemical agents. It is used here to reduce any inflammation not addressed by 40 / and the tissues.
- Treatment time: Use this combination for 4 minutes.

81, 49 / 142
- 81Hz is used for increasing secretions. / 142Hz is used for the fascia. The fascia secretes the ground substance necessary for repair of the fascia, ligaments and tendons.
- Treatment time: Use for 1–2 minutes or if you are sensitive to the feel of tissue softening and time allows, use the frequency as long as the softening happens.

Treatment application

- **Contact Placement** and **Treatment Application** are the same as for Chronic Facet Joint treatment except for the waveslope.
- **Use a gentle waveslope for acute injury treatment.** All other microcurrent and treatment parameters are the same.

- **Patient Position:** Use the recommended facet treatment positioning or any position that is comfortable for the injured patient.
- **Manual Technique:** The manual technique in acute facet joint injuries requires an even softer touch. Use very light contact and minimal pressure because the newly injured tissues are acutely inflamed. The patient can be treated with no manual contact at all for the first one or two treatments.

Box 5.2

Summary for treating acute facet joint injuries

Stop the bleeding
- 18 / 62

Treat the joint
- 124 / 59, 39, 783, 157, 480, 191, 142, 62, 100
- 294, 321, 9, 49 / 480, 157, 783
- 40 / 59, 39, 783, 396, 157, 480, 191, 142, 62, 100
- 40 / 116
- 81, 49 / 142

Treating facet joint pain week 1 to week 5 after injury

The conditions affecting the tissues in week one to week five after a facet joint injury are different than those used acutely and different than those used in week six and in chronic facet joint injuries.

Hydration

- The patient must be hydrated to benefit from microcurrent treatment.
- Hydrated means 1 to 2 quarts of water consumed in the 2 to 4 hours preceding treatment
- Athletes and patients with more muscle mass seem to need more water than the average patient.
- The elderly tend to be chronically dehydrated and may need to hydrate for several days prior to treatment in addition to the water consumed on the day of treatment
- *DO NOT* accept the statement, "I drink lots of water"
- *ASK* "How much water, and in what form, did you drink today before you came in?"
- Coffee, caffeinated tea, carbonated cola beverages do not count as water.
- Water may be flavored with juice or decaffeinated tea.

Channel A: condition frequencies

The frequencies listed are thought to remove or neutralize the condition for which they are listed except for 81, 49 / which are thought to increase secretions and vitality respectively

- Inflammation   40 /
- Calcium influx, hardening   91/
- Chronic inflammation   284 /
- Increase secretions   81 /
- Restore vitality   49 /

Channel B: facet joint tissue frequencies

- Bone: ___/ 59 and ___/ 39
  - ○ It is presumed that one is for cortical bone and one is for cancellous bone but it is not known which is for what tissue. When treating bone both frequencies are used.
- Periosteum: ___/ 783
  - ○ The periosteum lines the bone and is very pain sensitive.
- Cartilage: ___/ 157
  - ○ Cartilage lines the facet joint and becomes damaged, degenerated, calcified and inflamed when traumatized by acute or chronic compression of the joint surface.
- Joint Capsule: ___/ 480
  - ○ The joint capsule surrounds the joint and becomes scarred and inflamed when over stretched by trauma.
- Tendons:___ / 191
  - ○ The tendons attach the muscles and fascia to the posterolateral joint capsule and periosteum.
- Ligament: ___/100
  - ○ The spinal ligaments connect bone to bone and connect the adjacent joints.
- Nerve: ___/ 396
  - ○ This refers to the dermatomal nerves that may be irritated by the facet joint inflammation and the recurrent nerves that innervate the joint capsule and infiltrate the joint in response to chronic inflammation.
- Fascia: ___/142
  - ○ The fascia is the thin connective tissue covering surrounding the muscles and virtually all visceral tissue.
- Artery and Elastic Tissue in the Muscle Belly: ___/ 62

- ○ 62Hz is the frequency used for the artery and the elastic tissue in the arterial walls. The muscle belly responds to this frequency either because it is full of small arteries or because the elastic tissue in the muscle belly is somehow related to the artery wall.
- Immune System: ___/ 116
  - ○ Animal research in mice demonstrated a 62% reduction in swelling as a measure of inflammation when the frequency 40/116 (reduce inflammation in the immune system) was delivered to the tissue.

Treatment protocol for facet joint pain week 1 to week 5 after injury

- Use this protocol for acute exacerbations of chronic facet conditions.
- Use between week one and week six after an injury.

When a patient presents within the first to the sixth week after a fall, auto accident or any trauma in which the joint has been hyperextended, pain can be much reduced and recovery much accelerated by using FSM for the subacute injury. The channel A condition frequencies are different than for the chronic or acute conditions. It is important to remember that the body needs fibrosis to repair the newly injured tissue and no frequency thought to remove fibrosis should be used in the six weeks immediately following an injury.

40 / 116
- Reduce Inflammation in general.

40 / 59, 39, 783, 396, 157, 480, 191 142, 62, 100
- Inflammation, / bone, periosteum, nerve, cartilage, capsule, tendon, fascia, artery, muscle belly, ligament.
- Treatment time: Use these combinations for 2 to 4 minutes each. 40Hz is used for reducing inflammation. Research has shown 40Hz to have a time-dependent response in a mouse model of inflammation. 50% of the reduction in inflammation was present at 2 minutes. The full response was present at 4 minutes.

284 / 59, 39, 783, 396, 157, 480, 191 142, 62, 100
- Chronic inflammation / bone, periosteum, nerve, cartilage, capsule, tendon, fascia, artery, muscle belly, ligament.

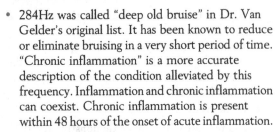

- 284Hz was called "deep old bruise" in Dr. Van Gelder's original list. It has been known to reduce or eliminate bruising in a very short period of time. "Chronic inflammation" is a more accurate description of the condition alleviated by this frequency. Inflammation and chronic inflammation can coexist. Chronic inflammation is present within 48 hours of the onset of acute inflammation.

91 / 142, 480, 783, 157

- Calcium ions and hardening / fascia, joint capsule, periosteum, and cartilage.
- Within 2 weeks of a new injury, especially if it is an acute exacerbation of the chronic injury 91/ seems to reduce joint pain and soften the tissues very effectively. It is a safe transition between the subacute and chronic treatments that can be used from the second week up through the chronic treatment phase.

81, 49 / 142

- 81Hz is used for increasing secretions. /142Hz is used for the fascia. The fascia secretes the ground substance necessary for repair of the fascia, ligaments and tendons.
- Treatment time: Use for 1–2 minutes or if you are sensitive to the feel of tissue softening and time allows, use the frequency as long as the softening happens.

NOTE: In acute exacerbations of a chronic facet problem do NOT use the 58/'s or 13/ or any frequency to remove or soften scar tissue. Scar tissue is needed to repair the recent injury. The 58/'s may be used after the injury is 6 weeks old to soften the repair tissue and make the joint and soft tissues more flexible and help prevent future re-injury.

Treatment application

- **Contact Placement** and **Treatment Application** are the same as for Chronic Facet Joint treatment except for the waveslope.
- **Use a gentle waveslope for acute injury treatment.** All other microcurrent and treatment parameters are the same.
- **Patient Position:** Use the recommended facet treatment positioning or any position that is comfortable for the injured patient.

- **Manual Technique:** The manual technique in facet joint injuries from the second week through the six week allows more soft tissue mobilization than the acute phase but a little less than the chronic condition. The myofascial tissues may be addressed as discussed in the chronic facet patient.

Box 5.3

Summary for treating sub-acute facet joint injuries

- 40 / 116
- 40 / 59, 39, 783, 396, 157, 480, 191, 142, 62, 100
- 284 / 59, 39, 783, 396, 157, 480, 191, 142, 62, 100
- 91 / 142, 480, 783, 157 (with movement)
- 81, 49 / 142

Chronic facet joint patient case report

The patient was a 47-year-old man who worked as a security driver for an armored car company. His job included driving and lifting boxes that weighed up to 40 pounds. When he arrived at the clinic he was scheduled for disc surgery in 4 weeks. The surgeon had proposed doing a three level disc replacement and fusion and told the patient that he would be back to work in 6 weeks. His symptoms were 8 years chronic low back pain and leg pain only down to the knee. He could not lay prone; extension and sitting made his pain worse. His sensory examination was normal.

He had had physical therapy, massage and chiropractic treatments. He rated his pain as varying from a 5–7/10 on a 0–10 VAS. He was treated in the clinic 5 days a week with FSM, supine manipulation on a drop table specific for facet joint mobilization. He was pain free at the end of each visit and his pain at each subsequent visit declined consistently over a 2-week period. He was sent to physical therapy specifically for a home exercise program for core strengthening and spinal stabilization. He purchased an FSM unit to treat himself at home as needed. He remains pain free after 2 years with home FSM treatment and exercises.

Bibliography

Beaman, D.N., Graziano, G.P., Woitys, E.M., Chang, V., 1993. Substance P innervation of lumbar spine facet joints. Spine 18, 1044–1049.

Cavanaugh, J.M., Ozaktay, A.C., Yamashita, H.T., King, A.I., 1996. Lumbar facet pain; biomechanics, neuroanatomy and neurophysiology. J. Biomech. 29, 1117–1129.

Cavanaugh, J.M., Lu, Y., Chen, C., Kallakuri, S., 2006. Pain generation in lumbar and cervical facet joints. J. Bone Joint Surg. Am. 88 (Suppl. 2), 63–67.

Chen, C., Lu, Y., Kallakuri, S., Patwardhan, A., Cavanaugh, J.M., 2006. Distribution of A-delta and C-fiber receptors in the cervical facet joint capsule and their response to stretch. J. Bone Joint Surg. Am. 88, 1807–1816.

Gerwin, R.D., Dommerholt, J., Shah, J., 2004. An expansion of Simons' integrated hypothesis of trigger point formation. Current Pain and Headache Reports, 8, 468–475.

Hoppenfeld, S., 1976. Physical examination of the spine and extremities. Appleton-Century Crofts, Division of Prentice Hall, New York.

Huckfeldt, R., Mikkelson, D., Larson, K., Hammond, L., Flick, B., McMakin, C., 2003. The use of micro current and autocatalytic silver plated nylon dressings in human burn patients: a feasibility study, Pacific Rim Burn Conference.

Lewis, C., 2004. Physiotherapy and spinal nerve root adhesion: a caution. Physiother. Res. Int. 9, 164–173.

McMakin, C., 1998. Microcurrent treatment of myofascial pain in the head, neck and face. Topics in Clinical Chiropractic 5 (1), 29–35.

McMakin, C., 2004. Microcurrent therapy: a novel treatment method for chronic low back myofascial pain. Journal of Bodywork and Movement Therapies 8, 143–153.

McMakin, C., 2005. Cytokine changes with microcurrent treatment of fibromyalgia associated with cervical spine trauma. Journal of Body Work and Movement Therapies 9, 169–176.

McMakin, C., 2007. Private communication.

Netter, F., 1991. Atlas of human anatomy. Plate 159. Ciba-Geigy, New York.

Phillips, T., 2000. Unpublished data, private communication.

Souza, T., 2009. Differential diagnosis and management for the chiropractor: protocols and algorithms, fourth ed. Jones & Bartlett Publishers, Sudbury, MA.

Travell, J.G., Simons, D.G., 1983. Myofascial pain and dysfunction: the trigger point manual. Williams & Wilkins, Baltimore.

Travell, J.G., Simons, D.G., 1992. Myofascial pain and dysfunction: the trigger point manual, vol. 2. Williams & Wilkins, Baltimore.

Treating ligaments and sprain injuries

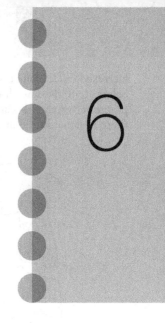

Ligaments connect bone to bone in virtually every joint in the body. Ligamentous instability or laxity is caused by repetitive microtrauma or a one-time injury in which the ligament is stretched beyond its limits of integrity or torn (Dodds 2004). The persistent inflammation and immune system response in chronic inflammatory conditions such as rheumatoid arthritis disrupts the integrity of ligamentous structures and causes ligamentous laxity. Ligamentous laxity and joint hypermobility contribute to further joint degeneration and inflammation (Konttinen 1989).

Ligamentous laxity negatively affects the function and stability of every joint in which it occurs. Functional instability in the ankle following an acute ankle sprain is more due to ligamentous laxity and proprioceptive deficits in the joint than to any lack of muscle strength (Lentel 1995). Ligamentous laxity and apophyseal arthritis in the cervical spine leads to destruction of the disc, cartilage and the vertebral endplates due to inflammation and hypermobility of the spinal segments (Martel 1977).

Not all stresses at a joint cause ligamentous damage. Repetitive physiologic stresses at high strain such as those created while running or doing other repetitive load activities produce significant ligamentous laxity while a relatively few stresses at low strain rate such as those created doing squats do not (Steiner 1986).

In general, ligaments are slow to repair and healing requires a balance between stabilization sufficient to prevent re-injury and motion sufficient to provide adequate circulation, and forces sufficient to organize the repair tissue along functional lines. It is important to maintain proprioceptive input to the joint, the healing ligament and the surrounding muscle tissue during the healing process. Healing ligaments are weaker and more lax than normal ligaments and care must be taken to prevent re-injury during the repair process (Hart 1987).

It is outside the scope of this text to provide a comprehensive exploration of the pathology of ligamentous injury and repair. The clinician using FSM for pain management needs to know how to recognize ligamentous laxity and how to treat it successfully with FSM and adjunctive therapies.

Diagnosing ligamentous laxity

The index of suspicion for ligamentous injuries is created by the history and mechanism of injury. The definitive diagnosis for ligamentous laxity is made with a stress x-ray. A standard x-ray taken with the spine or extremity joint supported in a neutral position or with the patient supine is not useful in determining ligamentous stability. In the cervical spine and lumbar spine the "stress" for the stress x-ray is provided by gravity and positioning the body so the weight of the head or trunk stresses the spinal segments thought to be injured. The ribs and spinal architecture make ligamentous injuries in the thoracic spine extremely rare and their diagnosis and treatment is not addressed here.

Cervical ligamentous laxity

The lateral cervical flexion–extension x-ray is three views taken from the side first with the head in neutral, second with the head flexed forward as far as possible and third with the head extended back as far as possible. This series is used to discover

© 2011, Elsevier Ltd.
DOI: 10.1016/B978-0-443-06976-5.00006-X

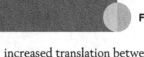

increased translation between a vertebra and the one below it. If the line drawn along the anterior and posterior vertebral bodies is not smooth and linear there is some degree of ligamentous laxity.

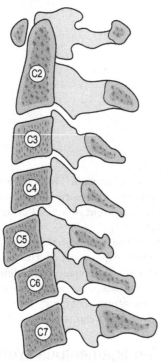

Figure 6.1 • When the lateral cervical spine flexion x-ray shows the posterior and anterior margins of the vertebral body of C5 forward of the margins of C6 it indicates ligamentous injury to and laxity in the posterior ligaments that should stabilize the segment. If the segment slides posterior during extension it indicates that the anterior ligaments have also been injured. If total translation exceeds 3.5mm the segment is considered unstable and a surgical consult is advised.

The transverse ligament connects the lateral masses of C1 passing behind the odontoid process stabilizing it in the arch of C1. The transverse ligament is evaluated by judging the space between the dens and the arch of C1 in lateral view flexion extension x-rays.

The odontoid or dens is stabilized in the lateral plane by the alar ligaments. The alar ligaments attach the odontoid tip at lateral angles to the occiput at the foramen magnum – like a tent stays holding a post in neutral. The alar ligament is often injured when the head is rotated at the time of impact. Injuries to the alar ligaments allow excess translation between C0, C1 and C2 in lateral flexion and rotation creating symptoms of severe sub-occipital headache, pressure and pain in the distribution of the occipital nerve and referred pain from the C2 facet joint. The C2–3 facet joint becomes a pain generator when the ligamentous laxity at the dens allows abnormal movement of C1 on C2 placing abnormal biomechanical strain on the C2–C3 facet joint creating inflammation in the joint. The manifestations are severe myofascial trigger points in the sub-occipital muscles, hyperesthesia at C2 dermatome, joint pain and peri-orbital referred pain from the C2–C3 facet joint and a constant relentless headache.

This alar ligament injury can be diagnosed by identifying the mechanism of injury and symptom pattern and by appropriate imaging. The relationship between C0, C1 and C2 is assessed by the APOM (anterior to posterior open mouth) x-ray view. The APOM side bending view assesses ligamentous stability at this level. The APOM neutral view is compared to left and right APOM side bending views. The side bending APOM is collimated as for the APOM but the patient is asked to bend the head as far to the left and then to the right as possible. The patient should be warned that this important evaluation will increase symptoms and should be pre-medicated if necessary. The imaging is positive when the lateral mass C1 overhangs the vertebral body of C2 unevenly from side to side. Some slight translational movement at this level may be normal but it should be symmetrical. Any excessive or uneven translation of C1 on C2 combined with the characteristic symptoms and a history of trauma to the head or neck with the head in rotation is diagnostic. A thin slice high resolution MRI of the upper cervical spine (occiput to C3) can clearly visualize and demonstrate the ligamentous injury if performed and read properly.

Lumbar spinal ligaments are evaluated with six x-rays. Three views are taken from the front in an anterior–posterior (AP) view with the patient standing first with the low back in neutral, second with the patient side bending to the left and third with the patient side bending to the right. The lateral views show the low back vertebra first in neutral, then in flexion and last in extension. X-ray views are available to evaluate most joints with gravity or weights being used to assess the length of the ligament when it is stressed by weight. The reader is referred to their preferred radiology text to identify which views should be ordered to assess the joint in question.

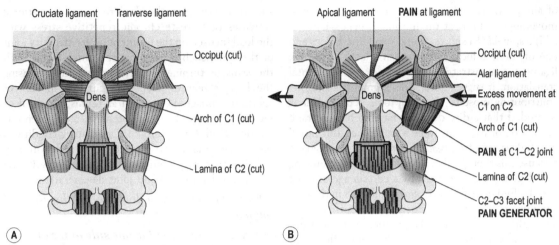

Figure 6.2 • A) C1 is held in place by a series of important ligaments. (1) The posterior view of the occiput, C1 and C2 – the occipital – atlanto – axial complex – shows the posterior osseous structures removed. The transverse ligament is the horizontal component of the cruciate ligament and is the most important stabilizer of C1 on C2 in flexion and extension. Injuries to this ligament are found on lateral view flexion – extension x-rays when the space between the anterior dens and the arch of C1 increases. The apical and alar ligaments stabilize C1 on C2 during rotation and lateral flexion. B) When the alar ligaments are injured the dens is not stable during lateral flexion and rotation. The excess movement creates inflammation and the ligaments, periosteum, nerves and facet joints become pain generators. Injuries to this ligament are discovered only in an APOM side bending x-ray.

Those skilled in manual therapy and diagnosis have been taught to evaluate the injured and the uninjured side to detect subtle excessive joint movement as part of their clinical training (Grieve 1981, White 1978).

The tools to diagnose a ligamentous injury are therefore easily available. The challenge for the clinician is in knowing when to look for and how to assess ligamentous injury. In general, if a patient is still in pain 12 weeks after an injury to the neck or any joint, then the injury involves something more than the soft tissues such as the muscles. The original physical diagnosis may have targeted the sprain strain injury to the muscles and ligaments but after 12 weeks these soft tissues should have healed.

In the cervical and lumbar spine, the primary suspects as cause of persistent pain are the facets and discs and ligaments that have been torn or stretched beyond their ability to heal. Injury to any or all three of these structures may contribute to neuropathic inflammation and activation which in turn creates biomechanical dysfunction, myofascial pain and trigger points. The lax ligaments allow excess motion at the injured spinal segment and the excess motion causes constant microtrauma and inflammation to the discs and facet joints and the nerves at that segment. Abnormal segmental motion stimulates proprioceptors that activate muscles to splint the joint protectively. Neuropathic pain secondary to inflammation from the disc and facet joint also creates pain and muscle splinting.

The splinted muscles constantly contract to stabilize the joint and may contain either latent or active trigger points making them taut and painful. These tissues are the most obvious pain generators and are likely to be the first treated because they are assumed to be the primary pain generators (Travell 1992). If treatment of the muscles with any therapy, including FSM, successfully reduces the pain and splinting, the patient will feel better for several hours but the joint will lose its stabilizing support and the patient will complain that the segmental pain and muscle tenderness is worse when it returns within hours of treatment. This reaction to treatment, while inconvenient is a valuable signal to evaluate the spine or extremity joint for ligamentous injury with a stress x-ray.

Flexion–extension x-rays or stress x-rays of any joint ordered and taken when the injury is less than 4 weeks old may not accurately represent the condition at the joint because the soft tissues around the injured ligaments swell for up to 4 weeks from the onset of an injury and create an artificial splint for the ligaments. The practitioner is advised to check the dates of injury and compare them to the dates of any previous imaging read as negative for excess movement and repeat the imaging if necessary.

If a spinal MRI shows several small disc bulges and one of them is located at the same level as the lax ligament demonstrated on x-ray by excess segmental translation, it suggests that this segment is the one contributing most to the symptoms. The reader is reminded that a disc does not have to have a frank herniation or fragment to be a pain generator. Small disc bulges are often read as normal by a radiologist because it is thought that a certain amount of bulging and degeneration is normal by a certain age in most people. End plate fractures and small tears in the disc annulus are invisible on imaging but sufficient to allow diffusion of the inflammatory material from the nucleus pulposus out into the spinal fluid and the lateral foramen where it can irritate both the spinal cord and the nerve (Olmarker 1993, 1995, Ozaktay 1995, 1998, Taylor 1993).

The findings on a flexion–extension spinal x-ray will show increased translation or sliding of the upper vertebra on the lower one moving forward or back or both when the head is flexed or extended. If the vertebra moves a total of 4mm in one direction, the joint may be medically unstable and a surgical consult is advisable especially in the cervical spine. Translation of the vertebra of more than 4mm can compromise the safety of the spinal cord especially if the patient is subject to additional trauma such as a fall or auto accident.

Ligamentous laxity in the peripheral joints such as the ankle, knee, elbow, wrist or shoulder has similar indicators. If the joint does not respond in 12 weeks to therapies that would be expected to repair the injury, then stress x-rays or a specific evaluation for joint ligament stability should be performed. In some joints suspected ligamentous tears require an arthrogram to determine the extent of the ligamentous and joint damage. Dye is injected into the joint in an arthrogram and if it leaks out this indicates that the capsular ligaments are ruptured.

History questions specific to ligamentous laxity

How were you injured?

If there is a specific mechanism of injury and the patient can identify a specific time when the pain started after the injury, then look for forces sufficient to damage the ligament in question. Auto accidents and falls commonly cause ligamentous injuries in the spine, especially the cervical spine. If there is no specific injury onset, then look for job or recreational activities that create chronic repetitive stress with the load focused on the ligament in an extremity joint or the spine such as running, repetitive lifting with the arms or turning the arm or shoulder or using the legs or feet to push. Participation in contact sports or impact sports such as tennis, handball or racquetball may be associated with ligamentous injuries. Look for systemic inflammatory conditions such as rheumatoid arthritis, lupus or inflammatory arthritis that may compromise tissue integrity by creating inflammation and joint degeneration.

Which way were you looking at the time of impact?

Was your head turned to one side or the other at the time of impact?

Did your head turn as you landed?

These three questions will tease out a mechanism of injury that would reasonably be expected to damage the alar ligaments and create ligamentous laxity and instability at C1–C2. The symptom picture of sub-occipital muscle tension and headaches, C2–C3 facet joint pain and periorbital referred pain and C2 hyper-esthesia suggest this line of questioning.

What makes the pain worse?

Injured ligaments allow more segmental movement and any activity that stresses them will create excess movement at the injured joint and increase inflammation and pain. Look for increased pain with repetitive movement or activities that stress the joint in question. The pain may begin during the activity but it is more likely to increase 60 to 90 minutes after the activity.

Is neck pain worse when you read or use a computer?

Sometimes general questions are not adequate to prompt an accurate report and the questions need to be specific to the exact activity associated with increased pain. When ligaments in the neck are injured the pain will increase when bending the head or neck forward while typing or reading. Pain may increase during the activity or 1 to 2 hours after it.

Is the pain worse after you lift or do physical therapy exercises?

Cervical ligaments will be stressed and become painful after lifting the arms overhead or lifting a load out in front of the body during some work activities and during most exercises prescribed to strengthen muscles in the cervical spine. In general, if standard physical therapy exercises make the pain worse it indicates that the ligaments have been injured. Injured ligaments in the wrists or elbows become inflamed and painful after being stressed by lifting, pulling or rotating the wrist during exercise. The ligaments in the ankles and knees become inflamed and painful after walking or running or any activity that stresses them during exercise. The key here is that the pain may not start during the loading exercise but will start 1 to 2 hours after it.

Is the pain worse after massage or myofascial therapy?

If the tight muscles splinting the injured segment relax after massage or myofascial therapy then lax ligaments and the hypermobile segment will become more painful within 1 to 2 hours following the massage. This reaction is diagnostic and can be discovered in the history.

Is the pain worse in certain postures?

Certain postures put gravitational stresses on the ligaments and joints. Leaning even slightly forward while sitting to read or use a computer puts the head forward of the shoulders and stresses the vertebral ligaments of the cervical spine. Bending forward at the waist or leaning to the side stresses not only the lumbar discs but the ligaments as well.

Imaging

- Cervical spine: flexion–extension x-rays, APOM side bending, upper cervical MRI.
- Lumbar spine: flexion–extension and side bending x-rays.
- Extremity joints: stress x-rays.

Physical examination

Most practitioners reading this text have been trained to perform a physical examination to evaluate ligamentous laxity. This brief description is meant to be a reminder rather than a comprehensive or definitive instruction. The reader who desires more complete instruction is referred to any professional text on physical examination of the spine or extremities.

Gently palpate the area suspected of having injured ligaments. If the ligaments are lax there will be tenderness at the ligament–periosteum junction where the ligaments attach to the bone.

It is possible to detect subtle excessive joint movement by comparing the motion created by stressing the joints on both the injured and the uninjured side of the body if that has been part of your clinical training. Stabilize one side of the joint and gently press the other side of the joint away from the stabilized side. If the joint on the symptomatic side of the body moves more than the joint on the non-painful side this suggests a ligamentous injury. If this testing procedure has not been part of your clinical training or if you are not proficient in evaluating ligamentous injuries do not attempt to evaluate the joint by stressing it. It is beyond the scope of this text to provide instruction in physical examination and the reader is referred to any professional text of physical examination techniques.

Muscle involvement

Biomechanical abnormalities of a spinal segment or the extremity joint created by ligamentous injury contribute to muscle splinting and the formation of taut bands and myofascial trigger points in the muscles and fascia around the injured joint by both central and peripheral mechanisms. Neural feedback from the injured joint feeds back into the spinal cord and upregulates impulses going out to the joint from the spinal cord to increase muscle tension. The constant tension creates myofascial trigger points in the muscles. Trigger points cause the muscles to be short and taut and contribute to the compression and abnormal loading of the joints and ligaments creating further inflammation and biomechanical dysfunction. Myofascial trigger points sensitize pain nerves that feed back into the spine. This neural input from the muscles compounds the nociceptive sensitization of the nerves from the dorsal rami and amplifies the pain response in the area of the injured ligaments. Palpation of the muscles in the area around the injured ligament, whether in the spine or the extremity joints, will almost always reveal splinting, trigger points and tenderness in these muscles. As the ligaments are successfully treated and begin to stabilize the taut bands should soften and disappear as treatment progresses.

Movements that use trigger point laden muscles will create both local and referred pain from the myofascial trigger points. The same injuries that traumatize and damage the ligaments can also damage extremity joints, the facets and discs.

The practitioner treating ligamentous laxity may of necessity end up treating the extremity joint, or the disc, the nerve and the muscles associated with the injured ligament.

Treating ligamentous laxity

Hydration

- The patient must be hydrated to benefit from microcurrent treatment.
- Hydrated means 1 to 2 quarts of water consumed in the 2 to 4 hours preceding treatment
- Athletes and patients with more muscle mass seem to need more water than the average patient.
- The elderly tend to be chronically dehydrated and may need to hydrate for several days prior to treatment in addition to the water consumed on the day of treatment
- *DO NOT* accept the statement, "I drink lots of water"
- *ASK* "How much water, and in what form, did you drink today before you came in?"
- Coffee, caffeinated tea, carbonated cola beverages do not count as water.
- Water may be flavored with juice or decaffeinated tea.

Channel A: condition frequencies

The frequencies listed are thought to remove or neutralize the condition for which they are listed except for 81, 49 / which are thought to increase secretions and vitality respectively

- Inflammation   40 /
- Chronic inflammation   284 /
- Calcium ions   91 /
- Scarring   13 /
- Increase secretions   81 /
- Restore vitality   49 /
- Something torn or broken   124 /
- Remove trauma   294 /
- Restore function   321 /
- Remove histamine   9 /

Channel B: tissue frequencies

- Bursa ___ / 195
  - The bursa is a gel filled sac that forms a cushion between adjacent tendons and between tendons and the periosteum.
- Connective tissue: / 77
  - This frequency appears to influence the connective tissue that creates the matrix for the muscles, ligaments, tendons and fascia.

- Fascia ___ / 142
  - The fascia is a layer of specialized connective tissue that surrounds every muscle and all of the viscera. The fascia secretes the ground substance that is required to repair itself and ligaments and tendons.
- Ligaments ___ / 100
  - The ligaments are specialized connective tissue linking bone to bone at the periosteum often in the vicinity of the tendons, bursa in the extremity joints.
- Nerve ___ / 396
  - Any dermatomal or peripheral nerve including proprioceptive and nociceptive nerves to the joints and musculoskeletal structures.
- Periosteum ___ /783
  - The periosteum is the very well innervated fibrous outer layer of the bone to which the ligaments attach.
- Tendons ___ / 191
  - Tendons are specialized fascia that connect muscle to the bone at the periosteum.

Treatment considerations

The conceptual framework for treatment of chronic ligamentous laxity with FSM is different than it is when treating any other chronic condition. The repair tissue laid down in the area of chronic ligamentous injuries is ineffective and disorganized due to chronic inflammation and constant aberrant motion. In most chronic injuries the first FSM strategy is to remove scar tissue but this is not done casually when treating chronic ligamentous injuries. Even though the pain and injury is chronic, the body needs to be encouraged to lay down scar tissue to repair the ligaments as if the injury was new. This is contrary to the treatment rationale for every other chronic condition treated with FSM.

The treatment rationale with ligamentous laxity is to treat the ligament to reduce or remove the impediments to healing. Frequencies are used to remove the pattern of being "torn or broken", to reduce inflammation, chronic inflammation and calcium hardening and to increase the secretions of ground substance to enhance tissue repair and to increase vitality in the injured tissues. When the ligaments have been injured, the periosteum to which the ligaments attach, the tendons that connect muscle to the joint, and the bursas beneath the tendons in the extremity joints are usually collaterally inflamed or have been traumatized by the same mechanism of injury.

The desire on the part of the practitioner to soften the painful muscle tissue around the ligament by removing the scar tissue and disorganized ineffective repair tissue must be resisted. It will worsen the ligamentous pain and compromise joint stability. Treatment two or three times a week for 4 to 6 weeks while the patient is doing exercises designed specifically to strengthen the small inter-segmental muscles supporting the spinal joints or the stabilizing muscles in the peripheral joints will enhance the beneficial effects of exercise on ligamentous healing. This is not a simple or guaranteed outcome. Stabilizing injured ligaments is challenging and difficult. Use of FSM has been shown to make the process more effective.

Box 6.1

Summary for treating extremity joint ligamentous laxity

Treat the Ligament
- 294, 321, 9, / 100
- 124 / 100, 191, 142

Reduce Inflammation
- 40 / 116
- 40, 284 / 100, 191, 195, 783, 142, 77, 396

Support Healing
- 81, 49 / 142, 100, 191

Treat the muscles
- 91 / 142, 62, 396, 77, 191, 783
- 81 / 49 / 142

If anesthetics or narcotics present
- 43, 46, 19 / 396

Treatment protocol for chronic or acute ligamentous laxity

294, 321, 9, / 100
- Trauma, Paralysis, Allergy Reaction / ligament.
  - These three frequencies – the basics – do not tend to change symptoms but they appear to be important in restoring normal function to injured tissue. If you think of a time when you have suffered a physical injury you may notice that it is

possible to distinguish between the symptoms from the injury and the effect of the "fact" of the trauma, the shock of it to your system. 294 / is thought to address the "fact of the trauma" or the shock to the system created by the trauma.
- When a tissue is traumatized it sometimes behaves as if it has "lost" a line of instructions not unlike a computer when it freezes for the same reason. 321 / is thought to "reboot" the tissue and is described as being used to neutralize "paralysis" moving it past the lost instruction and on to the next step to facilitate return to function.
- When any tissue is traumatized the first response is the secretion of histamine to initiate the inflammatory response. When treating to arrest the immediate effects of a new injury removing the histamine from the injured area seems to stop the inflammatory progression.
- These frequencies don't necessarily change symptoms but they seem to help speed recovery.
- Treatment time: Use for 1 to 2 minutes or if you are sensitive to the feel of tissue softening and time allows, use the frequency as long as the softening happens. Use these frequencies only on the first two to three treatments.

124 / 100, 191, 142
- Something torn or broken / ligament, tendon, fascia.
- 124Hz is thought to remove the "fact of being torn or broken" from the injured tissue. This is a conceptual shift to the medically trained mind. In an energetic model, conditions have a physical consequence in the tissue – the ligament is "torn or broken" – and at the same time there is also an energetic or vibrational pattern that impresses itself on the semiconductor field that is the injured tissue. It is as if the pattern of being "torn or broken" has impressed itself on the ligament's field, interferes with the normal healing processes and prevents tissue repair. In an energetic model it is thought that removing this pattern of being "torn or broken" enables the normal repair processes to become effective. This frequency rarely if ever changes symptoms but it seems to enhance tissue repair of "torn or broken" tissues.
- Treatment time: Use for 1 to 4 minutes each or if you are sensitive to the feel of tissue softening and time allows, use the frequency as long as the softening happens. Use this frequency only on the first two to three treatments.

40 / 116
- A/B pair for Inflammation.

40, 284 / 100, 191, 142, 783, 77, 396
- Inflammation, chronic inflammation / Ligament, tendon, fascia, periosteum, connective tissue and nerve.
- Treatment time: Use these combinations for 2 to 4 minutes each. 40 / 116 reduced inflammation in the mouse model regardless of what tissue had been painted with arachidonic acid. 40 / 116 is the frequency to reduce general inflammation. Research has shown 40Hz to have a 4-minute time-dependent response in a mouse model of inflammation. 50% of the reduction in inflammation was present at 2 minutes. The full response was present at 4 minutes.

91 / 142, 396, 783
- Calcium ions, hardening / in fascia, nerves and periosteum.
- Calcium crystals flow into the tissues in response to inflammation and chronic inflammation.
- Treatment time: Use these combinations for 2 to 4 minutes each. The response and relief will vary from patient to patient in different tissues.

81, 49 / 142, 100, 191
- 81Hz is used for increasing secretions. / 142Hz is used for the fascia, 100 addresses the ligaments and 191 the tendons. The fascia secretes the ground substance necessary for repair of the fascia, ligaments and tendons. The additional tissue frequencies are included in the event that 81Hz is actually increasing collagen release from these tissues.
- Treatment time: Use for 2 to 4 minutes or if you are sensitive to the feel of tissue softening and time allows, use the frequency as long as the softening happens. This frequency combination appears to increase collagen deposition for enhanced ligamentous repair.

Treating ligamentous laxity in an extremity joint

Treating ligamentous laxity in an extremity joint adds the bursa to the list of tissues being treated.

294, 321, 9, / 100
- Trauma, Paralysis, Allergy Reaction / ligament.
- Detail and treatment times as above.

124 / 100, 191, 142
- Something torn or broken / ligament, tendon, fascia.
- Detail and treatment times as above

40 / 116
- A/B pair for Inflammation.

40, 284 / 100, 191, 195, 783, 142, 77, 396
- Inflammation, chronic inflammation / ligament, tendon, bursa, periosteum, fascia, connective tissue and nerve.
- If the ligament being treated is in an extremity joint instead of the spine there will be a bursa associated. Ligamentous laxity in an extremity joint creates aberrant joint motion which usually inflames the bursa and associated joint structures.

81, 49 / 142, 100, 191
- 81Hz is used for increasing secretions. /142Hz is used for the fascia, 100 addresses the ligaments and tendons. The fascia secretes the ground substance necessary for repair of the fascia, ligaments and tendons. The additional tissue frequencies are included in the event that 81Hz is actually increasing collagen release from these tissues.
- Treatment time: Use for 2 to 4 minutes or if you are sensitive to the feel of tissue softening and time allows, use the frequency as long as the softening happens. This frequency combination appears to increase collagen deposition for enhanced ligamentous repair.

Treat the Muscles at the Spine and Extremity Joints Note: 58 / 00, 02, 32 and 13 / 142, 62, 396 are missing. Treating myofascial tissue is different when treating an area with ligamentous laxity. Do not use the 58/'s or any frequency to remove scar tissue until a treatment trial has been done without them. Unless it is carefully done, removing scar tissue will destabilize the joint and cause an increase in pain.

If the disorganized and ineffective scar tissue must be removed in the process of treating the myofascial pain and adhesions between the nerves and the fascia, the injured joint and weakened lax ligaments must be artificially splinted for 1 to 2 days after the treatment by some means such as tape or a brace or a cervical collar. The muscles will eventually splint again because of biomechanical dysfunction and segmental inflammation at the joint but when they re-splint they should not have or develop myofascial trigger points for about 3 to 4 weeks. This window gives the patient time to progress in physical therapy strengthening the supporting muscles to improve joint stability.

The practitioner is advised to prepare the patient for this process and to be considerate of the patient's schedule and priorities during the inevitable symptom increase during this project. It is prudent to inform all members of the treatment team about the treatment plan and to prepare them for the removal of scar tissue and the window of laxity that will follow. Physical therapists will need to adjust the exercise program to use lighter weights and more repetitions to increase vascularity and strengthen the supporting muscles without causing undue joint stress. Removing scar tissue or treating myofascial pain without these precautions can create significant exacerbations.

40 / 116
- A/B pair for reducing inflammation.

40, 284 / 100, 191, 195, 783, 142, 77, 396
- Inflammation, chronic inflammation / ligament, tendon, bursa, periosteum, fascia, connective tissue and nerve.
- These frequencies to reduce inflammation and chronic inflammation have already been used in the process of treating the ligamentous tissues and do not need to be repeated when treating the muscles.

91 / 142, 62, 396, 77, 191, 783
- Remove calcium ions and hardening from the fascia, the muscle belly elastic tissue, associated nerve fibers, the connective tissue, tendons and the periosteum where the tendon and ligaments attach.
- Treatment time: Use each frequency for 2 to 4 minutes each
- This frequency will produce softening in myofascial tissue. 91 Hz may be used with each tissue frequency for 2 to 4 minutes each in a manual microcurrent unit (one that allows manual selection of a three-digit frequency) or in a unit that automatically changes frequencies after a set time interval of 2 minutes. If a manual microcurrent unit is being used and the practitioner is sensitive to the softening in the muscle, the frequency can be used for as long as it is producing changes in muscle texture. The tissue response may last for up to 5 or more minutes depending on the patient and the chronicity. Athletes with myofascial dysfunction respond very well to 91 Hz and it may produce softening for up to 5 to 10 minutes with certain tissues.

- **Narcotics:** If patients are on high levels of narcotics or have had multiple injections with anesthetics it is sometimes necessary to run the frequencies to "remove" narcotics and anesthetics. It is not thought that these frequencies actually remove the narcotic or anesthetic. It is much more likely that they somehow influence the membrane in such a way as to make it more receptive to treatment.
- Use **43, 46, 19 / 396** if joint has been injected with anesthetics or if patient is on narcotics with contacts the same as for the rest of the treatment.

Note: Use of FSM with Prolo therapy

If the patient is planning to see a practitioner who uses prolo therapy to help stabilize the ligaments, FSM treatment should be suspended for 4 to 6 weeks after the prolo treatments while the desired scar tissue is being created. Prolo therapy involves the injection of an inflammatory sugar-based substance intended to create acute inflammation and stimulate healing and the formation of healthy scar tissue. If FSM treatment has not been effective in a 4 to 6 week treatment trial, prolo therapy is a reasonable next step and the two make a good combination.

If the pain is neuropathic pain instead of ligamentous pain, prolo therapy will increase nerve pain at least until the spinal ligaments that are contributing to the dysfunctional disc can be stabilized. FSM may be used to alleviate the neuropathic pain without compromising the result of the prolo therapy. Six weeks after the last prolo therapy injection when the ligament has been shown to be stable, FSM may be used to modify scar tissue and hardening in the fascia, muscle and nerve to normalize joint mechanics and function. The practitioner should avoid use of the frequencies for removing scar tissue (58/'s, 13, 3/) for more than 1 to 2 minutes each during the first few treatments after prolo therapy.

 Stenosis precaution

If there is dense scar tissue or bony stenosis of the nerve root or spinal cord or if a disc fragment is compressing the nerve root or cord at the involved level the patient's pain may increase when polarized positive current is applied. If the patient is positioned comfortably, it is the only time the pain will increase during polarized positive treatment for nerve inflammation. It may increase in the dermatome or at the

Continued

spine or both. Assess patient position to determine whether it is contributing to the pain increase.

Stop treating immediately if pain goes up during treatment. Move the patient to a seated position if possible. Move the contacts slightly up the spine superior to the nerve root being treated, reduce current levels and change the current from polarized positive to alternating. If this is going to reduce the reaction it will do so in 5 to 10 minutes. If the pain continues to increase, stop treating with current. The pain should go back down in a few hours although it may take up to 24 hours to reduce to base line.

This reaction is diagnostic. If physical examination findings of reduced sensation and deep tendon reflexes at the involved level or hyperactive deep tendon reflexes below the involved level are present this reaction suggests the need to x-ray or perform an MRI to confirm the presence of compression.

Treatment application for ligamentous laxity

- **Current level:** Use 100–300μamps for average patients. Use lower current levels, 40–100μamps, for very small or debilitated patients. Use higher current levels, 200–400μamps, for larger or very muscular patients. In general, higher current levels reduce pain more quickly. Do not use more than 500μamps as animal studies suggest that increases in ATP level off at current levels above 500μamps while current levels below 500μamps increase ATP up to 500%.
- **Current Polarization**
  - ○ ± **Alternating or biphasic Current:** Current is used in alternating mode for treatment of most tissues except nerves. "Alternating DC current" is actually DC (direct) current that alternates its polarity from positive to negative during the machine duty cycle.
  - ○ + **Polarized Positive Current:** Current is polarized positive for most nerve treatments and may be beneficial in treating other tissues in some patients. When the current is polarized positive the DC wave form alternates from the zero line to positive in a square wave pattern. Some patients simply respond better to polarize positive current and some respond better to alternating or biphasic current. There is no explanation for this difference in response.
- **Waveslope: Moderate to Gentle**
  - ○ The waveslope refers to the rate of increase of current in the wave as it rises in alternating mode from zero up to the treatment current

level every 2.5 seconds on the Precision Microcurrent. Other microcurrent instruments may have slightly different duty cycles and the wave form may change more or less frequently. A sharp waveslope has a very steep leading edge on the wave shape indicating a very sharp increase in current. A gentle waveslope has a very gradual leading edge on the waveform indicating a gradual increase in current.

- ○ Use a moderate to sharp waveslope for chronic pain.
- ○ Use a gentle waveslope for acute pain or new injuries. A sharp waveslope is irritating in new injuries.
- **Lead Placement**
  - ○ **Spinal Ligaments:** FSM typically uses graphite gloves to conduct the current. The graphite gloves need to be kept moist so they conduct the current comfortably. The graphite gloves can be placed in a small warm wet towel or fabric sleeve, or alligator clips connected to the leads can be clipped to the wet contact.
  - ○ Place the **positive leads** in wet fabric to ensure a broad contact on the posterior spine at the involved spinal segment where the ligaments are painful in the cervical or lumbar spine.
  - ○ Place the **negative leads** in wet fabric placed on the body anterior to the spinal contact.

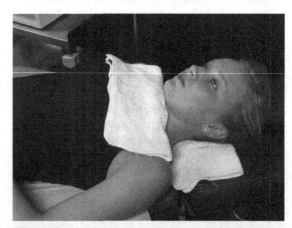

Figure 6.3 • Graphite gloves are placed in warm wet fabric contacts (face cloths). The graphite glove with the two positive leads in it is placed behind the neck and the graphite glove with the two negative leads in it is placed on the chest to allow current and frequencies to flow through the injured ligaments. This placement is used if there is no significant dermatomal nerve pain.

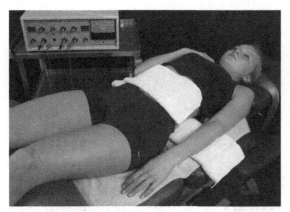

Figure 6.4 • Place the graphite gloves in separate warm wet fabric contacts (hand towel or face cloths). If there is no dermatomal nerve pain the lumbar ligaments can be treated by placing the positive leads glove fabric contact behind the back and the negative leads contact on the abdomen.

If two machines are being used to treat the ligaments and discs and the nerve and muscle simultaneously place the positive leads from both machines in the contact behind the back. Place the negative leads glove from the machine running the disc and ligament protocol on the abdomen and place the negative leads glove from the machine running the nerve and muscle protocol at the distal end of the affected nerve.

OR

Treating spinal ligament combined with nerve pain

* Wrap the **positive leads** contact around the spine to treat the ligaments of the cervical or lumbar spine.
* Wrap the **negative leads** around the limb at the end of the dermatomal nerve if there is nerve pain that must be treated at the same time.

OR

* **Adhesive Electrode Pads** may be used although the gloves seem to be more effective for reasons not understood. The electrode pads must be placed carefully so that the current and frequencies for the two channels cross in an interferential pattern through the area to be treated.
* Place the positive electrode from channel A on the skin over the injured spinal ligament. The negative electrode from channel A must be placed so that the current flows down an imaginary line diagonally through the body from the channel A positive electrode.
* Place the positive electrode from channel B on the skin over the contralateral spinal ligament or

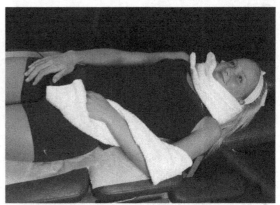

Figure 6.5 • If the nerve is to be treated at the same time as the cervical ligaments, wrap the positive leads glove in a warm wet fabric contact (hand towel) and wrap the contact around the neck so the current flows through the nerve from proximal to distal. Wrap the negative leads glove in a warm wet fabric contact (hand towel) and wrap the contact around the nerve root to be treated. The C5, C6, C7, C8, T1 and T2 nerve roots are being treating in this photograph. To treat the C3 or C4 nerve roots the negative contact would be placed up near the shoulder at those dermatomes.

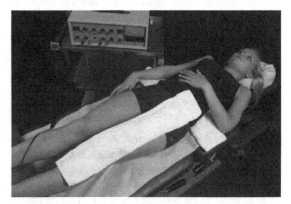

Figure 6.6 • If the nerve is to be treated at the same time as the ligaments the contact with the negative leads glove wrapped in it needs to be placed at the end of the nerve being treated in this case L3, L2, and L1. If all five nerve roots require treatment the towels can be connected to make one longer contact which is wrapped around the foot to treat L4, L5 and S1. The graphite glove with the positive leads is wrapped in the warm wet fabric contact (hand towel) and placed at the spine.

Box 6.2

Summary for treating spinal ligamentous laxity

Treat the Ligament
- 294, 321, 9, / 100
- 124 / 100, 191, 142

Reduce Inflammation
- 40 / 116
- 40, 284 / 100, 191, 142, 783, 77, 396
- 91 / 142, 396, 783

Support Healing
- 81, 49 / 142, 100, 191

Treat the muscles
- 91 / 142, 62, 396, 77, 191, 783
- 81 / 49 / 142

If anesthetics or narcotics present
- 43, 46, 19 / 396

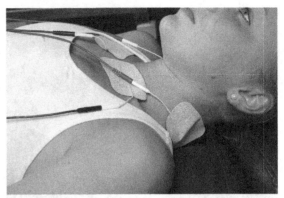

Figure 6.7 • Place the positive leads from channel A on the right side of the neck and the negative lead from channel A on the left upper chest just below the clavicle. Place the positive leads from channel B on the left side of the neck and the negative leads from channel B on the right upper chest just below the clavicle. The current and frequencies form an interferential pattern, crossing in three dimensions through the area to be treated.

adjacent to the first contact over an extremity ligament. The negative electrode from channel B must be placed so that the current flows down an imaginary line diagonally through the body from the channel B positive electrode. The current and the frequencies must pass through the area to be treated as an "X" in three dimensions. The negative electrodes may be placed directly anterior or anterior and slightly inferior to the spinal contacts. The negative electrodes may be placed at the ends of the nerve root affected by the injured disc.
A diagram for the placement would look like this:

Positive Electrode Channel A	Positive Electrode Channel B
Area to be Treated	
Negative Electrode Channel B	Negative Electrode Channel A

- **Extremity Joint Ligaments:** As a matter of habit the practitioner should wrap the contact containing the positive leads around the limb proximal to the joint in the event that the current may need to be polarized positive. The contact containing the negative leads should be wrapped around the limb and placed distal to the joint. If the practitioner is certain that the nerve is not involved and the current will not need to be polarized positive the contacts may be placed on opposite sides of the joint being treated.
- If wet towels are used, care should be taken to see that the towels do not touch each other. Current

will follow the path of least resistance and if the towels are less resistant than the patient the current will flow in the towels and avoid the tissue that needs treating. See the placement as shown in the photographs.

Adjunctive therapies

Ligaments are slow to heal and the muscles supporting the injured joint must be strengthened carefully to avoid overloading the injured area and exacerbating the instability. Comprehensive discussion of spinal and extremity joint stabilization exercises are beyond the scope of this text but the practitioner should be aware that such exercise protocols exist. In general, the exercises consist of small range, almost isometric muscle contractions using little or no weight. The muscle contractions increase vascularity and promote healing at the segment in addition to strengthening the muscles so they can assist in stabilization. The benefits of appropriate therapeutic exercises to train the muscles to compensate for the injured ligaments and stabilize the joint cannot be overestimated.

- **Nutrition:** Nutritional supplements to provide the building blocks for collagen repair are also helpful. Essential fatty acids, EPA/DHA, cold water fish oils at a dosage of one gram per day reduce inflammation and help ensure that repair tissues

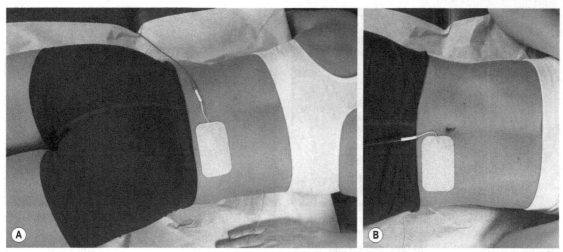

Figure 6.8 • To treat a lumbar ligament with no nerve involvement, place the positive lead from channel A on the right side of the low back. Place the negative lead from channel A on the left side of the abdomen at or below the same level as the disc being treated. Place the positive lead from channel B on the left side of the low back and the negative leads from channel B on the right side of the abdomen.

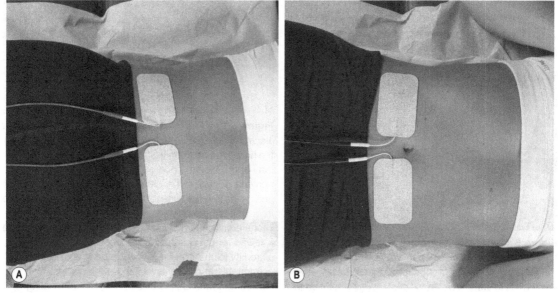

Figure 6.9 • Pads from both channel A and channel B in place on the lumbar spine and abdomen for treatment of lumbar ligaments without nerve involvement.

are flexible. Vitamin C provides one of the constituents of collagen and supplementation of one gram per day may help reduce inflammation and enhance collagen formation. The patient should have a source of high quality protein appropriate to individual nutritional requirements.

• **Skin Taping:** In some cases it may be useful to place adhesive, athletic tape on the skin overlying the injured joint. The tape on the skin inhibits

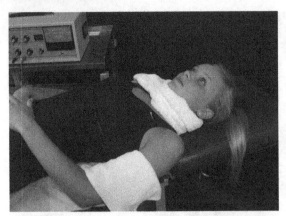

Figure 6.10 • When shoulder ligaments are injured and there is a component of C4 or C5 neuropathic pain, the graphite glove with the positive leads can be placed in a warm wet fabric contact wrapped around the neck and the graphite glove with the negative leads can be placed in a warm wet contact wrapped around the upper arm. The distal contact allows the current to flow through the ligaments and along the nerve so that both can be treated with the same set up.

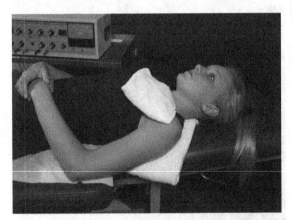

Figure 6.11 • If there is no nerve involvement, place the positive leads glove in a warm wet fabric contact behind the shoulder with the patient supine. Place the negative leads glove in a warm wet fabric contact (face cloth) on the anterior shoulder. The hands can be used to palpate and follow tissue changes under and around the towels.

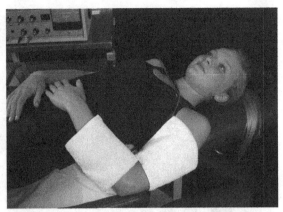

Figure 6.12 • Elbow: the fabric contacts are placed proximal and distal to the joint.

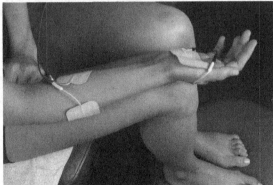

Figure 6.13 • Place the positive lead channel A adhesive electrode pad on the anterior surface of the forearm and the negative lead channel A pad on the posterior surface of the hand. Place the positive lead channel B pad on the posterior surface of the forearm and the negative channel B pad on the anterior surface of the hand. The current and the frequencies from channel A and channel B cross in an interferential pattern at the wrist. The same process is to be followed for using adhesive electrode pads on any extremity joint. Adhesive electrode pads are not usually comfortable at current levels above 100μamps. The current can be used polarized positive or alternating DC current and the proximal contact should always contain the positive lead.

muscle firing and serves to stabilize the joint below. Comprehensive description of skin taping is beyond the scope of this text but the practitioner treating ligamentous laxity should be aware that it is useful and pursue further training

or refer the patient to someone with this skill until the ligament is repaired.

• **Avoid:** The patient should avoid any activity or therapy that stresses the joint or disrupts connective tissue, including yoga, lifting heavy

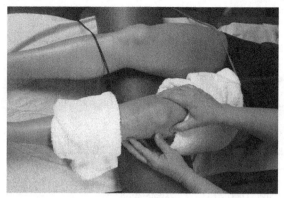

Figure 6.14 • Wrap the glove with the positive leads in a warm wet fabric contact (hand towel) and wrap the contact around the thigh just above the knee. Wrap the negative leads glove in a warm wet fabric contact (hand towel) and wrap that contact just below the knee or at the knee. The current can be used polarized positive or alternating DC current and the proximal contact should always contain the positive lead. Palpate the changes in the tender ligament being treated or mobilize the myofascial tissue by placing the hand under the towel during treatment.

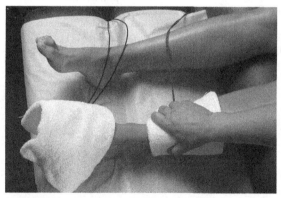

Figure 6.15 • Wrap the glove with the positive leads in a warm wet fabric contact (hand towel) and wrap the contact around the calf just above the ankle. Place the contacts higher on the calf if the gastrocnemius and soleus are involved in the ankle injury. Wrap the negative leads glove in a warm wet fabric contact (hand towel) and wrap that contact just below the ankle or at the ankle. The current can be used polarized positive or alternating DC current and the proximal contact should always contain the positive lead. Palpate the changes in the tender ligament being treated or mobilize the myofascial tissue by placing the hand under the towel during treatment.

weights, prolonged static postures that weight the lax joint, any ballistic movement that might tear fragile repair tissue, any movement that reproduces the mechanism of injury and any "deep" soft tissue therapy that might disrupt newly forming repair tissue. This caution applies to the use of FSM for myofascial therapy.

• **Expected outcomes:** The patient with a ligamentous injury should be warned that the process of repair will require 4 to 6 months of attention and effort even with the use of FSM as an adjunct. FSM can reduce inflammation, encourage enhanced tissue repair and speed up the repair process, reduce the number and severity of exacerbations and shorten the time required to achieve joint stability. The use of prolo therapy after a 4-month trial of FSM treatment may be helpful if healing is not proceeding as quickly as desired. In the author's opinion, "prolo" therapy should not be used until there has been a period of stabilization exercises to prepare the area.

A successful outcome will depend on the extent of the original injury, the severity of the ligamentous injury, patient compliance with exercise, the patient's overall health and nutritional status and, to some extent, good luck.

Case report

The patient was the 62-year-old female driver of a vehicle parked in icy conditions at the bottom of a steep driveway in front of a home that sat below the level of the roadway by 15 feet. Her vehicle was struck by a pickup truck that left the road way after losing control on the ice and was air born at the time of impact with the front quarter panel and door pillar on the driver side. She presented for treatment 4 months after the accident having been to a physical therapist, a massage therapist and a chiropractor for treatment previously. Her pain was worse after physical therapy, after massage and much worse after spinal manipulation so she discontinued both therapies after a short time. Her medical physician referred her for treatment with FSM.

The severity of the impact, the fact that she was still in moderate pain 4 months after the accident and the fact that her symptoms worsened after physical therapy and after massage and after spinal manipulation all suggested that her symptoms were due to ligamentous laxity. A full spinal series of x-rays including flexion–extension x-rays were taken. They demonstrated mild spinal degeneration consistent with her age and documented a total of 4mm translation of C4 on C5 and 3mm of translation at C5 on C6 in flexion and extension. She was placed in a cervical collar to be worn during any physical activity and referred to a spinal surgeon who saw no need for surgical treatment.

She was treated with FSM twice a week for 12 weeks and sent to physical therapy for spinal stabilization (STEP) exercises. At the end of 3 months the ligamentous laxity at C5 on C6 was 1mm and the ligamentous laxity of C4 on C5 was reduced to 1mm.

Bibliography

Dodds, S.D., Panjabi, M.M., Daigneault, J.P., 2004. Radiofrequency probe treatment for subfailure ligament injury: a biomechanical study of rabbit ACL. Clin. Biomech. 19, 175–183.

Grieve, G.P., 1981. Common vertebral joint problems. Churchill Livingstone, Edinburgh.

Hart, D.P., Dahners, L.E., 1987. Healing of the medial collateral ligament in rats. The effects of repair, motion, and secondary stabilizing ligaments. J. Bone Joint Surg. Am. 69, 1194–1199.

Konttinen, Y.T., Santavirta, S., Kauppit, M., Isomaki, H., Slati, S., 1989. Atlantoaxial laxity in rheumatoid arthritis. Acta Orthopaedica Scandinavica 60 (4), 379–382.

Lentell, G., Baas, B., Lopez, D., McGuire, L., Sarrels, M., Snyder, P., 1995. The contributions of proprioceptive deficits, muscle function and anatomic laxity to functional instability of the ankle. J. Orthop. Sports Phys. Ther. 21, 206–215.

Martel, W., 1977. Pathogenesis of cervical discovertebral destruction in rheumatoid arthritis. Arthritis Rheum. 20, 1217–1225.

Meyers, T., 2001. Anatomy trains. Churchill Livingstone, Edinburgh, pp. 9–49.

Olmarker, K., Rydevik, B., Nordberg, C., 1993. Autologous nucleus pulposus induces neurophysiologic and histologic changes in porcine cauda equina nerve roots. Spine 18, 1425–1432.

Olmarker, K., Blomquist, J., Stromberg, J., et al., 1995. Inflammatogenic properties of nucleus pulposus. Spine 20, 665–669.

Ozaktay, A.C., Cavanaugh, J.M., Blagoev, D.C., 1995. Phospholipase A_2-induced electrophysiologic and histologic changes in rabbit dorsal lumbar spine tissues. Spine 20, 2659–2668.

Ozaktay, A.C., Kallakuri, S., Cavanaugh, J.M., 1998. Phospholipase A_2 sensitivity of the dorsal root and dorsal root ganglion. Spine 23, 1297–1306.

Steiner, M.E., Grana, W.A., Chilag, K., Schelberg-Karnes, E., 1986. The effect of exercise on anterior posterior knee laxity. Am. J. Sports Med. 14, 24–29.

Taylor, J.R., Twomey, L.T., 1993. Acute injuries to cervical joints, An autopsy study of neck pain. Spine 18, 1115–1122.

Travel, J.G., Simons, D.G., 1992. Myofascial pain and dysfunction. The trigger point manual, vol. 2. Williams & Wilkins, Baltimore.

White, A.A., Panjabi, M.H., 1978. Clinical biomechanics of the spine. JB Lippincott, Philadelphia.

Treating muscles, fascia and myofascial trigger points

7

Myofascial pain is defined as pain arising from muscles or related fascia and comes from hyperirritable areas of muscle, ligaments and fascia known as myofascial trigger points (Bennett 2007). There are approximately 400 muscles forming the largest organ in the body amounting to approximately 40% of the body weight and there is no single medical specialty that is solely responsible for the study of their diagnosis and function. Myofascial trigger points have been associated with low back pain, neck pain, tension headaches, temporomandibular joint pain, forearm and hand pain and pelvic and urogenital pain syndromes in 44 million Americans and so a clinical practitioner in any specialty is likely to see patients with myofascial pain caused by trigger points (Borg-Stein 2006, Simons 1983, Fernandez-de-las-Penas 2006, 2007, Ardic 2006, Hwang 2005, Dogweiler-Wiygul 2004).

The first challenge for the practitioner is to recognize that myofascial trigger points may be causing the patient's pain; the second challenge is to locate, effectively treat and eliminate myofascial trigger points as pain generators; the third challenge is to eliminate the factors in the patient's biomechanics, physiology and lifestyle that perpetuate the myofascial dysfunction. Myofascial pain caused by trigger points must also be distinguished from the full body pain, central sensitization, sleep disturbances and neuroendocrine dysfunction characteristic of fibromyalgia.

Characteristics of myofascial trigger points

Active myofascial trigger points cause pain at rest, restrict muscle range of motion and have characteristic myotomal pain referral patterns that do not follow dermatomal nerve root patterns or scleratomal patterns emanating from joint structures. The original referral patterns were identified in the 1930s by injecting hypertonic saline into muscles (Kelgren 1938) and pain patterns for over 100 muscles have been documented in detail in the two-volume text, Myofascial pain and dysfunction: the trigger point manual (Travell 1983, 1992). Myofascial trigger points are found by gentle palpation across the direction of the muscle fiber to identify an indurated taut band of muscle and then specific palpation within the taut band to locate a painful nodule that feels like a hardened grain of rice or lentil. Firm pressure on the small nodule may cause the muscle to twitch and may recreate the patient's pain complaint in the myotomal referral area. Latent myofascial trigger points have taut bands that are tender to touch and restrict range of motion but do not cause spontaneous referred pain.

Calcium release

Myofascial trigger points are thought to arise from focal injury to muscle fibers caused by trauma or overuse. Biopsies of myofascial trigger points reveal a cluster of numerous microscopic foci of sarcomere "contraction knots" that are scattered throughout the tender nodule (Simons 2001, Gerwin 2004). These contraction knots are thought to be caused by calcium release from the sarcoplasmic reticulum and are maintained by an "energy crisis" in the now hypermetabolic muscle once the constant contraction is initiated. Muscle contraction requires the energy of four ATP; muscle relaxation requires

© 2011, Elsevier Ltd.
DOI: 10.1016/B978-0-443-06976-5.00007-1

two ATP (Adenosine triphosphate, ATP, is the chemical energy that fuels all physical processes; Guyton 1996). Once facilitated, the motor end-plates release increased amounts of acetylcholine to maintain the contraction, perpetuating the contraction knots and forming a self perpetuating cycle of activation, energy depletion and local metabolic stress (Mense 2003). Calcium release from the sarcoplasmic reticulum becomes relevant for FSM treatment of trigger points because the frequency thought to "remove calcium ions" is one that softens the taut band and usually eliminates the trigger points.

Nerve sensitization

Persistence of the trigger point leads to neuroplastic changes at the level of the dorsal horn in the spinal cord, leading to central pain sensitization and expansion of the pain beyond its original boundaries into the referred pain area (Arendt-Nielsen 2003). The central neuroplastic changes account for the characteristic trigger point referral patterns. Neuropathic pain sensitization at the level of the nerve root and the spinal cord accounts for the pain intensity seen during stimulation of the trigger point that often appears disproportionate to the stimulus (Curatolo 2006). The twitch response that occurs when the muscle is stimulated is a spinal reflex that can be abolished by transection of the spinal nerve that innervates the trigger point (Hong 1994, 1996).

The local biochemical milieu in an active trigger point is different from that of normal muscle fibers or latent trigger points. A microdialysis needle was used to take constant stream samples of the biochemical environment within an active trigger point before, during and after a twitch response and compared it to normal muscle and latent trigger points. Active trigger points show significantly elevated levels of the inflammatory peptides TNF-α, Interleukin-1(IL-1), calcitonin-gene-related-peptide (CGRP), substance P, bradykinin, serotonin, and norepinephrine (Shah 2005). Early biopsies of trigger points showed mast cells degranulating releasing histamine into the area around the trigger point (Simons 1983). The neural component of trigger point pain and perpetuation is relevant to FSM treatment because the most effective treatment protocols have evolved to include treating "inflammation in the nerve and the spinal cord" first with the FSM treatment protocols known to reduce inflammatory cytokines (McMakin 2005).

Treating myofascial trigger points

There is no form of drug therapy that alleviates myofascial trigger point pain or muscle dysfunction. Trigger point injections with saline and 1% lidocaine or procaine or dry needling are considered to be the most effective therapy but require a skilled well trained therapist to precisely localize the active trigger point by identifying a local twitch response in the taut band. Studies have shown problems with localizing the taut band and the active trigger point (inter-rater reliability) between therapists depending on their skill and training (Gerwin 1997, Hsieh 2000, Sciotti 2001). Needling or injection of single active trigger points limits effectiveness in muscular areas populated by multiple active, latent and satellite trigger points. Full length stretching of the muscle while using an ethyl chloride vapocoolant spray, called "spray and stretch", disrupts the focal contractions and stops the prolonged ATP consumption that perpetuates the contraction knots. Not all muscles are suitable for this intervention and environmental considerations have reduced its use in recent years. Postural and ergonomic corrections to modify factors that perpetuate trigger points are critical to successful management.

Diagnosing myofascial pain

Any patient who presents with a chronic pain complaint should have a focused neuromuscular evaluation that includes evaluation of reflexes and sensation and a palpatory evaluation to check for taut bands and myofascial trigger points. There are wall charts and diagrams in text books that illustrate the referred pain patterns for specific muscles (Travell 1983, 1992, Niel-Asher 2008). The diagrams give guidance as to what muscles are likely to be a source of the referred pain in a given area. The practitioner should match the patient's area of complaint with the pain patterns in the diagram and then check the muscles that refer pain to that area. Palpation of a taut band and the small painful nodule that is the trigger point, pressure on the nodule that reproduces the patient's pain and restricted range of motion due to muscle tightness are all diagnostic of an active myofascial trigger point.

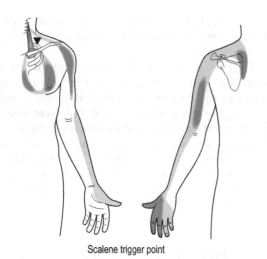

Scalene trigger point

Figure 7.1 • Myofascial trigger points refer pain to sites distant from the source of the pain in distinct patterns that do not follow dermatomal or scleratomal referral patterns. Pain in the arm, shoulder or hand may originate with a trigger point found in the anterior scalenes. The trigger points in the scalenes may in turn be a result of a disc injury or overuse caused by poor posture.

History of causation consistent with myofascial trigger points

The patient should have some history of overuse or trauma that would account for the formation of a myofascial pain problem. Chronic postural strain, repetitive muscle use, degenerative joint and disc disease, acute disc injuries, food allergies and other inflammatory conditions and emotional stress are among the conditions that contribute to trigger points. Look for some temporal association with activities or events and the onset of pain. If the pain started around June of 1999, ask what was happening in May of 1999.

Physical examination

Physical examination should include deep tendon reflexes, a dermatomal sensory examination and palpation of the muscles suspected to be the source of the pain. The presence of dermatomal hyperesthesia or numbness, or hyper or hypoactive reflexes suggests neuropathic involvement that may influence treatment.

Myofascial palpation should be guided by the patient's pain diagram and description. If the patient locates the pain at the "shoulder" the 12 muscles that can refer pain to the shoulder should be evaluated for the presence of taut bands and active and latent trigger points. Sustained pressure on the trigger point may reproduce the patient's pain but a trigger point that is already maximally referring may not increase its referral in response to pressure. Detailed descriptions and advice on how to conduct a myofascial palpatory examination are beyond the scope of this text but the reader is encouraged to pursue training in this skill.

The discs and facet joints should be considered and examined because myofascial trigger points can be created by and perpetuated by degenerative joint and disc disease and can in turn exacerbate degenerative joint disease when the taut muscle compresses the spinal segment.

Myofascial trigger points can create abnormal biomechanics in the peripheral joints – the shoulder, the elbow, the hip, the knee and even in the wrist and ankle when taut bands interfere with optimal joint motion. Conversely, inflammation in the peripheral joints, tendons and bursa can create muscle guarding and tightness that leads to taut bands and active trigger points. The dysfunction forms a feed forward and feedback cycle that perpetuates both the joint inflammation and the myofascial trigger points.

A visceral examination or abdominal palpation may be necessary if the patient has myofascial trigger points created by gastrointestinal or gynecological organ referral.

Treating myofascial trigger points with FSM

FSM was first used to successfully treat myofascial trigger points in 1996 and the first two articles published were collected case reports showing successful pain resolution in trigger points in the head, neck and face pain and in low back pain (McMakin 1998, 2004). FSM provides microamperage current known to increase ATP production by 500% in rat skin (Cheng 1982). The current alone would address the energy crisis that perpetuates the contracture knots allowing the knots to release by increasing ATP.

The frequencies used to "reduce inflammation in the nerve" have been shown to decrease inflammatory cytokines including IL-1, CGRP, substance P and serotonin – demonstrated by Shah to be increased in the active trigger point milieu (McMakin 2005, Shah 2005). FSM has been shown to down regulate spinal cord activation and reduce central sensitization in the treatment of fibromyalgia associated with spine trauma and could reasonably be assumed to perform the same function to reverse the central neuroplastic changes seen in myofascial pain. The observed effects of muscle softening, relaxation of the taut band and resolution of the trigger point occur as a response to specific frequencies meant to reduce inflammation in the nerve and reduce calcium ion deposits in the fascia. It is reassuring that these frequencies coincide with the pathologies now known to be associated with myofascial trigger points.

When FSM is used to treat myofascial trigger points the positive pair of electrodes are applied at the spine where the relevant nerve root exits and the other pair is applied at the end of the dermatomal nerve supplying the muscles being treated. The current flows through a regional area of biomechanically and neurologically related muscle tissue. The treatment does not require precise localization of the taut band or active trigger point which eliminates the reliability problems that have plagued dry needling and injection trigger point treatment methods and allows successful treatment by less skillful clinical assistants. The treatment can be applied to any muscle or muscle group and has no known negative environmental impact which gives it a distinct advantage over vapocoolant spray and stretch technique. When the dysfunctional muscle is treated at the same time as its related agonist and antagonist muscles in a functional region it provides biomechanical balance that enhances recovery and return to function.

The treatment is pain free, low risk and non-invasive and produces rapid reduction in pain giving it a distinct advantage over other methods in the treatment of myofascial trigger points.

Treating chronic myofascial pain and trigger points

Treatment of myofascial pain and trigger points has been developed over 12 years of clinical experience and literally tens of thousands of patient treatments.

The protocols have become so predictably effective that the response to treatment can be used diagnostically.

The myofascial protocol has three parts. It starts with the frequencies to treat the nerve then moves to the frequencies to treat the muscle and then to the frequencies to treat the facet joint, the disc or the peripheral joints that might be instigating or perpetuating factors. This treatment is so consistently effective that if it does not eliminate the taut band and reduce the pain then some visceral source for the trigger points should be considered.

Hydration

- The patient must be hydrated to benefit from microcurrent treatment.
- Hydrated means 1 to 2 quarts of water consumed in the 2 to 4 hours preceding treatment
- Athletes and patients with more muscle mass seem to need more water than the average patient.
- The elderly tend to be chronically dehydrated and may need to hydrate for several days prior to treatment in addition to the water consumed on the day of treatment
- *DO NOT* accept the statement, "I drink lots of water"
- *ASK* "How much water, and in what form, did you drink today before you came in?"
- Coffee, caffeinated tea, carbonated cola beverages do not count as water.
- Water may be flavored with juice or decaffeinated tea.

Channel A: condition frequencies

The frequencies listed are thought to remove or neutralize the condition for which they are listed except for 81, 49 / which are thought to increase secretions and vitality respectively. They are listed alphabetically and not in order of use or importance.

- Calcium, induration   91 /
- Chronic inflammation   284 /
- Inflammation   40 /
- Scarring   13 /
- Sclerosis   3 /
- Support Secretions: 81 /
- Restore vitality   49 /

Channel B: tissue frequencies

Neuropathic component

- Nerve: ___ / 396
  - Dermatomal nerve roots become inflamed and sensitized from constant input by the contracting myofascial tissue or from a nearby disc injury. The disc nucleus contains very concentrated levels of the inflammatory substance phospholipase A_2 (PLA_2). When the annulus is damaged by trauma or postural strain it allows diffusion of small amounts of PLA_2 to the nerve. This concentration is sufficient to cause nerve inflammation and muscle hypertonicity but insufficient to cause a classic dermatomal neuropathy.
- Spinal Cord: ___ / 10
  - The spinal cord becomes sensitized and facilitated by the constant neural input from the muscle and nerve.

Myofascial component

- Fascia: ___ /142
  - The fascia is the thin connective tissue covering surrounding the muscles and all soft tissues. The fascia becomes inflamed, calcified and fibrosed during the degenerative process.
- Artery and Elastic Tissue in the Muscle Belly: __ /62
  - 62 is the frequency used for the artery and the elastic tissue in the arterial walls. The muscle belly responds to this frequency either because it is full of small arteries or because the elastic tissue in the muscle belly is somehow related to the artery wall.
- Nerve: ___ / 396
  - Fine neural fibers travel between layers of fascia in a fascia–nerve–fascia sandwich to innervate the muscles. Constant contractures and local metabolic dysfunction create inflammation at the site of the trigger point. Inflammation leads to calcium influx and fibrosis. Fibrosis between the nerve and fascia restricts movement, creates neuropathic pain and muscle activation when the nerve is stretched as the fascia moves. Calcium ions flow into the nerve when it is inflamed and change the firing threshold.
- Connective tissue: ___ / 77
  - This frequency appears to influence the connective tissue that creates the matrix for the muscles and fascia.

- Tendons: ___ / 191
  - The tendons attach the muscles and fascia to the joint capsule and periosteum.

Joint component – facet joints, discs, and peripheral joints

- Periosteum: ___ / 783
  - The periosteum lines the outside of the bone, interweaves with tendinous and ligamentous attachments and is very pain sensitive. Inflammation and calcification in the periosteum are the most common chronic pain generators in facet and peripheral joint pain.
- Joint Capsule: ___ / 480
  - The joint capsule attaches to the periosteum, surrounds the joint and becomes fibrosed, calcified, scarred and inflamed when damaged by trauma or chronic mechanical stress.
- Cartilage: ___ / 157
  - Cartilage lines the facet and peripheral joint surface and becomes damaged, degenerated, calcified and inflamed when traumatized by acute or chronic compression of the joint surface (see Chapter 6: Treating Facet Joint Pain).
- Disc Annulus: ___ / 710
  - The disc annulus wraps around and contains the nucleus and is very well innervated and pain sensitive. It is the most common pain generator in chronic discogenic pain and in mild acute disc injuries that would create myofascial trigger points (see Chapter 4: Treating Discogenic Pain).
- Disc as a whole: ___ / 630
  - This frequency is thought to address the disc as a whole.
- Disc Nucleus: ___ / 330
  - The gel like disc nucleus fills the center of the disc and absorbs water to become a cushion for the vertebral bodies in the spine. It is very high in PLA_2 and very inflammatory.
- Bursa or tendon sheath: ___ / 195
  - The major tendons in the peripheral joints are cushioned by bursas that lie between the tendons and between the tendons and the periosteum. Bursas become inflamed and calcified by overuse and repetitive stresses.
- A/B pairs for Scar Tissue:
  - 58 / 00
  - 58 / 01
  - 58 / 02
  - 58 / 32

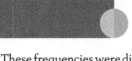

These frequencies were discovered in a list of frequencies published by Albert Abram's in Electromedical Digest in 1931. 58 / 00 was the frequency combination to remove "abnormal cellular stroma", probably meant to address the tendency of the cell to form scar tissue. 58 / 01 was used for scar in bony tissue. 58 / 02 was used for scar in soft tissue and 58 / 32 was used for scar tissue adhesions. When there is no bone involved 58 / 01 is not used. These are A/B pairs in which channel A is not a condition and channel B is not a tissue but both frequencies form a frequency pattern that appears to eliminate or lengthen scar tissue.

In treating chronic complaints the 58/'s are used in order as listed above for approximately 1 to 2 minutes each at the beginning of the treatment to soften the tissues. If there is no bone involved in the complaint it is customary to leave out 58 / 01. For those practitioners who can feel the softening produced by the frequency, it is often helpful to run the frequency until the softening stops and the tissue becomes relatively more firm. There may be some patients in whom one or more of these frequencies will produce softening for up to 3 to 4 minutes.

The 58/'s will increase range of motion but do not change pain.

Caution: 58 / 00, 01, 02, 32

- Do not use these frequencies on injuries newer than 5 to 6 weeks old.
- Newly injured tissue must form scar tissue in order to repair itself.
- Removing the scar tissue seems to undo the healing by weeks in a new injury.
- The 58/'s can be used very briefly (15 seconds) to modify scar tissue as it is forming after the first four weeks.
- Never use this combination before the injury is 4 weeks old

This precaution is the result of trial and uncomfortable error. A patient was being treated for facet joint and soft tissue injuries caused by an auto accident that had occurred 3 weeks previously. She was pain free after four treatments in 21 days and was treated on a Tuesday. She returned on Thursday complaining that whatever had been done on Tuesday had "undone" 2 weeks worth of healing and she felt as much pain as she had 2 weeks previously. Review of the Tuesday treatment notes revealed that the 58/'s had been used in addition to the protocols that had been reducing the pain for the preceding three weeks. She was so much improved that it seemed as if the injury was much older and the date of injury was not checked before treatment. When the symptoms increased the presumption was made that the 58/'s had removed repair tissue necessary to keep the joint and soft tissues pain free and stable. Treatment with frequencies to reduce inflammation and increase collagen eliminated her pain and she recovered as expected. The 58/'s were used again 4 weeks later to increase range of motion and there was no increase in pain.

Trial and error during the first year of treating with FSM in similar situations helped to determine that the 58/'s should not be used within 5 to 6 weeks of a new injury. They can be used briefly four weeks after the date of injury – for 5 to 10 seconds each – to thin out scar tissue as it is forming, especially in athletes who seem to heal faster than non-athlete patients. This reaction is predictable and reproducible. Take this precaution seriously.

Treating myofascial pain and trigger points

Treat the nerve – Treat the muscle – Treat the joint

Treat the nerve

Nerve protocol

40 / 396
- Reduce Inflammation in the nerve.
- Polarize current positive +.
- Treatment time: 5 minutes or as long as positive response occurs.
- The protocol to reduce inflammation in the nerve usually begins softening the muscles between the two contacts within one minute. At the end of 5 minutes the softening should have maximized and achieved whatever reduction in neural inflammation or sensitization that can be accomplished.

40 / 10
- Reduce inflammation in the spinal cord.
- Polarize current positive +.
- Treatment time: 2 minutes or as long as positive response occurs.

- The protocol to reduce inflammation in the cord is especially helpful in treating muscles in the cervical spine and shoulder that are especially tight bilaterally and seems to address spinal cord sensitization and upregulation. If this frequency combination is going to produce additional softening of the muscles it will do so within the first 2 to 3 minutes. If no change in muscle tone or texture becomes apparent in that time, change frequency to the next in the protocol. If the muscle softens in response to this frequency, the frequency combination can be used until no further softening is perceived which may take up to 5 to 10 minutes depending on the patient.

- Predicted Response: The frequencies for inflammation in the nerve and cord cause muscle relaxation in more than 80% of patients treated. As this response begins, use the manual techniques described below and wait for the tissue to stop softening before changing to the muscle protocol.

Stenosis precaution

If there is dense scar tissue or bony stenosis of the nerve root or spinal cord or if a disc fragment is compressing the nerve root or cord at the involved level the patient's pain may increase when polarized positive current is applied. It is the only time the pain will increase during polarized positive treatment for nerve inflammation. It may increase in the dermatome or at the spine or both.

Stop treating immediately if pain goes up during treatment. Move the patient to a seated position if possible. Move the contacts slightly up the spine superior to the nerve root being treated, reduce current levels and change the current from polarized positive to alternating. If this is going to reduce the reaction it will do so in 5 to 10 minutes. If the pain continues to increase, stop treating with current. The pain should go back down in a few hours although it may take up to 24 hours to reduce to base line.

This reaction is diagnostic. If physical examination findings of reduced sensation and deep tendon reflexes at the involved level or hyperactive deep tendon reflexes below the involved level are present this reaction suggests the need to x-ray or perform an MRI to confirm the presence of compression.

Treatment application

Lead placement: manual therapy

- The positive leads from channel A and channel B are placed in one glove.

- The negative leads from channel A and channel B are placed in the other glove.

- The two gloves will always be on opposite sides of the body part being treated during manual treatment of trigger points and myofascial tissue. The required interferential field forms in the space between the two gloves which should include the tissue being treated. The polarized positive current used with 40 / 396, 10 relaxes the tissue even if the contacts are not set up proximal distal.

- **Positive leads:** The positive leads are wrapped in or attached to a warm wet contact, such as a hand towel or long graphite electrode that is wrapped around the neck or placed along the spine where the nerve roots exit that innervate the involved muscle group.

- **Negative leads:** The negative leads are wrapped in or attached to a warm wet fabric contact or long graphite electrode that wraps around the end of the nerve root at the distal end of the muscle group to be treated.

Adhesive Electrode Pads may be used for convenience although the gloves seem to be more effective for reasons not understood. The adhesive electrode pads are especially useful for home treatment because they allow the patient to be active while being treated. The pads become "prickly" or sting when current levels are above 150µamps so may not be useful for larger patients or athletes.

When applying treatment with adhesive electrode pads, the current and the frequencies must pass through the area to be treated in an interferential pattern, forming an "X" in three dimensions. The positive electrodes are placed at the spine at the level of the disc to be treated. The negative electrodes may be placed directly anterior or anterior and slightly inferior to the spinal contacts if the disc alone is being treated or if the nerve is to be treated the negative electrodes may be placed at the ends of the nerve root affected by the injured disc.

A diagram for the placement would look like this:

Positive Electrode	Positive Electrode
Channel A	Channel B
Area to be Treated	
Negative Electrode	Negative Electrode
Channel B	Channel A

Manual therapy between the contacts: The practitioner's hands can palpate, mobilize, and manipulate

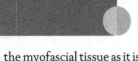
the myofascial tissue as it is treated by the current and frequencies being delivered by the stationary contacts. There should be some interference to prevent current flow through the practitioner. Latex or nitrile gloves can be worn on the hands or even on one hand to block the current or some form of massage oil can be applied lightly on the hands to serve as an insulator. Follow the directions for manual technique covered below.

Current level

- Average patients require 100–300µamps. Use lower current levels, 20–60µamps, for very small or debilitated chronically ill patients. Use higher current levels, 300–500µamps, for larger or very muscular patients. In general, higher current levels reduce pain and create softening more quickly. Do not use more than 500µamps as animal studies suggest that current levels above 500µamps reduce ATP production (Cheng 1982).
- **Note:** Current levels over 150µamps make it difficult to use the graphite gloves directly on the skin because they dry out quickly and the current becomes uncomfortable easily. It becomes cumbersome and tedious to continually moisten the graphite gloves. If higher current levels are required due to the patient's size using wet towel contacts is recommended.

Waveslope

- Use a moderate to sharp waveslope with a ramped square wave pulse.
- The waveslope refers to the rate of increase of current in the ramped square wave as it rises from zero up to the treatment current level every 2.5 seconds on the Precision Microcurrent and the automated family of FSM units. Other microcurrent instruments may have slightly different duty cycles and the waveslope may be different but any unit which provides current flow with a square wave pulse should produce the desired effect. A sharp waveslope has a very steep leading edge on the square wave indicating a very sharp increase in current. A gentle waveslope has a very gradual leading edge on the waveform indicating a gradual increase in current.
- Use a moderate to sharp waveslope for chronic pain. Use a gentle waveslope for new injuries. A sharp waveslope is irritating in new injuries.

- Different microcurrent devices may provide different wave shapes and waveslopes but the reader may find them to be equivalent.

Manual technique: let the frequencies and current do the work

For those trained in manual therapies treating the muscles while using FSM requires some adjustment of technique. The key is to let the frequency do the work and to use the hands with gentle but firm pressure and minimal muscle contraction allowing maximal sensitivity to the softening affect created by the frequencies. The hands should lie gently on the skin allowing the pads of the finger tips to glide across the muscle. Ideally the hands will be almost limp with just enough tone in the distal finger muscles to allow the finger pads to gently assess the state of the tissue. This gentle touch allows the muscles being examined to relax and avoids the resistance created by overly aggressive palpation. The therapist may use body weight translated through the shoulder muscles and serratus anterior to advance the arm and increase the pressure of the hand and finger pads rather than use tension in the forearm and finger flexors to increase pressure.

The hands are sensing the change and softening in the muscles being created by the current and frequencies and helping it along but not forcing it. The frequencies will create the desired change of state in the muscle; it is not necessary to use force. The patient's muscles will relax and allow deeper palpation if the practitioner's hands are relaxed and will defensively tense if the contact is too firm or if the palpating fingers are too tense.

Move the fingers slightly every two to three seconds across the region, using gentle but firm pressure and a gentle pulling motion as if trying to warm, soften and elongate a piece of nougat or soft taffy. Pressure can be directed both along and across the muscle fiber direction. A gentle kneading motion is sometime effective. Small circular scrubbing motions are less effective and should be avoided especially in the anterior cervical spine near the sensitive baroreceptors and neurovascular structures.

Manual myofascial therapy using graphite gloves

- See Figures 7.2 to 7.9.

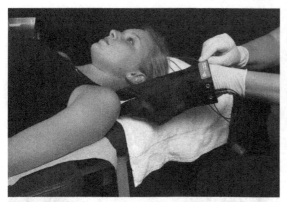

Figure 7.2 • A latex or nitrile glove is worn under the graphite glove to block current conduction to the practitioner. The graphite conducting gloves are placed on the practitioner's hands over the insulating glove. Two positive leads are connected to one glove, usually the right. Two negative leads are connected to the other graphite glove. The interferential field where the current and frequencies mix is created between the two gloves.

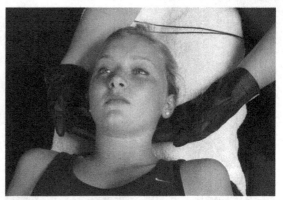

Figure 7.4 • The starting position for the manual treatment of the cervical spine with the practitioner wearing the graphite gloves is shown. RELAX the wrists and lay backs of the wrists on the treatment table. RELAX the fingers and raise them so the pads of the finger tips contact the skin in the suboccipital area. DO NOT let the graphite gloves touch the patient's ears as this will conduct current through the brain.

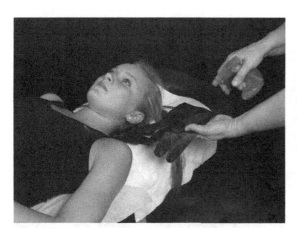

Figure 7.3 • The graphite glove must be moist or wet to conduct current comfortably. The gloves may be sprayed with water at regular intervals during the treatment. Or the practitioner may dip the fingers of the graphite glove into a small plastic dish at regular intervals, usually when a frequency is changed or when the patient complains of a prickling or stinging sensation when the gloves become dry. It is best to avoid the stinging by wetting the gloves at regular intervals before they become dry.

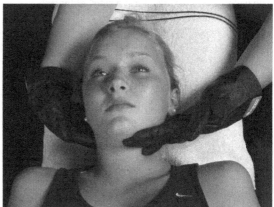

Figure 7.5 • Keep one hand still at the sub-occipitals. Bring the other hand around the neck, under the ear, and just below the jaw, allowing the finger tips to glide over the skin, Let the finger tips glide over the skin moving several centimeters at a time, not breaking contact but gliding in a smooth motion applying gentle pressure, moving the finger tips every 2 to 3 seconds. The fingers are sensing change rather than forcing it, inserting themselves gently in between adhered tissues as they soften and separate. The contact can become more firm as the tissues become very soft, later in the treatment.

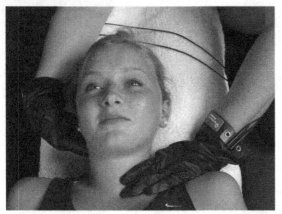

Figure 7.6 • Using the same smooth gliding gentle pressure move the finger tips down the anterior cervical spine. Move the fingers every 2 to 3 seconds, not breaking contact with the skin, using gentle relaxed finger tip pressure to sense the changes being created. Do not "scrub" using little circles; this movement is annoying to the patient and can have inconvenient effects if done over the carotid sinuses. If the tissue is softening and time allows, stay on the frequency that is producing softening changes. If 1 to 2 minutes have passed and no changes have occurred, change to the next frequency on the list. When the gloves are lifted off the patient's skin to change the frequency, it is a good opportunity to wet the gloves by spraying them with water or by dipping them in a small water dish.

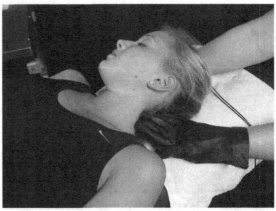

Figure 7.8 • As the fingers move up the posterior cervical spine the soft tissues should be softening, especially after the second or third circuit. The softening of the superficial fascia allows easy palpation of the facet structures and makes the taut bands containing trigger points or fibrosis stand out against the "smooshy" relaxed superficial tissues. The amount of cervical rotation is exaggerated for photographic clarity; the neck should be slightly rotated and each segment is rocked from side to side as facet joint tissue frequencies are used.

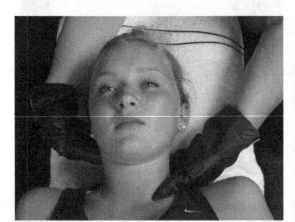

Figure 7.7 • Relax the fingers and the wrists so they can change orientation easily and move comfortably around the supraclavicular space towards the muscles, discs, and facet joints of the posterior cervical spine. Keep the fingers relaxed and the pads of the fingers placed with gentle and firm upwards pressure. Move the fingers, gliding the fingers with gentle firm pressure every 2 to 3 seconds, up the posterior cervical spine towards the occiput. As the hand is being moved the frequencies are being changed every 1 to 3 minutes.

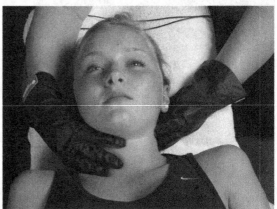

Figure 7.9 • Place the hand that just finished the circuit of one side of the cervical spine at rest at the suboccipital muscles. Move the other hand down the neck, under the jaw, down the anterior cervical muscles, around the supraclavicular space to the posterior cervical muscles and facet joints.

Box 7.1

Technique for treating the cervical muscles

- RELAX the wrists and lay backs of the wrists on the treatment table.
- RELAX the fingers and flex them gently so the pads of the finger tips contact the suboccipital muscles.
- GLIDE them across the skin to contact the other muscles.
- DO NOT let the graphite gloves touch the patient's ears as this will conduct current through the brain.
- DO NOT "scrub" or apply prolonged directed pressure over the carotid sinuses

Treat the muscle

A/B pair for scar tissue:

58 / 00, 02, 32

- Remove scarring and adhesions from soft tissues and reduce the tendency to create scar tissue. These frequencies will produce the most pronounced change in tissue texture if the muscle has been injured by trauma.
- **Polarize current positive + or alternating ± (see note below*).**
- Treatment time: Use each frequency for 1 to 2 minutes each or as long as positive softening response occurs.
- If fibrosis or adhesions are involved in the muscle dysfunction the frequencies will begin to soften the muscle within the first minute. Use each frequency for 1 to 2 minutes. If the practitioner is sensitive and can feel the softening in the muscle, the frequency can be used for as long as it is producing changes in muscle texture or discontinued as soon as the softening stops even within seconds. If there has been significant muscle trauma from an accident, a crush injury or surgery each one of the 58/'s may produce softening for up to 5 or 10 minutes each. If there has been no muscle damage the frequency will have virtually no effect on muscle texture and may be useful for only a few seconds.
- Application: The lead placement, current level and waveslope do not change for the muscle portion of the treatment protocol.
- ***Current Polarization May Change:** Current polarization may change for the muscle portion of the treatment. For reasons that are not

understood, about one half of patients treated will respond best if the current remains polarized positive during the muscle portion of the myofascial protocol and one half will respond best if the current is changed to alternating. If the patient responds to one or the other polarization while the 58 / 00, 02, 32 frequencies are being used then that polarization is to be used for the remainder of the treatment.

91 / 142, 62, 396, 77, 191, 783

- Remove calcium and hardening from the fascia, the muscle belly elastic tissue, the interfascial nerve fibers, the connective tissue, the tendons and the periosteum where the tendon attaches.
- Treatment time: Use each frequency for 2 to 4 minutes each.
- This frequency will produce softening in myofascial tissue. 91 Hz may be used with each tissue frequency for 2 to 4 minutes each in a manual microcurrent unit (one that allows manual selection of a three digit frequency) or in a unit that automatically changes frequencies after a set time interval of 2 minutes. If a manual microcurrent unit is being used and the practitioner is sensitive to the softening in the muscle, the frequency can be used for as long as it is producing changes in muscle texture. The tissue response may last for up to 5 or more minutes depending on the patient and the chronicity. Athletes with myofascial dysfunction respond very well to 91 Hz and it may produce softening for up to 5 to 10 minutes with certain tissues.

Manual technique – place the fingers on the tissue type being treated

- Think of muscle anatomy as tissue types.

The tissues treated respond very specifically to the frequency. Gentle manual pressure at the tissue being treated seems to assist the frequency effect. For example, when the "fascia" is being treated with 91 / 142 placing the fingers where the fascia is known to be most dysfunctional or hardened and gently separating the fibers as they soften will speed the softening process. When the muscle belly is being treated with 91 / 62 placing the fingers at the muscle belly and using them to follow the softening will assist the changes and allow more detailed assessment of them.

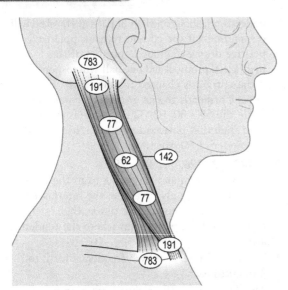

Figure 7.10 • When using a frequency to address a certain tissue place your fingers where you know that tissue to be. In the example above the sternocleidomastoid (SCM) muscle has a tendon (191) that attaches to the periosteum (783) at the mastoid process behind the ear. The tendon gives way to the fibrous distal end of the muscle, which contains a higher percentage of connective tissue (77) than the more central muscle belly (62). The muscle cross-section thins out again as it moves toward the distal attachment and once again contains a higher percentage of connective tissue (77) which coalesces into the tendinous attachment (191) at the periosteum (783) of the sternum and clavicle. The fascia (142) covers the entire muscle. Begin to think of anatomy as tissue types. Use a visual anatomy reference such as Netter (1991) and move your fingers to where you know these tissues to be.

The small interfascial nerve fibers that run the length of the muscle between the fascial layers are probably most affected at the motor end plates. As this tissue is being treated with 91 / 396 allow the fingers to find the areas of softening and gently probe them. Connective tissue (77) runs throughout the muscle but is a proportionally greater portion of the structure near the tendinous portion of the muscle. Focus manual pressure at the part of the muscle where connective tissue is most concentrated while using 91/77.

Tendinous trigger points are usually the last to disappear and respond well to manual pressure directly on the tendon during treatment with 91 / 191, 195. Tendons interweave with the periosteum at their attachment and this junction becomes painful from the constant tension of the taut and shortened muscle band. The tender nodule on the periosteum usually softens and appears to "melt" when 91 / 783 is applied.

To enhance the process of treating specific tissues the practitioner can envision the familiar anatomy as tissue types. For example from an anatomical perspective the sternocleidomastoid (SCM) muscle has its origin on the mastoid process and its insertion at the clavicle and sternum creating cervical flexion and contralateral rotation when activated. From a "tissue type" perspective the SCM attaches tendon (/ 191) to periosteum (/ 783) at the skull, becomes concentrated connective tissue (/ 77) just distal to that attachment and then becomes predominantly fascia (/ 142) that envelops the elastic muscle belly (/ 62) and the neural motor endplates (/ 396). From midline to distal attachment the connective tissue becomes more pronounced leading into the tendon that attaches again to periosteum.

For the practitioner who has less training in palpation or anatomy, the hands may simply traverse the area being treated and apply pressure to the tissues that are softening in response to the frequency being used. Use of an illustrated anatomy text, such as Netter's Illustrated Atlas that provides a detailed visual reference for location of tissue types within the muscles speeds up the learning process for the manual therapist (Netter 1991).

13 or 3 / 142, 62, 396, 77, 191, 783

- Remove scarring or sclerosis from the fascia, the muscle belly elastic tissue, the interfascial nerve fibers, the connective tissue, the tendons and periosteum.
- These frequencies will produce the most pronounced change in tissue texture if the muscle has been injured by trauma or physical injury.
- Treatment time: Use each frequency for 1 to 2 minutes each.
- 13Hz: If fibrosis or adhesions are involved the 13Hz will begin to soften the muscle within the first minute. Use 13Hz for 1 to 2 minutes with each tissue. If the practitioner is sensitive and can feel the softening in the muscle, the frequency can be used for as long as it is producing changes in muscle texture or discontinued as soon as the softening stops even within seconds. If there has been significant muscle trauma from an accident, a crush injury or surgery or if the muscle dysfunction is very chronic, 13Hz will produce pronounced softening in the area of the muscle

most injured. Athletes respond particularly well to 13Hz in most tissues treated.

- 3Hz: It is virtually impossible to verbally describe the difference between the changes created by 13Hz as compared to those created by 3Hz. Tissue affected by "sclerosis" feels stiffer, stringier and tighter to palpation before treatment than tissue more likely to respond to "scar tissue" or 13Hz. Ultimately, "sclerosis" is what goes away when the frequency 3Hz is used and "scar" is what goes away when the frequency 13Hz is used. The timing for 3Hz will be similar to that described above for 13Hz if the tissue responds to it by softening. Use one or both frequencies and compare their effects; they will be slightly different depending on the patient's physiology, the history of injury and the chronicity. One is usually more effective than the other in a given patient and each produces a distinct change in tissue texture.

81, 49 / 142

- Support secretions and vitality in the fascia.
- If the muscle is completely soft and pain free and in the unlikely event that there is no spinal or peripheral joint involvement, the treatment should be finished at this point. The fascia secretes ground substance that helps repair itself and the associated tendons and connective tissue and clinical use of 81 / 142 suggests that this frequency pair stimulates and supports this process.
- Treatment time: Use each frequency for 2 minutes each.
- There is no specific manual technique required while these frequencies are being used although it is interesting to feel the tissue change texture as these frequencies are having their effect.

Treat the joint

In most cases of myofascial pain there is some dysfunction in the spinal discs or facet joints or the peripheral joints associated with the formation or perpetuation of myofascial trigger points. The joint dysfunction may be a cause of the trigger points or its result. Comprehensive treatment requires that the joint component be addressed.

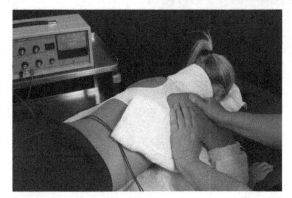

Figure 7.11 • Place the positive leads glove in a warm wet fabric contact (hand towel) that is wrapped around the neck. This allows all of the cervical nerve roots and the spinal cord to be treated. Place the negative leads glove in a warm wet fabric contact (hand towel) that is draped across the lateral thoracic spine, across the lower scapula, along the lateral chest wall, under the axilla and around the upper arm. This placement allows all of the cervical nerves, all of the brachial plexus and all of the muscles of the cervical spine and shoulder to be treated simultaneously. Move the hands every 2 to 3 seconds using the finger pads with relaxed fingers to assess and treat any muscle. Move the hands under the towels to treat the anterior and posterior cervical muscles (scalenes, SCM, trapezius), the subscapularis, the infraspinatus, the serratus anterior, the levator scapulae. Even the pectoralis muscles can be addressed by reaching forward under the shoulder. Block the current from flowing through the practitioner by using a latex glove or some sort of oil on the hands. Do not get oil on the graphite gloves as it ruins their conductivity.

Treat the disc

40 / 710, 630, 330

- **Remove inflammation from the spinal discs: the annulus, the disc as a whole and the nucleus pulposus**. 40 / 710 will produce the most noticeable softening in the surrounding fascia if the disc is involved. Use this frequency for 2 to 4 minutes. If the mechanism of injury involves flexion or combined flexion and rotation, or if flexion exacerbates the pain, the disc is almost certainly involved. Use 40Hz on channel A combined with all three disc tissue frequencies on channel B if 40 / 710 (annulus) produces a very strong response.
- Treatment time: 2 to 4 minutes for each frequency combination. Time will vary for each frequency combination depending on patient

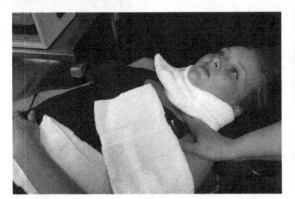

Figure 7.12 • Place the positive leads glove in a warm wet fabric contact (hand towel) and wrap it around the neck where it can treat the outflow of every cervical nerve. Place the negative leads contact in a warm wet contact (hand towel) that is draped across the abdomen, along the chest wall, under the axilla and around the upper arm and onto the chest. Position the patient's hand and forearm so it lays on the wet contact. This placement allows every cervical nerve root (C4–C8), the entire brachial plexus and every muscle in between to be treated simultaneously. Move the relaxed hands every 2 to 3 seconds allowing the finger pads to assess and treat the muscles in between and under the towels. This position allows easy access to the anterior scalenes, the pectoralis major and minor, subscapularis, serratus anterior, deltoid, biceps, triceps, corico-brachialis, SCM, forearm flexors and extensors. Block the current from flowing through the practitioner by using a latex glove or some sort of oil on the hands. Do not get oil on the graphite gloves as it ruins their conductivity.

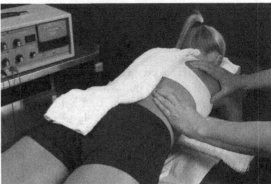

Figure 7.13 • With the patient prone, place the positive leads glove in a warm wet fabric contact (hand towel) lengthwise down the spine. Place the negative leads glove in a warm wet fabric contact (hand towel) lengthwise under the trunk from clavicle to pubic bone. This placement allows all of the thoracic nerves, discs, and facets and all of the thoracic muscles to be treated simultaneously. Move the hands every 2 to 3 seconds using the finger pads with relaxed fingers to assess and treat any muscle. Move the hands between and under the towels to treat the thoracic paraspinals, the latissimus, the trapezius, the rhomboids, and the thoracic intercostal muscles and nerves. Block the current from flowing through the practitioner by using a latex glove or some sort of oil on the hands. Do not get oil on the graphite gloves as it ruins their conductivity.

response. If time allows, continue using a given frequency as long as the tissue continues to soften. If the tissue stops softening and firms up, change to the next channel B frequency. Animal studies show 40 Hz produced maximal reduction in inflammation at 4 minutes.

91 / 710

- **Remove hardening from the disc annulus**. The disc annulus becomes hardened and calcified in chronic degeneration. When myofascial trigger points are associated with degenerative changes the muscles soften and the disc appears to become more flexible when 91 / 710 are used. This frequency combination prolongs the effect of the myofascial treatment.
- Treatment time: 2 to 4 minutes. The spinal joint will become more flexible as this combination is used. Gentle side to side rocking to mobilize the joint in extension and segmental rotation will help

maximize this affect. Change to the next frequency when the frequency does not produce any further improvement.

Treat the spinal facet joint

40 / 783, 157, 480

- **Remove inflammation from the spinal facet joint tissues: the periosteum, the cartilage and the joint capsule**. If the mechanism of injury involved extension or compression combined with extension as in a fall or rear-end auto accident, or if spinal extension exacerbates the pain, then inflammation in the facet joint tissues is almost certainly involved. This is not meant to be a comprehensive treatment of the facet joint but is meant to address the role of the facet joint as a perpetuating factor in the myofascial trigger points.
- Treatment time: 2 to 4 minutes for each frequency combination. Time will vary for each frequency combination depending on patient response. If time allows, continue using a given frequency as long as the tissue continues to soften.

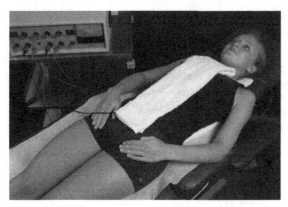

Figure 7.14 • The exact same process is used for treating the anterior thoracic muscles except that the patient is supine. Positive contacts are at the spine so the nerves can be treated with polarized positive current. Negative leads are placed midline on the trunk. This placement and patient position allows treatment of the thoracic intercostal muscles and nerves, the pectoralis major and minor, the abdominal obliques and rectus abdominus, the ilio-psoas, and even the glute medius and minimus. Glide the finger pads across the skin moving them every 2 to 3 seconds feeling for softening and mobilizing adhesions. Think of the anatomy as tissue types. When the frequency for "connective tissue" (77) is being used focus the fingers at the linea alba and the connective tissue bands in the rectus abdominus. When treating the thoracic intercostals remember to include the periosteum (783) among the frequencies used and place the fingers at the attachments between the periosteum and the intercostal fascia while it is running.

If the tissue stops softening and firms up, change to the next frequency. Animal studies show 40Hz produced maximal reduction in inflammation at 4 minutes.

91 / 783, 480

- **Remove hardening from the periosteum and joint capsule.** The joint capsule and periosteum become hardened and calcified in chronic facet joint degeneration. These two frequency combinations soften the joint capsule and reduce the tenderness where the capsule attaches to the periosteum. These two combinations usually produce significant improvement in joint function.
- Treatment time: 2 to 4 minutes. The spinal joint will become more flexible and less painful as this combination is used. The periosteum is very pain sensitive and 91 / 783 usually produces the best improvement in facet joint pain. 91 / 480 usually produce the best improvement in joint flexibility

and motion. Gentle side to side rocking with the finger tips to mobilize the joint capsule in segmental rotation will help maximize this affect. Change to the next frequency when the frequency being used does not produce any further improvement (see manual technique note below).

13 / 480, 396 with movement

- **Remove scarring from the joint capsule and its nerve.** Chronic inflammation in and around the joint creates fibrosis and scarring in addition to the calcium influx seen in chronically inflamed tissues. The joint capsule and its recurrent nerve become adhered to each other by scarring. When the capsule stretches during flexion or rotation the nerve is stretched and produces pain with movement. The pain produced by scarring in the nerve tends to be sharp and occurs only with movement. Releasing the scarring between the nerve and the capsule alleviates the pain fairly quickly and usually produces significant increase in motion.

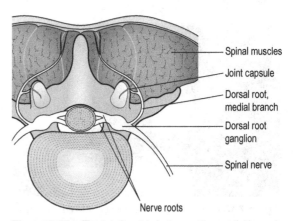

Figure 7.15 • The relationship between the medial branch of the dorsal nerve root that innervates the facet joint capsule and the paraspinal muscles. Inflammation of this nerve mediates facet joint pain and chronic inflammation leads to adhesions between the nerve and the facet joint capsule and between the nerve and the muscle. Branches of the ventral root stimulate muscle hypertonicity. Adhesions between the fascia and sensory and motor nerves cause pain with muscle contractions and joint motion. 13 / 396, 142 soften these adhesions and increases comfortable joint motion. Visualize gently teasing the nerve away from the capsule and the paraspinal muscles.

- **Manual Technique:** When using the frequencies for removing scar tissue from the joint capsule and its nerve, create slight segmental rotation to move the capsule through a small range while the frequencies for calcium and scarring are being used.

When treating the cervical spine supine this is accomplished by lifting the joint line a few centimeters on one side and then the other with the finger pads. Move the joint line in such a way as to reproduce this joint motion when the patient is prone. In the thoracic spine gentle pressure may be applied by using the thumbs to rock the joint in slight rotation at the capsule line. When treating the lumbar spine supine, the patient is positioned with the knees flexed and the back flat. If tolerated, the lumbar joints can be mobilized by rocking the knees a few inches from side to side to produce lumbar rotation. If rotation is not tolerated, the practitioner can place the finger pads on the joint line and lift the joint line about a centimeter, rocking the joint capsule from side to side. The use of such movements generally reduces pain and increases range of motion in the joint capsule more quickly. This manual technique can be beneficial when using 91 / 480 to remove calcium from the joint capsule.

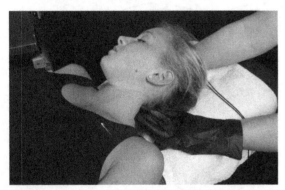

Figure 7.16 • Visualize the relationship between the facet joint capsule and nerve adhered to it. Visualize gently dissolving the scar tissue between the nerve, the joint capsule and fascia with 13 / 396, 480, 142 and gently rock the joint to tease the nerve away from the fascia and the joint capsule. The movement should be very small to start, perhaps 2–3mm, and should stop and go back to neutral at the first sign of restriction. Move the joint again by lifting the segment at the capsule; this time the movement may be easier and should move about 3–4mm and perhaps 10 to 20 degrees of rotation. Move the joint back to neutral at the first sign of pain, muscle splinting or resistance. Keep the backs of the hands on the table, keep the fingers relaxed and use the pads of the finger tips to lift the joint at the lamina / joint capsule juncture which can be identified by bony landmarks or by the presence of taut muscles over the capsule. This photo shows the very end range of this process. The technique applies to mobilizing any spinal joint and the surrounding muscles.

Treat the peripheral joint

40 / 191, 195, 783, 157

- **Remove inflammation from the peripheral joint tissues: the tendon, the bursa, the periosteum and the cartilage.** When there is a regional myofascial problem the peripheral joint will often be adversely affected. Abnormal biomechanics caused by hypertonic muscles in the shoulder will often create an impingement of the supraspinatus tendon and bursa. The diagnosis may be "impingement syndrome" but the cause will be trigger points and taut bands in the subscapularis and teres because they are not performing the function of pulling the humeral head down and away from the tendon, bursa and acromion during abduction. In the absence of direct trauma or specific overuse, all of this dysfunction may occur because the disc has inflamed the nerve, making the muscles taut and unresponsive. The same principle holds true for every peripheral joint. As always the cause must be treated in order to create lasting improvement.

- Treatment time: 2 to 4 minutes each. Time will vary for each frequency combination depending on patient response. Continue using a given frequency as long as the tissue continues to soften. Animal studies show 40Hz produced maximal reduction in inflammation at 4 minutes.

91 / 783, 480, 195, 191

- **Remove hardening from the periosteum, the joint capsule, the bursa and the tendon.** Inflammation leads to chronic inflammation which leads to induration or hardening in the soft tissues and joint surfaces. 91Hz softens the tissue being treated and in the case of peripheral joints reduces the pain in the periosteum and bursa in particular.

- Treatment time: 2 to 4 minutes on each combination. The joint will become more flexible and less painful as these combinations are used. The periosteum and bursa are very pain sensitive and 91 / 783, 195 usually produces the best improvement in peripheral joint pain. 91 / 480 usually produces improvement in joint flexibility and motion. Gentle rocking of the joint in a small range with the finger tips to mobilize the joint capsule will help maximize this affect. Change to the next frequency when the frequency being used does not produce any further improvement (see manual technique note above).

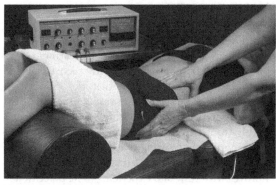

Figure 7.17 • Place the positive leads in a warm wet contact under the low back using either a graphite glove or alligator clips (see Chapter 11). Place the negative leads in a warm wet towel on the thigh above the knee. This placement allows polarization of the L2, L3 and L4 nerve roots and treatment of every tissue between the contacts. Lay the relaxed hand gently on the abdomen; palpate the muscle by increasing the pressure slowly to minimize guarding. If the abdominal muscles splint with very light pressure some visceral perpetuating factor is almost certainly involved. See "When is myofascial pain not myofascial pain?". If the trigger points are coming from the muscle, the nerve, the disc or the joint this position will allow simultaneous treatment of all of the agonists and antagonists, pain generators and perpetuating factors.

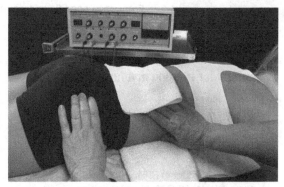

Figure 7.19 • The patient will be more comfortable lying prone if the discs are involved and the facet joints are not pain generators. Place the positive leads contact in a warm wet towel across the low back. Place the negative leads contact under the abdomen. This position focuses the current and frequencies on the lumbar spine alone. If there is referred pain or associated myofascial pain in the hamstrings or gluteals the negative leads contact may be placed under the knees so the current flows through the tissue in three dimensions. Using gloves or alligator clips in towels frees the practitioner's hands to focus on, assess or treat any muscle or joint.

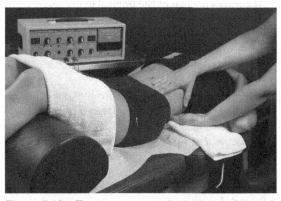

Figure 7.18 • The same contact placement can be used with modified manual technique to treat the anterior and posterior low back muscles and to increase motion in the lumbar facet joints when the pain is purely musculoskeletal. Patients with low back pain from myofascial trigger points and facet joint degeneration are most comfortable in a supine position with the back flat and knees bent. Treat the psoas and lumbar paraspinals first using the "treat the nerve – treat the muscle" strategy. When the protocol progresses to the "treat the joint" frequencies lay one hand under the arch of the low back and use the finger tip pads to lift and gently mobilize the facet joints as described in Fig. 7.16. Move the joints incrementally with a very slow gradual rocking motion while using 91, 13 / 396, 480, 783, 710.

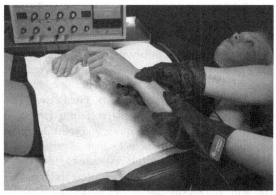

Figure 7.20 • Extremity muscles can be treated with the practitioner wearing the gloves, as shown here. Or any extremity muscle can be treated by wrapping the positive lead contact at the spine where the relevant nerve exits and wrapping the negative leads contact distal to the area of involved muscle and using the hands in between the two contacts to treat the desired muscles. The frequency protocols remain the same – treat the nerve, treat the muscle, treat the joint. Think of the muscles being treated and think of the anatomy as tissue types. Forearm and lower leg flexors and extensors have very long tendons, tendon sheaths and proportionally high concentrations of connective tissue that can become inflamed, calcified and adhered (40, 91, 13 / 191, 195, 77). The nerves in the extremities can become adhered to the surrounding fascia by trauma or inflammation (58/'s, 13 / 396, 142).

Box 7.2

Summary for treating myofascial pain

Treat the Nerve
- 40 / 396
- 40 / 10

Treat the Muscle
- 58 / 00, 02, 32
- 91 / 142, 62, 396, 77, 191, 783
- 13 or 3 / 142, 62, 396, 77, 191, 783
- 81, 49 / 142

Treat the Joint
- 40 / 710, 630, 330
- 91 / 710
- 40 / 783, 157, 480
- 91 / 783, 480
- 13 / 480, 396 with movement
- 40 / 191, 195, 783, 157
- 91 / 783, 480, 195, 191

Customize treatment

The frequency response is very condition and tissue specific and efficient treatment requires that the pain generators (fascia, nerve, periosteum) and the pathologies affecting them (inflammation, hardening, scarring) be accurately assessed. Different patients will respond differently to each portion of the myofascial protocol. This response becomes instructive. The frequency response, the tissue softening (smoosh) created when a correct frequency is used, happens so quickly and so predictably that eventually the practitioner learns to use this response to guide treatment and frequency choices. The successful frequencies will address the pathologies associated with the formation or perpetuation of trigger points.

For example, the mouse research demonstrated that the frequency to reduce inflammation functioned in a 4-minute time dependent fashion. All of the anti-inflammatory effect was present at 4 minutes and half of it was present at 2 minutes. In general this time dependent response seems to apply to humans as well.

In the interest of efficiency the joint portion of the treatment should focus on the tissues most affected by the pathology being treated. Every tissue may be treated with 40Hz for 4 minutes each but this increases treatment time considerably and not all of the tissues may actually be inflamed enough to require 4 minutes of treatment. Determining which tissues are most likely to be inflamed can be done according to the history and the mechanism of injury or by palpation of the painful area. If treatment time is limited 40Hz may be used with each tissue for only 2 minutes in the hope that the cumulative effects will create an optimal response. Ideally the manual therapist will note which tissue frequency has the strongest softening response to 40Hz and will spend more time treating that tissue.

The sensitivity needed to make this determination improves with time and experience. The practitioner is advised to use a relaxed hand during treatment in part because transmission of sensory information is enhanced when motor output is minimized. The practitioner is advised to be patient as this skill develops.

Customize by history and examination

If the mechanism of the original injury includes only flexion or flexion combined with rotation then the disc is most likely to be involved. If the pain increases when the patient flexes the painful area then the disc is most likely to be involved. If the injury was fairly minor, the disc annulus may be the only compromised tissue and the other two disc components may not respond to or require treatment.

If the mechanism of the original injury, even years earlier, involved extension (joint compression) and then flexion as is seen in a rear end impact auto accident or some falls, then the facet joint tissues may be the most inflamed but the disc annulus will be involved too.

If the mechanism of injury involves only chronic joint extension and compression or ballistic traumatic extension during a fall, then the spinal facet joint tissues are most likely to be inflamed and to respond to treatment.

If the history and examination suggests that the peripheral joint tendons, bursa and periosteum are inflamed due to impact, overuse or because the pain is localized directly over these structures then the treatment may reasonably be focused on inflammation and hardening in these tissues.

Customize by palpation

Once the nerve and muscle have been treated the texture of the soft tissues will have changed dramatically. Most of the soft tissue will be "smooshy" as if the ground substance within has changed from a solid to a gel or even to a liquid. The feeling is unlike anything produced by traditional myofascial therapy or any intervention short of general anesthesia and has to be experienced to be appreciated.

When the spinal discs or the facet joints or the peripheral joints are inflamed the muscles overlying these structures will not be "smooshy" but will remain stiff or taut after the surrounding tissues have become soft. The difference in texture and tone is dramatic to the practitioner experienced and adept at palpation and draws attention to the area needing attention.

If the taut muscles are just lateral to the spinous processes and include the multifidi or the iliocostalis group that overlie the spinal facet joints, and if they become stiffer with even minimal joint compression then reducing inflammation and hardening in the facet joint structures is most likely to produce the best response in the muscles.

If the taut muscles are more lateral to the spine and slightly anterior to the facet joint then the disc is more likely to be involved. In the cervical spine, the posterior and lateral scalenes, levator scapulae, and SCM will be tight and tender. In the thoracic and lumbar spine, the paraspinal muscles or the quadratus lumborum directly over the involved disc, but lateral to the lamina, will be taut when the surrounding muscles have relaxed from treating the nerve and muscle pathologies. In the cervical spine with the patient supine, the anterior scalenes and longus coli will remain taut and tender directly over the anterior portion of the involved cervical disc when the other muscles have relaxed. In the lumbar spine the psoas will remain tender and taut directly anterior to the involved disc. The muscle tension indicates that treating the disc should be the next step.

If the peripheral joint is inflamed the muscles directly over the tendon or bursa will be taut and there will be point tenderness to pressure directly over the inflamed periosteum, bursa and tendon.

Customizing treatment by either palpation or history makes treatment more efficient. The frequency response helps train sensitivity because the softening occurs when the frequency is correct. The practitioner can treat by the script provided above until the sensitivity to the softening affect develops.

Side effects of FSM myofascial treatment

Detoxification reaction

The most common side effect that occurs with myofascial treatment is a detoxification reaction similar to that seen after a deep tissue massage. The patient may feel flu-like symptoms including fatigue, brain fog, nausea, headache, generalized malaise and body aches or increased pain. The symptoms start about 60 to 90 minutes after the treatment and very rarely will progress to include vomiting.

The symptoms are presumed to come from incomplete processing of toxic metabolites released from the muscles as they pass through the liver so they can be excreted. There are two liver detoxification enzyme pathways that perform this function. The phase-one liver detoxification pathways perform hydrolysis reactions in which a water molecule is broken in half and the polarized particle is attached to the substance being processed so it can be shipped out of the liver as an inactive polarized metabolite. The phase-two detoxification pathways break the toxin apart and attach a cap, called a substrate to its active end. The substrate is said to be "conjugated" to the toxin and makes it inactive so it can be safely excreted as an inactive metabolite. Under normal conditions phase-one and phase-two detoxification pathways co-ordinate function and toxins are excreted at a steady rate.

When the liver is processing toxins at the normal rate, water and the substrates are recycled in time to meet the steady demand. When large quantities of toxins are released in a short time from the fascia by either deep massage or an FSM treatment, the liver detoxification pathways can become overwhelmed and run out of either water or substrate or both. With insufficient material available to complete the detoxification processes the liver enzymes release the half finished metabolites prematurely and these may, in many cases, be more toxic than the original product. These half-processed metabolites are the source of the symptoms experienced in a detoxification reaction.

This reaction is most often a problem in the first one to two myofascial treatments. Liver enzymes will proliferate in number and become more active in response to increased demand. The patient easily remembers to drink extra water after even one "detox" episode and this side effect is rarely seen more than once or twice.

- **Prevention:** The first myofascial treatment should not exceed 20 minutes. A short treatment on a smaller muscle group will limit the amount of toxins released. Patients with known liver disease or known problems with detoxification should be treated for an even shorter period of time. Patients should be instructed to drink up to one

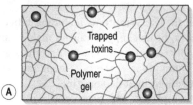

Polymer network with trapped toxins

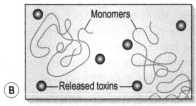

Depolymerized network releases toxins

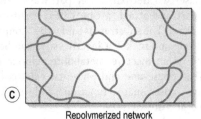

Repolymerized network

Figure 7.21 • Waste products trapped in the fascia are released during treatment as the fascia unwinds and can overwhelm liver detoxification processes if the liver has inadequate water or enzyme substrate (from Oschman 2008).

quart of water in the 90 minutes following treatment to supply the additional water needed for hydrolysis reactions in the liver. The patient may also be given an in-office dose of a complex low dose anti-oxidant supplement containing such substrates as vitamin C, vitamin E, n-acetyl-cysteine, lipoic acid and other liver friendly nutrients. If this is not possible the patient can be instructed to take a dose of a commonly available multiple vitamin supplement of their choosing when they reach home.

• **Treatment:** If the patient calls and describes a detoxification reaction recommend immediate consumption of water containing a bit of lemon if it is available and provide reassurance about the source of the symptoms and their temporary nature. Alcohol, Tylenol (acetaminophen) and caffeine occupy the same detoxification pathways used by the muscle metabolites and should be avoided after treatment. The reaction rarely lasts more than 4 to 12 hours when these steps are taken.

Nerve pain

When treatment for myofascial pain produces a significant increase in range of motion, as it often does, bone spurs near the neural foramen in the spine, primarily in the cervical spine, can impinge on the nerve because of the increased motion and irritate the nerve. The patient experiences improved neck pain but a new onset of pain in the distal nerve root. The patient may comment, "My neck feels great but my thumb and forearm really hurt."

• **Prevention:** This reaction is hard to prevent but can often be predicted which is almost as useful. If the patient is older than 45 or has a significant history of spine trauma, the presence of bone spurs in the cervical spine is somewhat predictable and can be confirmed by a standard x-ray series that includes oblique views which best demonstrate bony encroachment on the neural foramen. This reaction is uncommon but diagnostic and never happens except when range of motion allows bone spurs to move into the nerve. If the patient refuses or cannot have the x-ray the practitioner can proceed on the assumption that bone spurs are present. In treating patients who experience this reaction it would be advisable to end every future myofascial treatment by treating the nerve to see if it can be prevented.

• **Treatment:** The nerve pain is easy to treat by using 40 / 396 with the current polarized from the neck to the end of the irritated nerve root. The pain should be reduced within 10 minutes and eliminated within 20 minutes. The cerebellum and proprioceptive system react to the nerve irritation and restrict range of motion in the cervical spine within a day or two of treatment so the bone spurs will stay well away from the nerve in the future. The muscles will remain trigger point free and pain free for some period of time and it may be 3 to 6 months before the muscle need to be re-treated. If the muscles are less taut and the neck is more mobile there is some suggestion that the bone spurs can be reabsorbed.

Increased joint pain

When myofascial treatment increases range of motion and degenerated joints are allowed to move farther than they have in years, joint surfaces can become inflamed after the unfamiliar movement. It is similar to sliding a drawer open for the first time in years and hearing the screech as it scrapes across the sticky and stiff drawer glide. The unlubricated cartilage surface of the facet joint is the sticky drawer guide and the "screech" causes inflammation of the joint surface from the unfamiliar motion. The irritation in the capsule and recurrent nerves as they stretch beyond their normal range can also create increased joint pain following myofascial treatment.

- **Prevention:** This reaction can be prevented by remembering to treat the spinal joint for inflammation, hardening and scarring in the cartilage, the nerve and the joint capsule at the end of the myofascial protocol. 40, 91, 13 / 157, 480, 783, 396 used for 2 to 3 minutes each will usually minimize or prevent this reaction.
- **Treatment:** This reaction can be treated by applying 40 / 116, 157, 783, 59, 39, 480, 396 for 4 minutes each. See Chapter 5 for more detail on treating

Increased segmental pain from ligament laxity

If myofascial tissue has been tight to form a splint to stabilize a joint with lax ligaments and the FSM treatment loosens the muscles and increases the range of motion, the lax joint is no longer splinted or stable. The joint will translate instead of gliding properly, as described in the ligamentous laxity chapter, allowing the facet joints to crash into each other and creating stress on the discs and causing local inflammation. The patient will feel wonderful for about 2 to 4 hours following myofascial treatment but will report point tenderness over one or more joints at the spine after that.

The patient will often comment that the "treatment made my pain worse" in these cases. The reply should be, "When and where did your pain increase?" This reply reassures the patient that there is a reason for the pain which can be determined by knowing exactly when and where it increased. If the pain increased within 2 to 6 hours of the treatment and palpation localizes the tender area to the posterior joints or ligaments of the spine it is diagnostic of ligamentous laxity.

The suspicion should be confirmed by performing a stress x-ray view such as a flexion–extension x-ray in the cervical spine or a flexion–extension or side bending view in the lumbar spine. Measurement is taken from the line of the anterior and posterior vertebral body of the segment above compared to its position relative to the vertebral body below in neutral versus flexion and extension. The vertebral bodies should remain aligned as the spine curves with motion. If the line of the vertebral body moves forward or back relative to the vertebral body below, the segment is said to translate.

Translation is an abnormal motion. Slight translation of 1–2mm may not be significant if it is compensating for segments above or below do not move at all. But if the patient's painful segment is the same segment that translates on the x-ray the diagnosis is complete. Medical radiologists do not generally consider joint translation to be a problem until it reaches 4mm or more in a spinal joint, at which point the joint is considered to be unstable and may constitute a risk to the spinal cord. Chiropractic radiologists are trained to read segmental translation more carefully and such a consultation might be worthwhile if the reaction produces significant or prolonged segmental pain.

- **Prevention:** There is no way to prevent this reaction and no certain way to predict it. If there has been chronic pain lasting more than 6 months following trauma ligamentous laxity should be considered in the differential diagnosis. The reaction itself is diagnostic and so is not an entirely negative event. Ligamentous laxity is often occult creating smoldering chronic pain that erupts into acute painful events with any spinal stress. The muscles are often thought to be the source of the pain because they are so obviously tight and tender over the joint. In fact the muscles are tight and tender because they are subject to constant strain and overuse from compensating for the injured ligaments. When the FSM treatment relaxes the muscles it allows the lax ligaments to be discovered and paves the way for diagnosis, appropriate treatment and eventual recovery.
- **Treatment:** The increased pain can be reduced by treating for inflammation using 40 / 116, 100, 783, 191, 710. Treat for ligamentous laxity as discussed in Chapter 6 and rehabilitate the muscles using small range isometric specific spinal stabilization exercises.

When is myofascial pain not myofascial pain?

The final section of this chapter presents the protocols to treat myofascial pain and trigger points that are not in the strictest sense due to myofascial pathology but rather are due to some visceral condition or to side effects of lipid lowering medication. Travell & Simons (1983, 1992) describe trigger points in the rectus abdominus that are caused by or perpetuated by food allergies. This description came to mind when a patient with multiple trigger points in the rectus abdominus did not respond to the treatment for myofascial pain. Treating the nerve, the muscle and the joint did not change the myofascial tissue at all – which was very unusual. Ultimately we discovered that myofascial pain from trigger points never fails to respond to the protocols above as long as the cause is musculoskeletal. Time and experience led to the discovery of simple visceral treatments that resolve trigger points caused by visceral referral at least temporarily. Comprehensive treatment of these visceral issues is beyond the scope of this text but the response to treatment is so predictable that the practitioner can use it as an indicator of the need for more comprehensive treatment by whatever means are consistent with their training and scope of practice. FSM protocols for more comprehensive treatment of visceral conditions are presented in the FSM seminars and are available from trained practitioners.

Box 7.3

Summary for treating trigger points from visceral referral

When is myofascial pain NOT myofascial pain?

Treat Trigger Points from Statins or Other Toxins
- 57, 900, 920, 40 / 62, 142

Treat Trigger Points in the Rectus Abdominus from the Gut
- 40, 9 / 22

Treat Trigger Points in the Psoas and Obliques from the Ovary
- 40, 284 / 7

Treat Trigger Points in the Obliques from the Colon
- 40, 9 / 65, 85

Treat Full Body Trigger Points by treating the Spinal Cord
- 40 / 10 (+)

Treat trigger points from statins or other toxins

Patients who are taking the commonly prescribed lipid lowering agents called statins often develop muscle pain sometimes months after beginning to take the medication. Statins interfere with muscle metabolism by blocking the synthesis of co-enzyme Q10 that is required for normal muscle function. The patient will have trigger points and taut bands in the muscles and the trigger points will be tender to touch and cause referred pain. The muscles feel turgid, stiff and "gummy" and respond very slowly or not at all to the myofascial protocol listed above. It may be useful to treat the muscle for toxicity and inflammation but even this has not proven to be universally effective in statin myopathies. The patient can take 200–400mg per day of a CoQ10 supplement and see if it improves the pain. If the pain complaint and the inactivity it causes are sufficiently concerning the patient should consult the prescribing physician and ask about some alternative method of lowering cardiovascular risk. This protocol is also affective for trigger points that appear following exposure to organic chemicals such as pesticides, herbicides or solvents. Patients should take care to drink at least one to two quarts of water following use of this protocol to help flush out any toxic metabolites released from the fascia.

57, 900, 920, 40 / 62, 142
- Reduce toxicity and inflammation in the muscle belly and fascia.
- Set the patient up as you would for treating the region affected by the trigger points in question. Place the positive leads at the level where the nerves to these muscles exit the spine. Place the negative leads distal to the muscles being treated.
- Use alternating current and current levels appropriate to the patient's size.
- Children and small or debilitated patients use 40–100µamps.
- Average well hydrated patients use 100µamps. Larger or very muscular patients use 200–300µamps. Use the same manual technique used for treating any myofascial tissue. Treat for 20 to 30 minutes or until pain is reduced and the muscle tone is relaxed.

Treat the rectus abdominus – Treat the gut

Travell & Simon's comment about food allergies suggested that perhaps the frequencies to "reduce inflammation and histamine from small bowel" might help reduce the neural drive perpetuating the muscle tightness and trigger points. And that was exactly the case. When these frequencies were applied, the trigger points simply disappeared, melted and went "smoosh" in about 10 minutes after stubbornly persisting through 30 minutes of myofascial treatment. These protocols were developed clinically when the patient failed to respond to the myofascial protocol and had some visceral pathology that came to light with questioning or a more thorough physical examination.

The protocols for more comprehensive visceral treatment are presented in more detail in the FSM seminars.

40, 9 / 22

- Remove inflammation and allergy reaction from the small bowel.
- With the patient lying supine, place one graphite glove or both positive leads in adhesive electrodes on the back and place the negative leads on the abdomen.
- Use alternating current and current levels appropriate to the patient's size.
- Children and small or debilitated patients use 40–100µamps.
- Average well hydrated patients use 100µamps. Larger or very muscular patients use 200–300µamps. If inflammation in the small bowel is causing or perpetuating the myofascial pain, these frequencies will soften the muscle and relax the taut bands within 20 minutes. This reaction is diagnostic. If these frequencies soften the abdominal muscles and alleviate the pain then assessment of food allergies or sensitivities would be worthwhile.

Treat the psoas – Treat the ovary

One of the seminar practicum sessions teaches how to treat low back pain by treating the psoas. The psoas is a large muscle that attaches to the anterior surface of the vertebral bodies and discs from T12 to L3 and inserts onto the lesser trochanter on the medial surface of the femur. It flexes and externally rotates the hip and refers pain to the low back when it develops trigger points. The long muscle belly portion of the psoas joins the iliacus portion of the psoas as it lines the pelvic bowl, forming the iliopsoas, before it passes through the pelvis to attach to the femur. Palpating the psoas is done with the patient supine by laying the hand flat on the abdomen at the anterior superior iliac spine and pressing the fingers obliquely downward toward the spine and into the pelvic bowl. If the patient is asked to bring the knee towards the chest by flexing the hip, the psoas contracts and can be easily palpated and treated with the myofascial protocols.

During a seminar, a 26-year-old woman volunteered to be the model for this demonstration because she had low back pain and had been told that there were trigger points in her psoas. Palpation of the psoas proved to be impossible because the woman flinched and braced her abdominal muscles to the lightest palpation of the abdomen and pelvis. The psoas could not even be palpated because the left lower abdomen was so painful and 20 minutes of treatment for the nerve and muscle did not change the tenderness at all. Then she mentioned that she also had an ovarian cyst on the left side. The frequency for "reducing inflammation and chronic inflammation in the ovary" was applied. The pain and guarding in the abdomen was reduced immediately and then eliminated with 20 minutes of treatment with these frequencies. The psoas trigger points and her low back pain resolved. She was examined the next day during a subsequent practicum session and the abdominal tenderness and low back pain had not returned and the psoas could be easily and painlessly palpated.

This scenario has been repeated 20 or more times in seminars and in hundreds of clinical settings across the country. It is included in this text because only the frequencies for reducing inflammation and chronic inflammation in the ovary will resolve this "myofascial pain" that is not actually musculoskeletal in origin. Using the protocols for the nerve the muscle and the joint will not reduce the pain or eliminate the trigger points.

The protocols for more comprehensive visceral treatment are presented in more detail in the FSM seminars and are beyond the scope of this text.

40, 284 / 7

- Reduce inflammation and chronic inflammation in the ovary.
- With the patient lying supine, place one graphite glove or both positive leads in adhesive electrodes

on the back and place the negative leads on the abdomen with either a glove contact or adhesive electrode pads. Use alternating current and current levels appropriate to the patient's size. If an ovarian cyst is causing or perpetuating the abdominal tenderness these frequencies will soften the muscles and eliminate the pain within 20 minutes. Scarring in the fallopian tubes or ovary can create pain with abdominal palpation and if this problem is present the practitioner is advised to refer to an FSM practitioner trained in visceral treatments who can address this problem.

Treat the abdominal obliques – Treat the colon

During a seminar a 58-year-old physician was being treated during the supine low back practicum portion of the FSM seminar. Twenty minutes into the practicum the students treating him called out to say that he wasn't responding to the myofascial treatment frequencies. This non-response is unusual and closer examination revealed sheets of dozens of tiny trigger points in the abdominal oblique muscles and rectus abdominus in the lower left quadrant. The patient was asked if he had embarked on a fitness program that involved doing hundreds of sit-ups or if he had any sort of trauma or overuse to these muscles and replied that he had not.

The muscles in the lower left abdominal quadrant overlie the descending colon, a common site for diverticulitis. When asked if he had any history of descending colon pathology he said that he had some diverticuli that occasionally gave him problems. The frequencies to "reduce inflammation and chronic inflammation in the descending colon" were applied and all of the trigger points, muscular taut bands, abdominal tenderness and low back pain disappeared with 20 minutes treatment with these frequencies.

The descending colon was treated in this case because the protocol for myofascial trigger points did not change the tissue and because the presence of dozens of trigger points in the abdominal muscles did not make sense given the absence of any overuse or trauma. The resolution of the trigger points and pain when the frequencies for reducing inflammation in the colon were used confirmed the diagnosis and the choice of frequencies. This response has been consistent in all patients with this symptom picture and these physical findings in both seminar and clinical settings.

40, 9 / 65, 85
- Remove inflammation and allergy reaction from the descending colon and large bowel.
- With the patient lying supine, place one graphite glove or both positive leads in adhesive electrodes on the back and place the negative leads on the left lower quadrant of the abdomen.
- Use alternating current and current levels appropriate to the patient's size.
- Children and small or debilitated patients use 40–100µamps.
- Average well hydrated patients use 100µamps. If inflammation in the colon is causing or perpetuating the myofascial pain, these frequencies will soften the muscle and relax the taut bands within 20 minutes. This reaction is diagnostic. If these frequencies soften the abdominal muscles and alleviate the pain then assessment of large bowel pathology and food sensitivities would be worthwhile.
- FSM frequencies and protocols for more comprehensive treatment of visceral conditions are presented in the FSM seminars and are available from trained practitioners.

Treat full body trigger points – Treat the spinal cord

A patient presented for treatment in the clinic with fascia exquisitely tender to even light touch and with sheets of myofascial trigger points in virtually every muscle in the body. Prior to the appointment, he sent in a list of trigger points identified by his physical therapist in 94 of the 100 commonly treated muscles. This list prompted the first suspicion that there was a central cause for the problem. His lack of response to the myofascial trigger point treatment confirmed this suspicion. His presentation simply did not make sense as a strictly myofascial diagnosis. If trigger points are created by overuse or trauma then regional myofascial trigger points are a reasonable diagnosis. If a patient is magnesium deficient or has a muscular reaction to lipid lowering agents then trigger points may be in several regions. But exquisitely tender trigger points in virtually every muscle in the body are not a reasonable result of any local or regional trauma or overuse.

When examined, this patient had hyperactive patellar reflexes, dermatomal sensory loss at the T8 dermatome, and dermatomal sensory hyperesthesia from T4 through T7 and T9 through T11. The examination findings suggested that there had been a disc injury in the thoracic spine. This led to a more probing and directed history. The full body pain and myofascial trigger points started one month after a martial arts injury that involved ballistic flexion and rotation of the thoracic spine at the T8 level. The picture became clear with this revelation. The disc nucleus is very inflammatory. A breach in the disc annulus caused by combined flexion and rotation would expose the nerve and the spinal cord to inflammation products from the annulus. Exposure to the nuclear material and phospholipase A_2 that it contains damages the nerve and eventually stops conductivity. If conductivity in the spinal cord is impeded the body reacts as if it is a deafferentation injury and tightens the muscles body wide.

The physical examination and history suggested that spinal cord inflammation following a thoracic disc injury was the most reasonable explanation for the widespread symptoms. When the frequencies to "reduce inflammation in the spinal cord" resolved the pain and caused all of the trigger points to disappear in 60 minutes with no myofascial manual therapy or treatment this confirmed the mechanism and diagnosis. In this way the frequency response becomes diagnostic (see Chapter 9).

This patient presented with a diagnosis of myofascial pain from trigger points not fibromyalgia associated with spine trauma but the lack of response to the myofascial protocol combined with the history, the physical examination, and the widespread nature and exquisite tenderness of the trigger points suggested that the pathology had to be in the spinal cord. The positive response to the frequencies to "reduce inflammation in the spinal cord" confirmed the theory even though there is no other clinical context or literature that associates widespread myofascial pain with spinal cord inflammation. The response to treatment is so frequency specific that it becomes diagnostic. If the myofascial protocols do not change the condition and the protocol for "reducing inflammation in the spinal cord" is effective then inflammation in the spinal cord is almost certainly involved.

The astute clinician can be guided by the response to the myofascial protocols, the symptom picture, the physical examination and some history of trauma such as a fall, lifting injury or auto accident or any episode that includes some degree of spine trauma usually within 3 months prior to the onset of body pain and trigger points. Physical examination will reveal hyperactive patellar reflexes demonstrating

inflammation in the spinal cord above the level of L3 that slows the descending inhibitory impulses necessary to dampen reflexes to their normal level.

FSM is very specific and the response to treatment is equally specific. The standard treatments for myofascial trigger points will not affect myofascial tissue in the cases described above. As always with FSM treat the cause.

Myofascial trigger points – Case reports

The patient was a 46-year-old female referred from a pain clinic for treatment of chronic persistent moderate to severe low back pain of 3 years duration. She had been very physically active prior to her injury and was still riding her bicycle to work during the week and taking long rides on the weekends even though it exacerbated her low back pain. She reported that the pain began in a single episode when she lifted a trash can. Since the original injury she had been treated unsuccessfully with prescriptions for anti-inflammatory and pain medication by her medical physician, with twice a week chiropractic adjustments for one year, and with massage and acupuncture which made it worse.

The physical examination revealed multiple myofascial trigger points in the psoas, the rectus abdominus and the lumbar paraspinal muscles referring pain in the expected patterns. The lumbar facet joints were painful to joint compression at L4–5 and L5–S1 bilaterally. Reflexes and sensation were normal.

The patient was treated twice a week for three weeks. Treatment with FSM for myofascial trigger points resolved the myofascial trigger points in four treatments. The facet joints responded to treatment for chronic facet joint pain in an additional two treatments. The patient returned once a week for 2 weeks for treatment of trigger points in compensatory muscles and for mild recurrence of trigger points in the original painful muscles. She returned for a closing examination after 2 weeks with no treatment and no pain and was instructed to return if there was any recurrence. She remained pain free after 2 years with no recurrence.

Collected case reports 1997

Data was retrieved from the charts of 100 new patients seen between January and June of 1997. There were 50 patients with head, neck or face pain resulting from chronic myofascial complaints. There were five acute cervical pain patients and 21 chronic low back pain patients. The rest were shoulder, other extremity or thoracic myofascial pain cases. Most of the patients were referred to the clinic by a medical physician, chiropractor, naturopathic physician or another patient. Chronic pain was defined as pain lasting longer than 90 days after the precipitating trauma. Patients were treated with FSM and chiropractic manipulation once or twice a week as needed. Treatment frequency was reduced as pain and function improved. Home exercises were recommended when appropriate and as tolerated.

50 cervical myofascial pain patients

All but two of the patients with chronic cervical pain experienced significant and lasting pain reduction. Six patients returned for occasional maintenance two to three times a year. The chronic cervical myofascial pain patients required an average of 11.2 treatments, minimum of 1 and maximum of 34. The average duration of treatment was 7.9 weeks, minimum of 1 day, maximum of 5 months. The pain was reduced from an average of 6.8 to an average of 1.5. The average length of chronicity was 4.7 years, minimum of 1 year and a maximum of 28 years. A large number of these patients had pain chronicity of 2 to 5 years. The one patient who didn't benefit significantly had her pain reduced from an 8 to a 5/10 during treatment but the improvement wouldn't hold. After 33 treatments in 12 weeks, treatment was abandoned. Her injury was 4 years old and she had been refractory to all other methods of treatment including injections and other mechanical and electro-therapies. She was ultimately found to have cervical ligamentous laxity that was missed during her initial evaluations.

Range of motion was increased in all patients. Increases in flexion/extension of 20 to 30 degrees after the first 20-minute session were common. Approximately 80% of this increase persisted until the patient was seen again four days later and eventually the improved range became permanent.

88% (44/50) of these patients had failed with some other therapy. 75% (33/44) of them had failed with Medical care, 54% (24/44) had failed with Chiropractic, 38% (17/44) had failed with Physical Therapy, 11% (5/44) with Naturopathic, and 6% (3/44) with acupuncture. Many patients had used two or more of these therapies with minimal to no permanent effect.

21 low back myofascial pain patients

The low back pain patients had an average pain chronicity of 8.4 years with a range of 3 months to 20 years. The majority had been in pain between 5 and 10 years. The average incoming pain level was 6.8/10 on a 0–10 visual analog scale. 87% of the patients had failed with some other therapy. 19/23 (83%) had seen a medical physician; 7/23 (30%) had failed with chiropractic treatments; 6/23 (26%) had failed with physical therapy and 4/23 (17%) had failed with some other therapy such as naturopathic medicine or acupuncture. Many patients had used two or more of these therapies with no lasting positive effect.

Patients were treated twice a week with FSM and some with chiropractic manipulation using "drop table" technique where appropriate and treatment frequency was reduced to once a week as symptoms improved. Patients required an average of 5.9 treatments in 6 weeks. Removing one chronic facet joint patient from the list reduced the averages to 5.1 treatments in 5.1 weeks. Average outgoing pain score was 1.5/10 on a 0–10 visual analog scale. There were no recurrences or exacerbations in the low back group and follow up contacts showed lasting improvement over the next year.

Bibliography

Ardic, F., Gokharman, D., Atsu, S., et al., 2006. The comprehensive evaluation of temporomandibular disorders seen in rheumatoid arthritis. Australian Dental Journal 5 (1), 23–28.

Arendt-Nielsen, L., Graven-Nielsen, T., 2003. Central sensitization in fibromyalgia and other musculoskeletal disorders. Curr. Pain. Headache. Rep. 7, 355–361.

Bennett, R., 2007. Myofascial pain syndromes and their evaluation. Best Pract. Res. Clin. Rheumatol. 21, 427–445.

Borg-Stein, J., Wilkins, A., 2006. Soft tissue determinant of low back pain. Curr. Pain. Headache. Rep. 10, 339–344.

Cheng, N., et al., 1982. The effect of electric currents on ATP generation, protein synthesis and membrane transport in rat skin. Clinical Orthopedics 171, 264–272.

Curatolo, M., Arendt-Nielsen, L., Petersen-Felix, S., 2006. Central hypersensitivity in chronic pain: mechanisms and clinical implications. Phys. Med. Rehabil. Clin. N. Am. 17, 287–302.

Dogweiler-Wiygul, R., 2004. Urological myofascial pain syndromes. Curr. Pain. Headache. Rep. 8, 445–451.

Fernandez-de-las-Penas, C., Onso-Blanco, C., Cuadrado, M.L., et al., 2006. Myofascial trigger points and their relationship to headache clinical tension-type headache. Headache 46, 1264–1272.

Fernandez-de-las-Penas, C., Onso-Blanco, C., Miangolarra, J.C., 2007. Myofascial trigger points in subjects presenting with mechanical neck pain: a blinded controlled study. Man. Ther. 12, 29–33.

Gerwin, R.D., Dommerholt, J., Shah, J.P., 2004. An expansion of Simons' integrated hypothesis of trigger point formation. Curr. Pain. Headache. Rep. 8, 468–475.

Gerwin, R.D., Shannon, S., Hong, C.Z., 1997. Inter-rater reliability in myofascial trigger point examination. Pain 69, 65–73.

Guyton, A.C., Hall, J.E., 1996. Textbook of medical physiology, ninth ed. WB Saunders, Philadelphia.

Hsieh, C.Y., Hong, C.Z., Adams, A.H., et al., 2000. Inter-examiner reliability of the palpation of trigger points in the trunk and lower limb muscles. Arch. Phys. Med. Rehabil. 81, 258–264.

Hong, C.Z., 1994. Persistence of local twitch response with loss of conduction to and from the spinal cord. Archives of Physical Medicine and Rehabilitation 75 (1), 12–16.

Hong, C.Z., 1996. Pathophysiology of myofascial trigger point. Journal of Formosan Medical Association 95 (2), 93–104.

Hwang, M., Kang, Y.K., Kim, D.H., 2005. Referred pain pattern of the pronator quadratus muscle. Pain 116, 238–242.

Kelgren, J.H., 1938. Observations on referred pain arising from muscle. Clin. Sci. 3, 175–190.

McMakin, C., 1998. Microcurrent treatment of myofascial pain in the head, neck and face. Topics in Clinical Chiropractic 5, 29–35.

McMakin, C., 2004. Microcurrent therapy: a novel treatment method for chronic low back myofascial pain. Journal of Bodywork and Movement Therapies 8, 143–153.

McMakin, C., Gregory, W., Phillips, T., 2005. Cytokine changes with microcurrent treatment of fibromyalgia associated with cervical spine trauma. Journal of Bodywork and Movement Therapies 9, 169–176.

Mense, S., Simons, D.G., Hoheisel, U., Quenzer, B., 2003. Lesions of rat skeletal muscle after local block of acetylcholinesterase and neuromuscular stimulation. J. Appl. Physiol. 94 (6), 2494–2501.

Netter, F., 1991. Atlas of human anatomy. Plate 22, Ciba-Geigy, New York.

Niel-Asher, S., 2008. The concise book of trigger points, second ed. Lotus Publishing, Chichester, UK.

Oschman, J., 2008. Energy medicine: the scientific basis. Churchill Livingstone, Edinburgh.

Sciotti, V.M., Mittak, V.L., DiMarco, L., et al., 2001. Clinical precision of myofascial trigger point location in the trapezius muscle. Pain 93, 259–266.

Shah, J.P., Phillips, T.M., Danoff, J.V., Gerber, L.H., 2005. An in vivo microanalytical technique for measuring the local biochemical milieu of human skeletal muscle. J. Appl. Physiol. 99, 1977–1984.

Simons, D.G., Travell, J.G., 1983. Myofascial origins of low back pain; Principles of Diagnosis and treatment. Postgrad. Med. 73, 66, 68–70.

Simons, D.G., Mense, S., Russel, I.J., 2001. Muscle pain: understanding its nature, diagnosis and treatment. first ed. Lippincott Williams & Wilkins, Baltimore, pp. 205–288.

Travell, J.G., Simons, D.G., 1983. Myofascial pain and dysfunction: the trigger point manual; upper extremity. Williams & Wilkins, Baltimore.

Travell, J.G., Simons, D.G., 1992. Myofascial pain and dysfunction: the trigger point manual; lower extremity, vol. 2. Williams & Wilkins, Baltimore.

Treating fibromyalgia associated with spine trauma

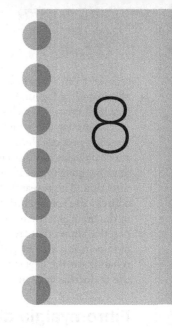

8

Fibromyalgia is a chronic pain condition associated with a complex of multi-system symptoms and has been characterized in recent years as a neuroendocrine disorder that includes characteristics of central pain sensitization and alterations in central hormonal function. There is no definitive laboratory test that will be positive in fibromyalgia and patients may or may not be diagnosed correctly.

55% of fibromyalgia patients report gradual onset of symptoms as middle aged adults. 55% could not recall a precipitating event. 24% report onset after some physical trauma such as an auto accident, fall or surgery. 14% report onset after some psychological stressor. Various studies report that up to 88% of fibromyalgia patients are female, 92–100% are Caucasian, average age at onset is 29–37 years old, average age at presentation is 34–53 years old (Moldofsky 1975).

Fibromyalgia patients have reduced levels of the branch chain amino acids, reduced serum levels of serotonin, epinephrine, norepinephrine and growth hormone and increased levels of substance P in the spinal fluid (Juhl 1998). Fibromyalgia is 13.3 times more common in patients following cervical injuries than it is in patients who have had lower extremity injuries. A study from Israel documented a 22% prevalence of fibromyalgia 1 year after auto accidents causing whiplash injuries in comparison with 1% prevalence after accidents involving leg fractures (Buskilla 1997).

Fibromyalgia patients process pain differently from normal patients. Patients with fibromyalgia have augmented central processing of nociceptive stimuli in comparison with pain-free controls. When measured by EEG, fibromyalgia patients have changes of greater amplitude on both sides of the brain in response to painful stimuli. Pain-free controls responded on only one side of the brain with smaller evoked potentials (Mountz 1995).

The nerves respond more strongly to painful stimuli and the response lasts longer than is normal. There was an increase in late nociceptive evoked somatosensory response in 10 FMS patients as compared to 10 controls (Bennett 1994). SPECT scanning of the brain of a patient with fibromyalgia shows reduced blood flow in the caudate nucleus of the thalamus, which is a site of central pain processing. Fibromyalgia patients have the characteristic pain of allodynia in which non-noxious stimuli such as light touch are processed as painful (Kandel 1985, Bennett 1999).

There is evidence that pain perception in fibromyalgia patients is different in quality from healthy patients; fibromyalgia patients are more sensitive to pain. In normal controls the pain threshold increases gradually between 80 and 160 pressure units and spikes dramatically at 160 units of pressure. Fibromyalgia patients show a linear increase in pain intensity with pressure intensity at every level from 80 to 200 units of pressure. Animal studies show this same pattern due to central sensitization and lowered firing threshold in the dorsal horn cells (Bendtsen 1998).

The most important thing you need to know about fibromyalgia is that it is curable. This chapter is intended to teach not only the frequency treatment protocols that are appropriate for treating fibromyalgia associated with spine trauma but also the conceptual framework for diagnosis and the adjunctive therapies that are necessary to help a patient to

DOI: 10.1016/B978-0-443-06976-5.00008-3

recover from fibromyalgia once the pain has been eliminated and to understand and address the cases in which recovery is elusive or difficult.

Eliminating the pain is only the first part of the recovery process. Returning the patient to full health is a challenging multidisciplinary project but has been done in enough cases to provide hope and therapeutic direction. The research shows that treatment must address the spinal cord, the pain processing centers in the brain and the neuroendocrine system. Clinical practice shows that treatment must reduce or eliminate pain as a way of reducing HPA stress and then rehabilitate the digestive system, the adrenals and the endocrine system.

Fibromyalgia diagnosis

Fibromyalgia (FMS) is a complex and still controversial diagnosis because it is a syndrome, a complex of symptoms forming a picture that must be diagnosed clinically. It cannot be diagnosed from an MRI, or by any imaging or blood test. There are more than 200 studies in the medical literature demonstrating neurologic and endocrine changes unique to fibromyalgia patients as compared to other chronic pain or depression patients. For the purposes of this chapter it will be assumed that the condition is real and can be diagnosed by a discerning, informed and educated clinician.

Patients are tested with an algometer to determine the point at which they report pain with pressure. The ACR criteria say that this threshold has to be reached at 4 pounds per square inch pressure or less. Using an algometer ensures that the testing is reproducible and will allow for repeat testing to document decreases in sensitivity as the patient improves. The report of full body pain, fatigue and non-restorative sleep lasting for more than 3 months fulfills the diagnostic criteria (Moldofsky 1975, Russell 1986).

What is not fibromyalgia

A careful history and laboratory blood work is required to ensure that the patient doesn't have one of the following conditions that cause symptoms similar to fibromyalgia. All too often a patient is mistakenly diagnosed with fibromyalgia (FMS) when the symptoms are instead caused by a treatable medical condition.

- **Chronic fatigue**: Fatigue, cognitive problems, pharyngitis, swollen lymph nodes, low grade fever,

substance P not elevated. Epstein–Barr viral titers and antibodies may be elevated.

- **Depression**: Check neurotransmitter profile by testing urine or using a questionnaire. Sleep disturbance with early morning awakening differs from fibromyalgia sleep disturbance and the cognitive dysfunction is different. FMS responds to smaller doses of anti-depressants. Rule out major depression.

- **Hypothyroidism**: Early hypothyroidism shows diffuse myalgia and fatigue. Laboratory values will be abnormal particularly TSH, T3, T4 and anti-thyroid antibodies. Body temperature is low in hypothyroidism but normal in FMS. Constipation, dry skin, and brittle hair are not characteristic symptoms of FMS. TSH is notoriously unreliable as a precise indicator of thyroid function. All parameters have to be taken into consideration.

- **Primary growth hormone deficiency and/or hypogonadism** (low testosterone in a male): When the complaint is muscle aches, fatigue, depression, exercise intolerance especially in a 20–40-year-old male, growth hormone and testosterone deficiency must be ruled out before a diagnosis of FMS or depression can be made. The history in growth hormone or testosterone deficiency may include a head injury, trauma or viral infection.

- **Sleep apnea**: Sleep apnea can cause fatigue and muscle aches. FMS can result from the stress response to sleep deprivation but if the patient has apnea the FMS can be easily resolved by correcting the apnea. Sleep apnea is at potentially fatal condition and proper diagnosis is crucial. Excessive daytime sleepiness, weight gain, reports of snoring or frequent nocturnal awakening should be followed up with a sleep study and CPAP prescription to correct the problem.

- **Inflammatory muscle disease**: While the symptoms of body pain and sleep disturbance (due to pain) are similar to FMS, muscle enzymes and sed rate will be elevated in this condition and are normal in FMS.

- **Lyme disease**: Lyme is reaching epidemic proportions in the US and is characterized by rapid symptom onset, rash, joint aches, positive antibody tests and may respond to doxycycline. The CDC diagnostic criteria requires that five out of five antibody markers be present for a definitive diagnosis but clinicians treating the condition report that if the patient has the symptoms and history characteristic of Lyme disease and have two or three of the antibody markers treatment is justified and useful.

- **Parkinson's**: The patient will present with stiffness often interpreted as mildly painful but myofascial pain due to age related arthritis and sleep disturbance may confuse the picture. Patient may have tremor, loss of spontaneous movements and loss of facial expression.
- **Polymyalgia rheumatica**: Pain and stiffness in shoulders, trunk and pelvis usually found in patients over age 50 are characteristic. Sleep disturbance may be age related or due to pain. Sed rate will be elevated in PMR and is normal in FMS.
- **Rheumatoid arthritis, lupus and systemic sclerosis**: Fatigue and myalgia occur before articular symptoms and can be mistaken for FMS. RA factor, sed rate, ANA titer will be normal in FMS, abnormal in these conditions.
- **Silicon breast implant reaction**: History will include breast implants – even saline. Symptoms include dry eyes and mouth, painful joints. 70% have positive ANA. Symptoms can persist even after removal of the implant.

Before a patient is diagnosed with fibromyalgia the following blood work must have been ordered and values must be in the normal range: complete blood count (CBC), chemistry screen to evaluate liver and kidney function, sed rate, ANA titer, muscle enzymes, CRP, salivary or serum hormone levels including cortisol, progesterone, DHEA and testosterone, IgF_1, TSH, T3, T4, anti-thyroid antibodies. A vestibular screening examination should be performed to rule out endolymphatic disorders.

If the patient reports symptom onset following spine trauma, a trial of treatment can be done to determine if the pain can be reduced. However the patient is entitled to more than one diagnosis and may have pain from fibromyalgia and one of the above conditions.

Different etiologies of fibromyalgia

In a clinical setting, fibromyalgia patients seem to sort into eight fairly clear although often overlapping etiologies. These are clinical distinctions based on patient histories and response to treatment developed during 12 years of treating hundreds of fibromyalgia and myofascial pain patients.

- **Stress**: One type of FMS seems to be associated with prolonged emotional or physical stress and physiologic sequelae of prolonged elevated cortisol

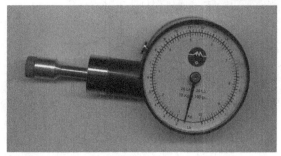

Figure 8.1 • The algometer allows delivery of a calibrated amount of pressure to assess pain sensitivity. The ACR criteria require that the patient report pain at 11 of 18 pressure points in response to 4 pounds per square inch pressure. There is also some mention of "the amount of pressure required to produce blanching of the examiner's thumb nail bed" which leaves room for considerable ambiguity. The algometer allows more precise and reproducible pressure.

and other stress hormones and the subsequent adrenal depletion (Maes 1998, Adler 1999). The section below describing the physiologic effects of severe prolonged stress explains the mechanism by which stress can create fibromyalgia (Dessein 1999).

- **IgG food sensitivities**: FMS can be associated with "leaky gut" and IgG food or environmental allergies. Mast cell overload from elevated IgG complexes causes the release of histamine causing "brain fog" and fatigue and stimulating class C pain fibers to create widespread aching.
- **Toxicity**: This etiology of FMS is associated with one-time acute or long-term chronic exposure to organic chemicals, heavy metals or pesticides that change nerve membrane firing characteristics creating generalized body pain, cognitive dysfunction and fatigue. Liver enzymes, especially GGT, may be elevated. GGT is so frequently positive that many labs no longer include it in a standard chemistry screen. It is the most sensitive marker for liver inflammation and must be ordered specifically. History questions regarding previous places of employment and residence, previous job descriptions such as hair dresser, landscape maintenance, printer, or painter will reveal exposures to organic chemicals (Baker 1997).
- **Genetic**: This type has a genetic link, seems to run in families and may be associated with food sensitivities, especially gluten, or may represent an increased need for enzyme substrate in the liver detoxification or serotonin pathways.

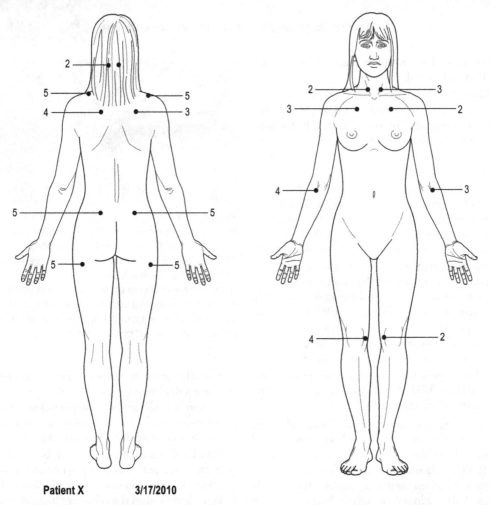

Patient X   **3/17/2010**

Figure 8.2 • When the tender points are evaluated with an algometer the number recorded on the diagram represents the number of pounds per square inch pressure that caused pain. Dating the record allows tender point evaluation to track progress.

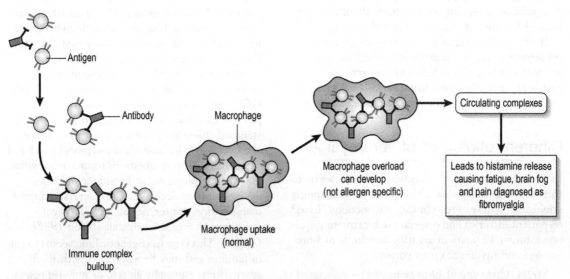

Figure 8.3 • When large numbers of IgG antigen–antibody complexes are ingested by macrophages histamine is released into circulation. Histamine stimulates class C pain fibers causing widespread diffuse aching and stimulates immune system responses leading to fatigue and cognitive dysfunction and a diagnosis of fibromyalgia.

- **Viral**: This type occurs after immunizations or viral illness. The symptoms may be from immune response to the virus or from nervous system response to the mercury preservatives in the immunizations.
- **Vestibular injuries**: This condition is not truly fibromyalgia but it is associated with the sleep disturbances and cognitive difficulties resulting from a vestibular injury or brain trauma. The sleep deprivation creates neuroendocrine stress eventually resulting in fibromyalgia. The patient will present with symptoms characteristic of FMS and the vestibular etiology has to be teased out during the history.
- **Peri-menopause and trigger points**: This type of FMS is associated with poorly managed menopause. Estrogen reductions cause sleep disturbance due to hot flashes and relative progesterone deficiency causes fatigue. Myofascial trigger points cause regional pain which can be in all four quadrants leading to central sensitization and a diagnosis of fibromyalgia. The solution for this etiology of fibromyalgia is proper hormone management and trigger point therapy using FSM (see Chapter 7) (McMakin 1998, 2004).
- **Spine trauma**: This type of fibromyalgia occurs after whiplash injuries, cervical or thoracic spine trauma, or after surgery and can be caused by any trauma that involves spinal flexion/rotation, spinal compression or ballistic segmental movement during a fall or impact (Bohlman 1979, Mendel 1989). The post-surgical cases are thought to occur when the neck is hyper-extended during intubation and constitute a cervical injury. Approximately 24–30% of fibromyalgia patients associate the onset of their condition with physical trauma although privately some clinicians have proposed the percentage to be closer to 50%. As a group they are the only FMS patients who complain specifically of pain in the hands and feet or describe their pain as burning.

All fibromyalgia patients, regardless of the etiology of their condition, have the same neuroendocrine and central sensitization features described in the fibromyalgia research but each etiology responds to different treatment strategies (Bennett 1999, Crofford 1998, Neeck & Reidel 1999). The model for the different types of fibromyalgia was developed when it was discovered that fibromyalgia could be successfully resolved when the treatment strategy addressed the specific cause or etiology of the pain or dysfunction.

Fibromyalgia associated with spinal trauma (cervical trauma fibromyalgia or CTF) represents a distinct etiology from fibromyalgia associated with other causes. The other types of fibromyalgia can be improved or cured without the use of FSM, although FSM helps accelerate the process. Fibromyalgia from spine trauma appears to respond only to FSM treatment and probably represents the 30% of non-responding fibromyalgia patients found in most fibromyalgia therapeutic studies.

Fibromyalgia from spine trauma – typical presentation and history

Treating fibromyalgia from spine trauma (CTF) is fairly easy; recognizing it can be more problematic because patients do not always associate their pain with the physical trauma but may attribute it to the emotional stress that accompanied the physical event. The patient who described her FMS as being due to the "emotional stress" of her divorce failed to recall falling off of a chair and hitting her head on the wall while painting the kitchen ceiling during her divorce until after treatment for CTF alleviated her pain and persistent questioning jogged her memory.

The pain diagram and symptom complaint describes aching burning midscapular pain, shoulder, neck, arm and hand pain that begins soon after the trauma and persists to varying degrees from the time of the injury to the date of presentation. Midscapular pain may represent referred pain from an injured cervical disc (Cloward 1959, Bogduk 1988). After some period of time, usually 1–6 months post-injury, the pain generalizes to the whole body, particularly down the thoracic and lumbar paraspinals, the gluteals and down both legs into the feet. The pain will be described as burning, aching, stabbing and sharp.

The patients generally rate the pain as varying between a 4 and a 9/10 on a visual analog scale. Most describe their hands and feet as feeling cold, burning or aching since the accident or injury. CTF patients have a characteristic affective response to the pain; it is particularly bothersome. Most have chronic headaches that can be quite severe. Many have been on narcotics, Neurontin or Lyrica for some time.

Imaging

MRI studies usually show a disc bulge or a contained herniation at C5–6 or C6–7 and less often at C4–5. In many cases the films have been read as normal by the original radiologist since degenerative changes and

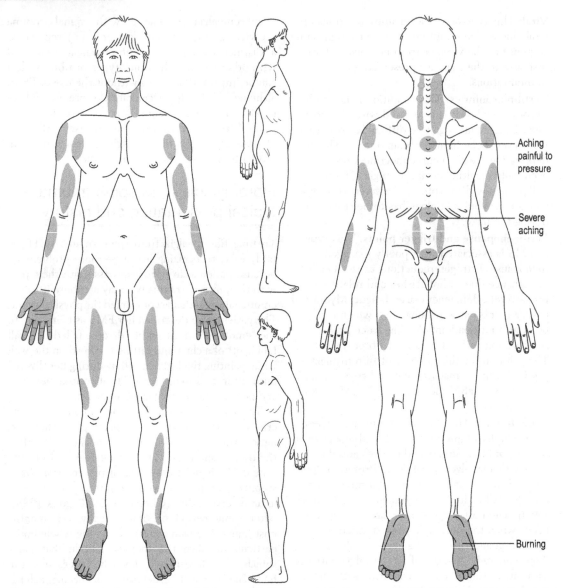

Figure 8.4 • The pain diagram for fibromyalgia associated with cervical spine trauma (CTF) differs from other fibromyalgia pain diagrams. As a group, CTF patients are the only fibromyalgia patients who describe their pain as burning and stabbing and report aching and burning in the hands and feet. This pain diagram is characteristic and predictive of a CTF diagnosis. It is virtually identical to pain diagrams characteristic of central pain except that central pain patients usually also report pain in the head and face (see Chapter 10).

small disc bulges are considered "normal" in a patient population. Many pain-free patients have disc bulges that do not produce symptoms. When the films were re-examined by a consulting radiologist specializing in spinal imaging the revised report described a central bulge or contained herniation.

The clinician is encouraged to review the films personally and not rely on the report when assessing fibromyalgia patients. The findings on the film must be correlated with the clinical assessment and physical examination as there is no way to tell from imaging alone whether a disc is causing symptoms.

Weight bearing flexion–extension MRI studies have recently become available in some facilities and will occasionally reveal a disc bulge that looks small in neutral but then extrudes in either flexion or extension causing spinal cord compression and myelopathic changes in the cord. The risk to the spinal cord requires a surgical referral for these patients.

Plain film x-rays cannot assess disc injuries but may reveal anterolisthesis or retrolisthesis near the abnormal segment. Flexion–extension lateral cervical spine x-rays may show increased translation, at the level of disc injury documented on the MRI.

In a very rare case the imaging may be completely normal but the mechanism of injury may involve force vectors that stretch the spinal cord and cause direct injuries to the spinal cord vasculature or neuronal tracts.

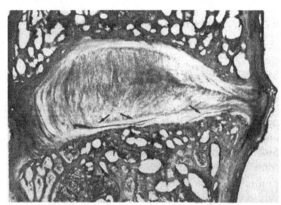

Figure 8.5 • This microscopic examination done at autopsy shows contained herniation and end plate fractures in a disc whose postmortem imaging was read as normal (reproduced with permission from Taylor & Twomey 1993). The patients in this study died from causes other than spine trauma during motor vehicle accidents.

Physical examination

The patellar reflex will be hyperactive, very brisk with a larger than normal amplitude. This is the hallmark diagnostic physical examination finding for fibromyalgia associated with spine trauma. In many cases, striking the patellar tendon on one side causes not only the hyperactive patellar reflex but also causes the adductors on the opposite leg to contract. In most cases the upper extremity and Achilles reflexes will be normal. Fibromyalgia that is not due to spinal trauma will demonstrate normal or even reduced patellar reflexes.

The sensory examination invariably shows hyperesthesia in one or more upper extremity dermatomes, usually C3, C4 or C5, and occasionally in a lower extremity dermatome.

Muscle strength will be normal in most cases. These patients are not generally surgical candidates

although some may be. Cervical compression, performed by applying axial pressure to the spine by pressing on the top of the head, will produce neck pain and an increase in shoulder pain in most cases.

Measurement of the 18 ACR defined tender points by algometer show at least the required 11 out of 18 necessary for a fibromyalgia diagnosis unless the patient was on narcotic medication that reduced sensitivity. Many of these patients will report pain with as little as 1–2 pounds per square inch of pressure.

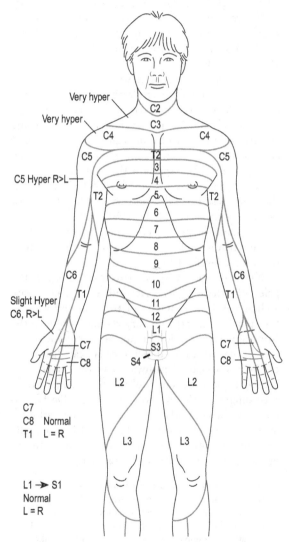

Figure 8.6 • CTF patients have specific dermatomal hyperesthesia in addition to the allodynia characteristic of all fibromyalgia patients. This patient had hyperesthesia to sharp in the right C3, C4, C5 and C6 dermatomes. C7, C8, T1 and all of the lumbar nerve roots had normal sensation.

How spine trauma leads to fibromyalgia

How could cervical spine trauma cause fibromyalgia and central pain sensitization? Trauma creates cracks in the disc annulus or the cartilaginous end plate and exposes the spinal fluid and spinal cord to the material in the disc nucleus. The disc nucleus contains neurotoxic concentrations of phospholipase A_2 (PLA_2) shown to cause nerve destruction in dogs, pigs and rabbits. PLA_2 has been shown to be so inflammatory and neuro-toxic that it destroys nearby nerves in a dose related response (McCarron 1987, Olmarker 1993, 1995, Ozaktay 1995, 1998, Cavanaugh 1997, Chen 1997, Marshall 1997).

The damage to the discs shown by Taylor & Twomey (1993) occurs in the postero-lateral portion of the disc which is directly adjacent to the antero-lateral portion of the spinal cord. The paleospinothalamic tract is the outermost of the two tracts in the lateral column of antero-lateral cord and carries diffuse deep pain information up the spine to the thalamus, caudate nucleus and the cortex (Lombard 1983). This tract is the one closest to the portion of the disc most likely to be damaged (Netter 1991).

The anatomic proximity of the cracks in the discs and endplates could expose this tract to very high neurotoxic levels of PLA_2.

If inflammation progressed to create damage in the paleospinothalamic nerves it would effectively create a chemical deafferentation of the pain pathways in the spinal cord. Inflammatory chemicals reduce the firing of nerves and slow or stop nerve conduction.

Trauma can cause direct mechanical disruption of the antero-lateral pathways and the spinal cord leading to deafferentation of these axonal pathways according to Taylor & Twomey (1993). Deafferentation in the antero-lateral ascending pain pathways in the spinal cord would produce what is essentially thalamic or central pain. Disruption of pain pathways in the spinal cord leads to central pain:

> "Central pain can arise not only from pathologic lesions in the thalamus but also from neurosurgical lesions placed anywhere along the nociceptive pathway from the spinal cord and brain stem to the thalamus and cortex. ... The sensations are unpleasant and abnormal, often unlike anything the patients had ever felt before: spontaneous aching and shooting pain, numbness, cold, heaviness, burning and other unsettling sensations that even the most articulate patients find difficult to describe. Central pain is particularly distressing emotionally."
>
> (Kandel & Schwartz 1985)

Fibromyalgia patients with a cervical trauma etiology use exactly the same pain descriptors, word for word, as central or thalamic pain patients. Patients with fibromyalgia that is not caused by cervical trauma do not have the same severity, quality or location of pain that cervical trauma patients describe. Their pain is diffuse and achy but it lacks the disturbing affective neuropathic intensity seen in the cervical-trauma mediated fibromyalgia patients. Post-traumatic fibromyalgia patients are the only group who complain of aching in their hands and feet and the only group that responds to the treatment protocol for inflammation in the spinal cord.

Treating fibromyalgia associated with spine trauma

Medical science accepts as a given that fibromyalgia is an incurable condition and the randomized controlled studies done so far have had that view as a starting point. Controlled trials by their nature can study only one intervention as it affects one or more symptoms. Since fibromyalgia is a collection of multiple symptoms affecting numerous systems each affected by multiple influences, the possibility that any one intervention will produce remission of all symptoms or cure the condition is extremely remote, especially if one starts with the presumption that the condition is incurable. The clinical strategies that have created recovery for so many patients operate within a framework in which recovery, while not inevitable, is thought possible because it has been observed to be so (Teitelbaum 2001). It is left to the reader to decide which viewpoint is most productive.

The treatment protocol in this chapter was developed by trial and error in 1999 and found to be effective in eliminating pain in over 200 FMS patients with spinal trauma onset. Pain has been reduced from an average of 7.4/10 to 1.4/10 in every patient with hyperactive patellar reflexes, dermatomal hyperesthesia, a history of trauma and pain in the hands and feet. Reducing the pain is relatively easy; achieving recovery is more involved because of the neuroendocrine and metabolic disturbances (McMakin 2005).

Pain is only part of the fibromyalgia diagnosis and symptom picture. Once the pain can be alleviated the patient still has the metabolic abnormalities characteristic of fibromyalgia. The neuroendocrine dysfunction in fibromyalgia patients is almost as disabling as the pain and it may be associated with alterations in central hormone function, primarily mediated corticotrophin releasing hormone or corticotrophin releasing factor (CRF or CRH).

Neeck & Reidel (1999) proposed, and it seems a reasonable hypothesis, that the pain itself serves as a chronic stressor elevating CRH in the hypothalamus. CRH in turn modifies levels of LHRH (luteinizing hormone releasing hormone), TSH (thyroid stimulating hormone), and GHRH (growth hormone releasing hormone) centrally contributing to disruptions in circulating hormones. Progesterone, growth hormone, thyroid hormone levels and thyroid receptor sensitivity are all affected. Chronic moderate neuropathic pain would be sufficient to cause the elevations in CRH found in fibromyalgia and the alterations in central pain processing common to fibromyalgia patients (Bennett 1999).

By the time the patient has been in moderate to severe pain for 1–2 years the symptoms generalize to include the classic neuroendocrine abnormalities seen in fibromyalgia caused by any etiology (Crofford, Demitrack 1996, Crofford, Engleberg, Demitrack 1996, Crofford 1998, Neeck & Reidel 1999). Understanding the neuroendocrine abnormalities is helpful when diagnosing fibromyalgia but it becomes crucial when attempting to resolve or cure it.

Understanding stress and neuroendocrine dysfunction

The key problematic central neuroendocrine hormone in fibromyalgia is corticotrophin releasing hormone or corticotrophin releasing factor (CRF or CRH). The stress response has its own evolutionary survival logic. When the body comes under attack it does not respond differently if the level 8/10 pain is caused by a tiger dragging you into the woods or by a disc bulge causing full body neuropathic pain. Certain stress responses go into effect mediated primarily by CRF/CRH and cortisol to keep the body alive until the attack is over. CRF stimulates the adrenals to increase cortisol levels and it acts centrally to modulate central regulatory hormones.

All repair systems and long-term physiologic processes are put "on hold" until the threat either kills you or resolves (Sapolsky 1994). This survival strategy is perfect for short-term attacks by tigers but creates problems when the stress persists in the form of moderate to severe pain lasting years.

Stress and thyroid

CRF suppresses thyroid stimulating hormone (TSH) centrally (Neeck & Reidel 1999). Primitive

survival logic dictates that the stress hormones are stimulating enough and additional thyroid hormone would be hyper-stimulatory. Elevated cortisol from the adrenal glands suppresses the peripheral conversion of the T4 storage form of thyroid hormone into the T3 active form of the hormone. Many fibromyalgia patients present as if they are clinically hypothyroid complaining of weight gain, constipation, dry skin, hair loss, fatigue and feeling cold. The patient becomes functionally hypothyroid because T4 cannot convert efficiently into T3 but TSH is almost always found to be in the normal or upper end of normal range when tested. TSH cannot rise in response to the relative peripheral insufficiency because it is suppressed centrally by CRF.

Stress and gonadal hormones

CRF suppresses FSH (follicle stimulating hormone) and LH (luteinizing hormone) centrally (Sapolsky 1994). The long-term projects of ovulation, sperm production, copulation and pregnancy are put on hold until the threat is gone. In women FSH and LH promote maturation of the corpus luteum and its increased production of progesterone to balance the estrogen produced by the ovaries during the post-ovulatory portion of the menstrual cycle. If production of progesterone by the corpus luteum is insufficient to balance estrogen the patient experiences the symptoms of premenstrual syndrome (PMS) caused by estrogen dominance. The patient complains of fatigue, irritability, water retention, sleep problems and emotional lability. These complaints are common to fibromyalgia patients.

Stress and growth hormone

CRF suppresses growth hormone releasing factor (GHRH) centrally interfering with growth hormone secretion (Bennett 1997). In an adult, growth hormone facilitates amino acid transport across the cell membrane to enhance tissue repair. Growth hormone in an adult is released during stage IV sleep and in a burst about 1 hour after vigorous exercise. Fibromyalgia patients do not experience stage IV sleep and they do not have the normal burst following exercise due to CRF suppression. Without adequate levels of growth hormone the normal exercises and activities of life and the minor tissue damage that follows are not easily repaired. This explains why fibromyalgia patients experience days or weeks of muscle pain after simple exercise or exertion.

Stress and the brain

CRF acts as a neurotransmitter and modifies cognitive processing to interfere with short-term memory and modulate long-term memory. In acute stress the only short-term information processing required is the answer to: "How do I get away from this tiger?" which leads the brain to focus on: "How did I get away from the tiger the last time?" Fibromyalgia patients complain of problems with short-term memory, processing and memory for details and sequencing of activities and information. And long-term memory is biased toward remembering unpleasant events and how they happened (Henley 2001).

Stress, digestion and IBS

Cortisol, chronic stress and sympathetic upregulation interfere with digestion. Digestive enzymes and stomach acid secretions are suppressed. Digesting meals is one of the short-term projects put on hold until the threat passes. Food can be digested tomorrow, if there is a tomorrow, but digestion is not as important as escape when the threat is present. If stomach acid secretions are suppressed, the stomach does not empty efficiently, leading to reflux of the semi-digested food and when it does empty the contents may not be as acidic as required for optimal digestion and absorption of minerals and protein.

The proper acidic pH of gastric contents creates the environment that supports proper bacterial flora in the intestines. Acid-loving bacteria decline and other bacteria proliferate in the more alkaline environment created by bicarbonate from the pancreas and relative decrease of acid. Intestinal bacteria help to digest food and create short-chain fatty acids that maintain intestinal health. If stomach acid and pancreatic digestive enzymes are both insufficient food may not be adequately digested or absorbed. Large undigested food particles may putrefy in the gut creating the local allergic responses and inflammation characteristic of irritable bowel syndrome commonly seen in fibromyalgia patients. Elevated cortisol levels cause thinning of the gut wall and when combined with inflammation caused by dysfunctional digestion, can contribute to the loss of gut membrane integrity sometimes called "leaky gut". Larger food molecules could leak across the membrane and encounter the immune system, contributing to food sensitivities commonly seen in fibromyalgia patients (Guyton 1986, Sapolsky 1994, Galland 1997).

Stress and insulin resistance

The stress response shifts the body to a short-term glucose economy to ensure that there is enough glucose available to fuel the muscles required to run away from the tiger. Insulin sensitivity declines as the body attempts to keep glucose out of storage and into the blood and muscles where it is needed emergently. This, combined with the exercise intolerance caused by growth hormone deficiency, leads to weight gain, insulin resistance and all of their associated health risk factors (Henley 2001, Sapolsky 1994).

Pain reduction and stress reduction

The key to resolving fibromyalgia appears to be keeping the pain below a 4/10 VAS level. When the pain is consistently kept below a 4/10, the neuroendocrine disturbances seem to resolve within approximately 4 months. It is intriguing to watch this transition. The neuro-hormonal and digestive disturbances common to fibromyalgia begin to improve within several weeks and may even resolve with no other intervention beyond pain relief. Reducing pain reduces stress and reducing stress allows the neuroendocrine system to return to normal function.

It is possible to provide adrenal support with FSM, nutritional supplements and herbs, to provide neuroendocrine support for cognitive function and mood with neurotransmitter precursors and FSM, and to support digestive system recovery with FSM, digestive enzymes, nutritional supplements, herbs and appropriate gut bacteria.

But if time allows and the patient is healthy enough to achieve it, it is intriguing to watch the body normalize function on its own with no other intervention except continuous pain relief.

Treating fibromyalgia associated with spine trauma

Hydration

- The patient must be hydrated to benefit from microcurrent treatment.
- Hydrated means 1 to 2 quarts of water consumed in the 2 to 4 hours preceding treatment.
- Athletes and patients with more muscle mass seem to need more water than the average patient.

- The elderly tend to be chronically dehydrated and may need to hydrate for several days prior to treatment in addition to the water consumed on the day of treatment.
- *DO NOT* accept the statement, "I drink lots of water".
- *ASK* "How much water, and in what form, did you drink today before you came in?".
- Coffee, caffeinated tea, carbonated cola beverages do not count as water.
- Water may be flavored with juice or decaffeinated tea.

Channel A: condition frequencies

The frequencies listed are thought to remove or neutralize the condition for which they are listed except for 81 and 49 / which are thought to increase secretions and vitality respectively

- Calcium ions   91 /
- Chronic inflammation   284 /
- Congestion   50 /
- Inflammation   40 /
- Remove anesthesia   19 /
- Remove opiates   43, 46 /

Reset basic functions:

- Remove nerve trauma   94 /
- Reset, reboot the nerve   321 /
- Remove histamine   9 /
- Scarring   13 /
- Sclerosis   3 /
- Increase secretions   81 /
- Restore vitality   49 /

Channel B: tissue frequencies

- Spinal Cord: ___ / 10
  - This frequency appears to affect the spinal cord but not the dura. Treating the dura is beyond the scope of this introductory text and is covered in the FSM Advanced courses.
- Midbrain: ___ / 89
  - The midbrain frequency appears to address the anatomical structures in the center of the brain including the thalamus and hypothalamus. The thalamus is involved in the central pain amplification and central

pain sensitization seen in fibromyalgia. In clinical applications, the use of this frequency on channel B combined with the frequency to reduce inflammation consistently reduces central pain and central pain amplification.

- Medulla: ___ / 94
- Forebrain: ___ / 90
- Hindbrain: ___ / 84
  - All parts of the brain are affected by prolonged pain. The medulla frequency is thought to address the entire brainstem including the reticular activating system which alerts the brain to threat. The forebrain modifies judgment to consider the affects of pain and the hindbrain modifies movement and activity to avoid pain. All of these parts of the brain are affected by chronic pain and central pain sensitization. Reduction of central pain amplification appears to be most effective when all parts of the brain are treated.
- Nerve: ___ / 396
  - Use for any dermatomal or peripheral nerve.

Treatment protocol

Prepare the cord for treatment

40, 50 / 10
- Remove inflammation and congestion / from the spinal cord.
- Alternating current: ±.
- Treatment time: 2 minutes each.

Alternating current minimizes the chance of a side effect thought to be caused by restriction of spinal fluid flow around a disc bulge near the spinal cord. Alternating current doesn't reduce pain as effectively as polarized positive current but it doesn't seem to increase the rate of spinal fluid flow. Use at the first treatment and in every treatment in any patient with known cord or thecal sac encroachment.

19, 43, 46 / 10
- Remove anesthesia, opiates / from the spinal cord.
- Current Polarized Positive +.
- Treatment time: 1 to 2 minutes each.

Response to treatment can be slow if the patient has had multiple injections or surgeries or is taking narcotics. Over time it was found that using the frequencies to remove "anesthesia" and "opiates" in the spinal cord improved the rate of response to treatment. It is not known whether these frequencies actually affect opiate levels or tissue storage of anesthesia metabolites or if they just make the receptors more sensitive to the frequency effect. These frequencies do not increase pain so it is unlikely that they have any direct effect on drug levels. Use at the first treatment and any time patients are taking narcotics.

94, 321, 9 / 10

- Remove trauma, remove "paralysis" and remove histamine /in the spinal cord.
- Current Polarized Positive +.
- Treatment time: 1–2 minutes each.
- Use these frequencies during the first and second treatments. They are not required during subsequent treatments.

Reduce the pain

40 / 10

- Remove Inflammation / from the spinal cord.
- Current polarized positive +.
- Treatment time: approximately 60 minutes
- Patient supine – well supported.
- Place patient hands on the skin of the abdomen.
  - Stay in the room with the patient during the first treatment for at least the first 20 minutes.

If there is going to be an adverse reaction to polarized current it will happen in the first 10 minutes. Pain will begin to recede upwards from the feet and lower legs within 10–15 minutes. If asked for a pain level after 15 minutes of treatment, the patient will usually report that their "neck hurts" but if asked how their legs feel they will usually notice that the pain in the legs is reduced or absent.

- Pain reduction proceeds upwards from the feet and legs and the neck and shoulder pain is reduced last.
- There is no manual technique involved. Set the patient up as shown and sit with them quietly for about 20 minutes.
- It takes approximately 60 minutes to reduce the pain to 0–2/10.
- If the pain is not reduced in the feet and legs by 50% within 30 minutes reassess hydration status, turn the current up or re-think the diagnosis.

Lead placement – Patient position

1. Patient should be supine with a bolster under the knees for low back comfort or seated in a recliner chair if one is available. The patient may be treated side lying if that is most comfortable but the head and torso must be well supported. The induced euphoria seen with this protocol during the first few treatments is profound and the patient must be in a well supported comfortable position. For subsequent in-office treatments and for treatments performed by the patient at home the patient may be in any comfortable position.

Table 8.1 Cytokine and neuropeptide changes produced with 40/10 treatment*											
Date	IL-1	IL-6	IL-8	TNF-α	IFNγ	SP	CGRP	VIP	NY	β Endorph	Cortisol	Serotonin
Baseline	392.8	204.3	59.9	299.1	97.2	132.6	100.8	8.5	18.1	5.2	15.5	285.6
#2	288.5	200.8	47.6	265.7	99.8	127.5	97.6	10.2	13.7	7.1	12.6	309.2
#3	103.2	121.7	21.3	96.5	73.7	82.4	61.3	32.9	7.2	21.4	33.7	202.1
#4	52.6	33.9	11.4	43.4	32.6	38.2	22.4	48.4	5.1	69.1	78.3	169.5
#5	21.4	15.6	4.8	20.6	11.4	10.5	8.6	69.9	6.6	88.3	169.9	289.6

*Cytokine data from MK, May 11, 2000.
This is the raw data from the first blood sample done on patient MK treated with the 40 / 10 protocol on May 11, 2000. Data analysis was performed by Terry Phillips, PhD a microimmunochemist at NIH shows dramatic changes in all parameters.

2. Wrap the glove attached to both positive leads in a warm wet hand towel and wrap the towel around the neck. The towel should be thoroughly wet and then firmly wrung out so it is not dripping.

3. Wrap the glove attached to both negative leads in a warm wet hand towel and wrap the towel around the feet.

4. The patient should be covered with a soft blanket from chin to toes to prevent chill as the towels cool off.

5. Place both of the patient's hands on the skin of the abdomen so the current flows through them during the treatment. This position improves the pain reduction in the arms and hands.

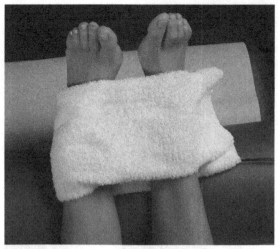

Figure 8.8 • The negative leads from channel A and channel B are attached to a warm wet fabric contact (hand towel) by alligator clips or by wrapping the graphite glove inside the towel that is folded lengthwise around the glove. The towel should be wet thoroughly and then wrung out so it is not dripping. Wrap the towel around both feet. If the patient is very large two towels can be joined by sliding one end into the other creating one longer contact out of the two towels.

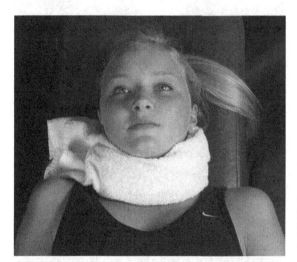

Figure 8.7 • The positive leads from channel A and channel B are attached to a warm wet fabric contact (hand towel) by alligator clips or by wrapping the graphite glove inside the towel that is folded lengthwise around the glove. The towel should be wet thoroughly and then wrung out so it is not dripping. Wrap the towel around the neck avoiding contact with the ears.

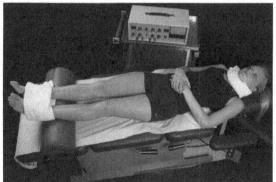

Figure 8.9 • Position the patient comfortably in a supine position. Position a bolster under the knees so the spine is comfortably flat. The patient should be covered with a soft blanket from chin to toes to prevent chill as the towels cool and should be well supported on the table or in a reclining chair since patients become very relaxed and many will fall asleep.

OR

• Place adhesive electrode pads on hands and soles of the feet. Channel A positive leads must be on opposite hand from the foot with channel A negative leads.

• **Current level:** 100–300µamps. Use lower current levels for very small or debilitated patients. Use higher current levels for larger or very muscular

patients. In general higher current levels reduce pain more quickly.

• **Waveslope:** Use a moderate to sharp waveslope for treating the spinal cord and fibromyalgia associated with spine trauma.

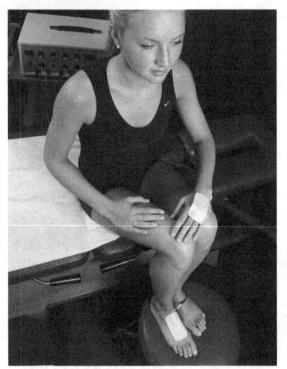

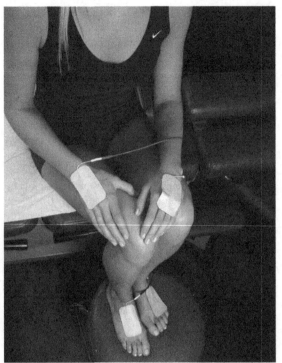

Figure 8.10 • When the patient is being treated at home or in a setting where use of towels is inconvenient adhesive electrode pads can be used on the hands and feet. Place the positive lead from channel A on the back of one hand and the negative lead from channel A on the top of the opposite foot. The photograph shows the patient seated for photographic convenience. The patient should be fully supported during treatments because many will fall asleep.

Figure 8.11 • Place the positive lead on one hand and the negative lead on the opposite foot. Larger pads conduct current more comfortably. If the pads become dry the current will sting or prickle and can be moistened with water.

Remedy: If mid-scapular pain and a headache occur despite the precautions built into the protocol, stop treating immediately and move the patient from supine to a sitting position. Place the negative leads on the floor under the feet and move the towel with the positive leads from the neck to the shoulders and change the current to alternating (±). Continue to run 40Hz and 10Hz using alternating current until the pain recedes. The entire treatment may be performed with alternating current but it takes more time to reduce the pain with alternating current.

Possible side effect – increased pain between the shoulder blades, headache

Some patients will experience an increase of pain between the shoulder blades and develop a headache within 5 minutes of treatment with current polarized positive from neck to feet. It is speculated that this effect is due to an increase in the rate of spinal fluid flow that first increases pressure on the disc annulus causing referred pain in the mid-scapular area, as shown in Chapter 5 from Cloward (1959), and then causing a headache as the spinal fluid pressure builds up into the ventricles. Using alternating current and the frequencies to reduce inflammation and congestion in the cord at the beginning of the treatment minimizes the chance of this side effect occurring and it should be rare.

Precaution – induced euphoria

Treating inflammation in the spinal cord has a curious effect on affect and cognitive function, especially in the first few treatments. Most, but not all, patients will experience an "induced euphoria" that is characteristic of this treatment. It is most pronounced while using 40 / 10 polarized positive and the practitioner may want to warn the patient that it is a normal effect as it begins. This is especially advisable for "type A" patients and for those who like to be in control of their surroundings.

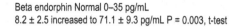

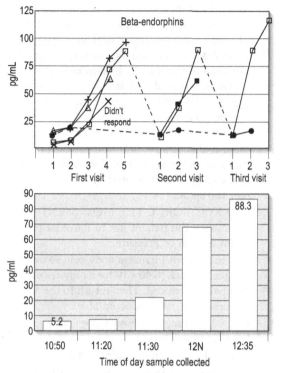

Beta endorphin Normal 0–35 pg/mL
8.2 ± 2.5 increased to 71.1 ± 9.3 pg/mL P = 0.003, t-test

Figure 8.12 • Beta-endorphin, in the first patient measured by micro-immunochromatography prior to treatment, was 5.2 pg/ml. Beta endorphin quadrupled in 45 minutes to 21.4 pg/ml and reached 88.3 pg/ml in 90 minutes, increasing endorphin levels by 17 times during the treatment period and causing the patient to ask drowsily if the treatment was "legal". The average endorphin levels published from six patients was 8.2 ± 2.5 increasing to 71.1 ± 9.3 pg/ml in a 90-minute period (P = 0.003).

Blood sample data shows endorphins increasing by 10 times in 90 minutes which quantified this response and provided a predictable timeline for its appearance. Endorphin levels double in the first 30 minutes in every patient for whom blood samples have been analyzed. The first sign will be a reduction in the rate of blinking, respiration and speech that starts within 10–15 minutes and corresponds to the reduction in lower extremity pain. Some patients fall asleep, all close their eyes and some become so "stoned" that they do not wish to or simply cannot speak. They can hear and should be reassured that the effect is normal and that it is temporary.

This dramatic effect usually appears at the 30–60-minute mark during the treatment as endorphin levels begin a very steep rise. This phenomenon will wear off as

the other frequencies are used at the end of the treatment protocol. The patient will remain relaxed and should come to full function within an hour or so after treatment. Most patients are in full possession of their faculties by the time they are ready to leave the clinic.

PRECAUTION: The practitioner should take care to ensure that the patient is safe to drive.

Side effect – agitation

The only side effect commonly encountered with this protocol is a sympathetic reaction that usually occurs 20–40 minutes into the treatment in about 10% of patients. The reaction is more likely to happen during the first few treatments and less likely with each successive treatment. The patient will become some combination of agitated, anxious, irritated, impatient or annoyed about something. As the pain and cytokines decline the blood chemistries show steep increases in cortisol and endorphins at about the same time that this reaction sets in and these changes in neuro-chemicals are assumed to be related to this phenomenon in some way.

The patient will not know that this reaction is caused by the treatment unless they have been warned about it and may ask to leave the room, stop the treatment, use the toilet or report feeling anxious about the time that has passed, the need to get home or make a phone call. It is wise to tell the patient at the beginning of the treatment that such a reaction is possible so the reaction will not concern or surprise them. The patient should be advised to inform the practitioner if any such symptoms occur.

If the patient has not been warned about this reaction before the treatment and it happens, the best approach seems to be to agree with whatever is concerning the patient and ask if they can delay responding to their urgent situation for just a few minutes. Patients have always agreed to this request. Change the frequencies to those used to quiet the sympathetics. Once the anxiety has passed, tell the patient that this reaction is not uncommon and explain the changes in brain chemistry responsible for it and ask the patient if they still need to do whatever it is that seemed so urgent a few minutes previously.

- Remedy: Change the frequency to 40 / 562.
- Reduce inflammation / in the sympathetics.
- Current polarized positive +.
- 2 to 5 minutes or as needed.
- Contact position does not change.

Once the patient is calm, resume treatment with 40 / 10 polarized positive. If the patient becomes agitated again repeat use of 40 / 562 until the patient is calm again and then resume treatment with 40 / 10 until the pain is gone.

Sustain pain reduction

The body pain should be reduced to 0–2/10 at approximately 60 minutes but may require as long as 90 minutes on the first treatment.

The treatment does not change local joint pain but will only change the full body neuropathic pain. The body pain will be eliminated but the patient may still have local facet joint pain in the neck or low back.

The pain relief achieved with just 40/10 would last between 2 and 12 hours. The shock and disappointment when it returned motivated the clinicians to find ways to make the pain reduction more lasting.

284, 91 / 10

- Reduce chronic inflammation, calcium ions / in the cord.
- Polarized positive + – for 2 minutes each. Treat with patient lying supine with contacts at the neck and feet. These frequencies seem to help make the pain reduction more lasting.

13 / 10 – Polarized positive +

- Reduce scar tissue / in the cord.
- Current polarized positive +.
- Patient seated – Contacts at neck and feet. Once treatment eliminated the pain patients wanted the relief to last longer. Questioning revealed that when the pain was reduced and patients began to exercise and increase range of motion, the pain returned with movement. In an effort to make the pain reduction more lasting it was hypothesized that the chronic inflammation in the spinal cord had caused adhesions in the spinal cord and that removing them would increase exercise tolerance and range of motion. The hypothesis was confirmed when it was discovered that forward trunk flexion of 20 degrees would cause pain or pressure between the scapula and that treating the cord to remove scarring resolved this problem. This protocol makes the pain reduction more lasting.
- Move the cord during 13 / 10 – until range of motion is normal.
    - Move the patient to a seated position with the positive leads glove in a warm wet towel that is wrapped around the neck and the negative leads glove wrapped in a warm wet towel placed under the feet.
    - Have the patient flex the trunk, not the neck, forward slowly until some tension is felt in the mid back usually between the shoulder blades.
    - Have the patient stop flexion and return to neutral upright position and wait 1 minute

while 13 / 10 continues to run. It's a nice time to chat with the patient about their hobbies and grandchildren.

- Have the patient flex forward again and there should be some increase in flexion. Stop movement at the first sign of tension or pressure in the mid back. This time the restriction should be felt lower down on the spine at about the T10 area. Return the patient to a neutral upright position and wait 1 to 2 minutes while 13 / 10 continues to run.
- Repeat this process until the patient can flex forward to between 70 and 90 degrees or to some range that is limited by the hips and not the spine.
- DO NOT FORCE THE MOVEMENT. Encourage the patient not to move past the point of pain or pressure.
- If a movement increases body pain switch the frequency back to 40 / 10 for 5 minutes or until the pain is reduced. Then return to the 13/ 10 process until range is acceptable.
- Use 3 / 10 if range of motion does not increase fully with 13 / 10.
- Reduce sclerosis / in the spinal cord.
- Some patients seem to respond better to 3 / 10 than they do 13 / 10. Use the same motion instructions and timing as described for 13 / 10.

81, 49 / 10 – Polarized positive + – for 2 minutes each

- Increase Secretions and vitality / Cord.
- Patients can remain seated for these frequencies. This protocol seems to improve motion and function and helps to make the pain reduction more lasting.

PRECAUTION: Patients treating themselves at home with automated individual units should be advised not to drive or operate dangerous equipment during the treatment. They should be seated or recline and should be physically safe if they fall asleep during treatment.

Reduce central amplification

It is common for the patient to be strongly affected by the endorphin levels and to appear almost disoriented once the pain is near 0/10, especially as the range of motion increases. One patient commented that, "I feel as if I should be in pain but I am not."

Treating Cord Fibrosis

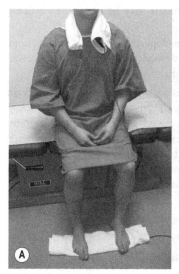
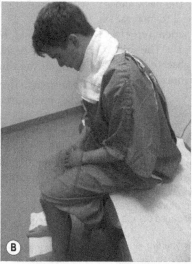
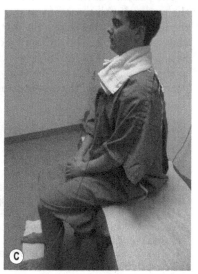

Treating CTF – Cord Fibrosis 13/10 + →

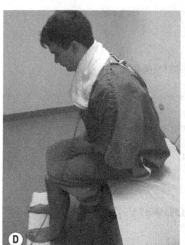
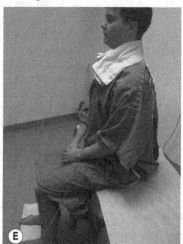
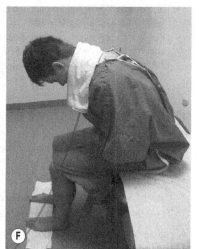

Figure 8.13 • A, B C: When the pain is reduced to 0–2/10, have the patient sit up on the edge of the table. With leads at the neck and feet – treat for adhesions in the cord with 13 / 10. Have the patient bend forward to the edge of pain or stiffness and then go back to neutral. Treat for 60 seconds with 13 / 10. D, E, F: Then have the patient flex the trunk forward again – the range will increase, then return to neutral. Each time the patient flexes forward to the edge of pain, the range should increase. Treat with 13 / 10 for 60 seconds then flex again. Treat for adhesions in the cord until forward flexion is normal and comfortable.

It was hypothesized that this disorientation was the result of central pain amplification that no longer had pain to amplify. The midbrain or thalamus shifts its function in fibromyalgia patients from pain suppression to pain amplification. When the pain is gone the amplification function has no object and the patient feels disoriented. Through trial and error, it was discovered that the protocols for central pain discussed in Chapter 10 would reduce or eliminate this feeling of disorientation.

40 / 89

- Reduce inflammation / in the midbrain.
- Current polarized positive +.
- Patient seated – Contacts at neck and feet.
- Treatment time 5–10 minutes.

The patient can remain seated for this portion of the protocol with the contacts still at the neck and the feet as they were during the protocol to increase range of motion. Run 40 / 89 until the patient reports having it feel more normal to be out of pain. The shift in the patient's affect can be easily observed. The dazed look clears and the eyes become more focused.

CAUTION: DO NOT run this protocol unless the patient appears disoriented by being pain free. If the patient does NOT have central amplification and the midbrain is performing its normal function of pain suppression, using frequencies to reduce the activity of the midbrain reduces central pain suppression and may cause pain to increase temporarily.

- The 40 / 89 protocol is only effective for central pain amplification.
- Do not use 40 / 89 for other types of pain.
- Do not use 40 / 89 before pain has been reduced to a 1–2/10 VAS by using 40 / 10.
- If use of 40 / 89 increases pain, switch back to 40 / 10 until the pain is reduced or use 81 / 89 for 1 to 2 minutes or until pain is reduced.

40 / 94, 90, 84 Polarized positive + – 1–2 minutes each

- Reduce inflammation / in the medulla, the forebrain and the hindbrain.
- Current polarized positive +.
- Patient seated – Contacts at neck and feet.
- Treatment time: 1 to 2 minutes each.

All parts of the brain are affected by prolonged pain. The medulla frequency is thought to address the entire brainstem including the reticular activating system which alerts the brain to threat. The forebrain modifies judgment to consider the affects of pain and the hindbrain modifies movement and activity to avoid pain. All of these parts of the brain are affected by chronic pain and central pain sensitization. Reduction of central pain amplification appears to be most effective when all parts of the brain are treated.

Address residual neuropathic pain

40, 284, 13 / 396

- Reduce Inflammation / in the nerves.
- Current Polarized positive +.

- Positive contacts at the neck – negative contacts at the hands may be needed to reduce arm pain.
- If patient has developed neuropathic irritation at L3 – place positive leads at low back and negative leads on the thighs.

If the patient does not or cannot place the hands on the abdomen during the treatment the arm pain may not be optimally reduced and may require specific treatment for the cervical dermatomal nerves with 40 / 396. This protocol usually eliminates the arm pain within 10 minutes. See Chapter 3 for details on treating neuropathic pain.

Box 8.1

Summary for treating CTF

Prepare the Cord
- 40, 50 / 10 – Current alternating
- 19, 43, 46 / 10
- 94, 321, 9 / 10

Reduce the Pain
- 40 / 10 – Current Polarized positive +
- 284, 91 / 10
- 13 / 10 – with movement
- 81, 49 / 10

Reduce Central Amplification
- 40 / 89
- 40 / 94, 90, 84

Making recovery possible

The most important thing you need to know about fibromyalgia is that it is curable. Not in every case or in every patient but it can be cured often enough that a cure should be the ultimate goal of therapy.

Practicalities

The long treatment times for this protocol are not possible for most practitioners and it is financially unfeasible for a clinician to spend 90 minutes with one patient. This treatment protocol requires a space for the patient but the patient does not require the clinician to be present after the first 15 minutes as long as the patient has been warned about the possible agitation side effect. The rewards and satisfaction that come with being able to help someone with this condition to become pain free make the time invested well worthwhile.

Treatment interval

There have not been any properly diagnosed patients to date in whom this treatment protocol has not produced pain relief. Patients will finish the treatment with pain levels between 0/10 and 3/10 on a VAS scale regardless of their incoming pain or chronicity.

The patient must be warned that the pain relief is temporary. The pain will return at a reduced level within 2 hours up to 2 weeks following the initial treatment. It is important to tell the patient that the pain relief is temporary: "When the pain comes back it will not be as bad as it was before but you will mind it more because it was gone for a while. There are two parts to pain. One is 'how much it hurts' and the other is 'how much you mind it or how bothersome it is'. The pain will be less intense but you will mind it more."

It is also important to tell the patient that if the treatment was effective the first time it will always be effective. **"If it worked the first time there will never be a time when it doesn't work and it is OK if you don't believe it."** Most patients with fibromyalgia from spine trauma have been in pain for so long and have been disappointed so may times that it is important to give them permission to be skeptical. Central sensitization is still an issue to some extent, even after 40 / 89 has improved the situation. Being out of pain is entirely foreign to the patient and it is going to take time for them to begin to trust that pain relief is possible and even longer for them to expect it as the norm. Repeated in-office treatment is important so that the practitioner can monitor and support the patient through this transition from pain patient to recovering patient.

Second treatment: The second treatment should be scheduled for 1–2 days after the first treatment so that the patient is treated a second time before the pain has had time to return to baseline pretreatment levels. The same procedure should be followed as in the first treatment and the same frequencies should be used. The "concussion protocol" discussed in Chapter 10 should be used once the pain has been reduced.

Follow-up

Subsequent treatments should be scheduled twice or three times a week. It is ideal if the patient's personal finances allow the purchase of a unit for home treatment. The HomeCare (Precision Distributing, Vancouver, Washington) is a preprogrammed automated microcurrent unit that provides the basic 40 / 10 protocol described above by sequencing automatically through the frequency sequences. If a patient has benefited from in-office care the HomeCare will provide the same pain relief and give the patient control of their pain.

The primary requirement for recovery from fibromyalgia is that the patient must keep the pain below a 4/10 level at all times for up to 16 weeks. For some patients this is a matter of four to six in-office treatments in 6 weeks. The neuropathic pain disappears and doesn't return but this is not the norm. Some patients need repeated treatments and using a HomeCare unit is often necessary to achieve this goal, especially if the patient cannot afford two or three in-office treatments per week. Any device can be used that provides microcurrent and delivers 40Hz on channel A and 10Hz on channel B.

It would be convenient if every patient benefited from the same adjunctive therapies for the neuro-endocrine and digestive dysfunctions but this is not the case. The same treatment protocol will produce pain relief in every patient and keeping the pain below a 4/10 is the primary requirement for recovery but reducing full body neuropathic pain is only a part of the recovery process. The practitioner will need every skill, experience, intuition and technique acquired in training and practice to produce recovery. Every patient treated to date with the 40 / 10 protocol has had pain relief but only 58% have recovered.

Orthopedic issues

Once the pain and pain amplification are reduced the patient becomes the same as any other orthopedic patient of a similar age discussed in the previous chapters. The injured disc that caused the cord inflammation must be repaired to prevent reoccurrence. If the disc has been separated from the end plate it may never recover and ongoing treatment or even surgery may be required especially if the segment is hypermobile.

Each patient will have unique combinations of orthopedic complaints that must be addressed. Every fibromyalgia patient has myofascial trigger points that will need to be treated. Facet joints, discs, muscles and extremity joints may all need treatment and reconditioning exercises if the patient is to recover full function. The reader is referred to FSM protocols in the preceding chapters for these conditions and to any of the many texts available in the area of spinal and physical rehabilitation. Some patients may require facet joint injections, epidural injections, spinal stabilization exercises and general reconditioning in order to recover.

Regardless of the orthopedic pain generators, if the neuropathic pain can be kept below a 4 / 10 the neuroendocrine system will right itself and the patient can recover from fibromyalgia.

Medication management and withdrawal

Medication management and withdrawal must be addressed if the patient is to achieve recovery.

Opiates and narcotics

Once the FSM protocol has reduced the pain, a patient taking narcotics is automatically over-medicated. Narcotic side effects which were not previously a problem may become problematic in some patients. It is essential that the patient begin reducing narcotic dosages within days or at most a week after the second successful treatment. The patient should trust through experience that the treatment will relieve pain predictably before they are asked to begin reducing pain medication. It is essential that patients taking high doses of opiates not stop their medication abruptly; narcotics withdrawal symptoms are stressful, unpleasant and can be dangerous.

Comprehensive medication management and withdrawal recommendations are beyond the scope of this text. In general, experience suggests that narcotics should be reduced first and that withdrawal should be gradual and adjusted to patient tolerance. FSM will manage the neuropathic cord mediated pain so that the patient doesn't require opiates for pain control but FSM doesn't help withdrawal symptoms. Patients should be warned against abrupt discontinuance of long-standing narcotic medication without medical supervision. It is prudent and completely acceptable to continue to take narcotics simply in order to avoid withdrawal symptoms. Patients may experience a range of withdrawal symptoms including but not limited to increased body pain and flu-like aching, sinus and nasal congestion, emotional agitation or depression, nausea and chills. The patient should continue to treat with FSM at home or

in the office to keep the body pain down while physician supervised medication withdrawal is accomplished during the weeks or months required.

Narcotic addiction becomes apparent when the patient stops using FSM at home or in the office, even though it reduces the pain, because taking the medication is easier or provides some comfort beyond pain relief. These cases account for some of the failures of FSM therapy in fibromyalgia recovery. To date, no patient using a fentanyl patch has persisted from pain free to full recovery. Frank conversation, counseling and drug rehabilitation have all been used successfully in a few cases but it is a challenging situation and success depends entirely on the patient's self awareness, motivation and personal support system.

It is important that common sense guide this process. Not every patient on narcotics is addicted or needs to be withdrawn. The case that comes to mind is the 76-year-old patient who had nerve damage in her left foot creating complex regional pain syndrome (CRPS) some 40 years previously. After years on various medications, she had been successfully managed on low dose methadone for 15 years and suffered no side effects from the drug even though her pain was still a 7/10 while taking it. When she became pain free and was able to walk she discontinued the methadone overnight because she felt it was wrong to take it if she had no pain. It caused significant withdrawal reactions. The patient had to be reassured that the practitioner had no judgment about her use of methadone and that it was completely acceptable for her to stay on a lowered dose of medication if only to avoid the stress of withdrawal at her age.

Anti-depressants

Anti-depressants are often used in chronic pain patients to help increase serotonin levels and modulate central sensitization or they may be used because clinicians have found them useful empirically or because the prescribing clinician feels that chronic pain problems are really caused by depression. For whatever reason they have been prescribed, many chronic pain patients will be taking one or more anti-depressants. Once the pain has been reduced, anti-depressants keep the patient from feeling pain but they also blunt all types of emotions. Patients don't feel bad when taking anti-depressants but in general they don't feel anything. Obviously if the patient had a problem with primary depression prior to the onset of pain then an appropriate psychiatric consultation should be performed before modifying anti-depressant medications. Depending on which medication or medications have been prescribed withdrawal may require weeks or months with careful monitoring and gradual reduction. Most but not all patients feel "more like themselves" when they have discontinued anti-depressant medication. Some patients feel best when they remain on a low dose. It is a completely individual response.

Other classes of medications that have been prescribed for various neuroendocrine or digestive symptoms may be withdrawn by the prescribing physician in collaboration with the patient as tolerated. Once the pain has been reduced the perpetuating factor for neuroendocrine and digestive complaints has been eliminated. In general the medications required previously to manage these symptoms will no longer be necessary. But it may take both the physician and the patient some weeks to recognize and act on this. Medication side effects should be evaluated and may become more prominent as the condition improves and the medication has fewer symptoms to control.

Digestive reconditioning

Digestion begins to improve on its own within a few weeks of pain reduction. The changes to digestion brought on by stress begin to resolve but occasionally direct therapeutic intervention will be helpful. This is a cursory review and practitioners are advised to explore the full range of information available on this topic (Galland 1997).

Digestive enzymes and hydrochloric acid are reduced by the stress response. Professional grade nutritional supplements containing digestive enzymes and hydrochloric acid taken just before the meal will help make digestion more comfortable. Proton pump inhibitors being taken for reflux or stomach bloating reduce stomach acid and should be discontinued. Once stomach acid and enzymes return to normal, digestion will improve and reflux should resolve.

Bacterial flora in the gut helps digest food and creates short chain fatty acids that repair the gut wall. The balance of beneficial bacteria and Candida maintained by proper digestive system pH and enzyme function is disrupted by stress. Replacement flora and suppression of excess Candida may help the gut recover more quickly.

Food allergy testing may help identify food intolerances and avoiding dietary allergens can help both the gut and the patient to recover more quickly. Serum allergy testing is more accurate and useful than skin testing which only identifies IgE reactions. Most food intolerances are IgG delayed sensitivities.

FSM can be used to reduce inflammation in the gut and to treat irritable bowel, leaky gut and constipation. These protocols are taught in the FSM Core seminar.

Adrenal rehabilitation

The adrenal glands which produce cortisol among other essential hormones can become depleted after years of sustained stress. Most professional grade nutritional companies provide supplements to assist with adrenal recovery. Some patients who are very depleted and exhausted may benefit from a low dose prescription adrenal replacement such as Cortef (Jeffries 1996).

Pain and stress disturb the normal diurnal rhythm in which we are awake and lively in the morning and quiet and ready for sleep after dark. Fibromyalgia patients are routinely exhausted in the morning and do not begin to feel awake until evening. As the pain and stress decline the normal diurnal rhythm begins to return. Nutritional supplements and herbs to quiet the adrenals may be used in the late afternoon and early evening. Supplements such as licorice root, vitamin B5, and vitamin C and combination supplements for adrenal support may be used in the morning. In the author's experience, glandular supplements or stimulants have never been successful in the long run (Henley 2001).

FSM protocols for adrenal support used in the morning increase salivary cortisol temporarily and seem to enhance adrenal recovery overall. FSM protocols to quiet adrenals may be helpful in quieting the adrenals, restoring diurnal rhythm and improving sleep. These protocols are included in the FSM Core seminar and are beyond the scope of this basic text.

Adrenal function will improve as the pain and stress remain reduced but adrenal rehabilitation may take a few years.

Neurotransmitter reconditioning

If patients are not on anti-depressants and the practitioner has or can acquire knowledge of how to measure, monitor and manipulate neurotransmitters using diet, exercise and selected amino acid and herbal supplements recovery can be enhanced. Neurotransmitters affect mood, sleep and cognitive function.

Physical reconditioning

Once the pain remains below a 4/10 for 2 weeks, on average, the neuroendocrine system begins to right itself. Patients start sleeping better, digesting their food better and begin to see a return of normal diurnal rhythm. They may comment that they are now tired earlier at night and awaken more rested in the morning. Patients begin to tolerate more exercise and may even crave it suggesting that the reduction in pain may lead to a reduction in CRF leading to a corresponding increase in growth hormone. Walking, swimming and gradual reconditioning are the safest way to begin physical rehabilitation and reconditioning. Resistance training should be undertaken gradually if at all, under supervision if possible and only to tolerance. Any activity that causes an increase in symptoms should be avoided. Over head lifting should be avoided because it stresses and compressed the cervical discs. If at all possible a specific program of spinal stabilization should be undertaken to strengthen the muscles in the neck and support and repair the injured disc. The physical reconditioning process may take several months and depending on the patient's age and length of illness may take up to a few years.

Psychological reconditioning

Prior to their first treatment many patients have finally accepted what they have been told by authority figures in white coats and support groups on the internet, "You will be in pain for the rest of your life. Fibromyalgia cannot be cured but you can learn to live with it." The greatest challenge most patients face when body pain is reduced from a 7/10 to a 0/10 during the first 90-minute treatment is the existential crisis that occurs when they need to answer the question, "Who am I if I am not in pain?" or "Who am I if I am not a pain patient".

This more than medication management and withdrawal, more than neuroendocrine recovery or reconditioning is the single most common source of treatment failures. Think about it. Who you are, who you think yourself to be, is by and large determined by what you do in our culture. If your activities and lifestyle have been defined by doctor's appointments and pain-limited activities for years and you have now been pain free for 2 weeks, "Who am I now?" is a reasonable question.

Some patients experience unexpected emotions that surprise them such as resentment, anger or grief. Why did I have to suffer? Why didn't I find you

sooner? What if it doesn't last? Why couldn't the other doctors help me? I am so sorry my family had to suffer along with me.

Some patients, especially those with a history of early childhood abuse or trauma and those raised in emotionally abusive environments, have internalized the abuse. They have a subconscious belief that they deserve to suffer, that life will always be difficult and painful. Studies show that their neuroendocrine system over reacts to threat and pain. The same stressor will produce a much stronger stress response in an adult abused as a child than it will in an adult raised in a non-abusive environment. Because the response is unconscious, the patient doesn't know that there is another way to be. It can be challenging to present this concept to the patient because it seems so personal. It is important that they not feel as if they have done anything "wrong."

Telling the story of the research done with baby mice may help because it externalizes the situation. It is easier to see the implications when the story is about mice than when it is personal. Two litters of genetically identical mice, born at the same time are put into two different situations. One litter is allowed to develop in a stress-free environment living in a large cage with adequate food and the comfort of their litter mates and mother. One litter is allowed to develop in the same environment but once a day, as soon as they are physically able to swim, they are placed in a beaker filled with cold water and made to swim for several minutes with no way of escape. This is an incredibly stressful situation for a mouse. After 2 weeks of this daily stressor the mice are left to mature normally in a stress-free environment. Then as adults both groups of mice are taught how to do a maze. Once mice learn a maze the drive to finish the maze and get the reward is very strong. The researchers put a blinking yellow light near the end of the maze. The yellow light, very similar to the yellow of an owl's eye and universally threatening to mice, caused all of the mice to immediately stop their progress along the maze and assess the threat. The stress-free mice considered the threat, saw that it wasn't really an owl and proceeded to the reward at the end of the maze. All of the stressed, cold-water swim mice stopped their progress, over-reacted to the threat and failed to finish the maze.

The early childhood stress had changed the way the brain was hard-wired to react to stress. This may explain why a large percentage of fibromyalgia patients have a history of early childhood abuse or trauma. Patients can usually understand how this applies to their situation.

Fortunately there is a difference between mice and humans in their ability to modify subconscious responses with conscious choices. If a patient is willing to explore this situation, hypnosis, cognitive behavioral therapy, relaxation therapy and mediation may all be helpful. Providing referrals and resources in this area is an important part of recovery.

There is no one answer or approach that will be appropriate for every patient. But in general the following guidelines have been useful:

- **Give permission:** Acknowledge the emotion by saying "I understand how you feel. You have suffered incredibly and no one really appreciates how much courage it took just to get through each day much less 14 years of days. It makes perfect sense that you would feel like this."

- **Encourage the patient:** You may be the one person in the patient's world who believes that recovery is possible. Support realistic expectation. Recovery takes about one month for every year of illness. They need to be patient and track improvements even amidst the setbacks. You are asking that they accept the diagnosis of fibromyalgia but reject the verdict.

- **Reframe the experience:** "Being ill has taught you a lot. You are different than you were when this started. The years were not 'wasted' you were just learning things that you didn't anticipate having to learn. You have learned that people will care for you just as you are, that the world will not end if you cannot clean the house every day or if a 7-year-old has to help you take out the trash, that you have resources around you to do what you have not been able to do, and that you can live within your limits and still have a life. You are wiser than you were when this started. Now, if we are lucky and all goes well, you get to get rid of the pain and keep the wisdom."

- **Living without pain:** "As inconvenient, uncomfortable, challenging and difficult as the pain has been it gave you certain benefits. It gave you an excuse not to do things you didn't want to do, go to Aunt Maude's party, clean the house, do certain projects. You found out that the world did not end if you did not do these things. Now that the pain is gone the world will still not end if you do not do these things. You can simply do or not do what you want to do or not do now that you no longer have the pain as

a reason. The world will still not end. Find other ways to do for yourself what the pain was doing."

- **During recovery:** "Pace yourself. You will have good days and bad days and then better days. Be patient with the process. Pay more attention to the good days and don't over do it. When you have a good day, give yourself permission to do something pleasant just for you. Take time to meet your own needs. If recovery is ahead then the time you spend on yourself is an investment in the future of your health."

- Every patient will require a different conversation depending on their personality and circumstances.

For the practitioner

A physician told his class of medical students, "It is the physician's job to hold the vision of the patient as healed until the patient can see it for himself."

Be persistent, positive and determined but never make promises or predictions. Cautious optimism is always safe. Hopeful skepticism is reasonable.

Use objective outcome measures such as the Oswestry functional pain inventory, fibromyalgia impact questionnaire, range of motion, tender point testing by algometer, VAS pain scales and pain diagrams to document patient progress. It is easy for a recovering patient to get engrossed in their current symptoms and forget how much their symptoms have improved. It helps if they can see an objective measure of their improvement.

As you become more adept at treating difficult patients, you will attract more difficult patients. Each chronic pain patient you help knows six patients with similar symptoms or worse. Eventually you will find a patient whose physical, emotional, financial, psychological or spiritual damage is so severe it cannot be repaired in this lifetime. You can still offer the patient compassion and understanding and some palliative care. FSM can be used to provide whatever degree of comfort can be achieved or that the patient will allow.

Treating very difficult emotionally wounded and sometimes demanding patients can be challenging for the practitioner and the staff. Boundaries, compassion and clear communication are important.

You can't want the patient's recovery more than the patient wants it.

Be fully engaged in the process; do not get attached to the outcome.

Case reports

- There are dozens of cases that could be presented here but these two are memorable.

Case #1

The patient was a 53-year-old disabled police officer diagnosed with fibromyalgia 4 years prior to his initial clinic visit. He had been a motorcycle patrolman making a routine traffic stop. Before he could dismount his motorcycle the traffic offender put his car in reverse and hit the officer, knocking him and the motorcycle up onto the sidewalk. The officer slammed into a power pole and fractured both of his forearms as he put them up to protect his face from the impact. He developed full body pain after his third arm surgery and was diagnosed with fibromyalgia several years later.

He was on narcotics, two anti-depressants, acid blockers and sleep medication. His pain level on the first day was rated as a 6–7/10 with the classic cervical trauma fibro pain diagram. His physical examination showed hyperactive patellar reflexes and strong neuropathic pain in the C4, C5 and C6 dermatomes bilaterally. He was treated with 40 / 10 and the concussion protocol (Chapter 10) on the first visit. At the end of the treatment his pain was 0/10. He returned 3 days later with his pain rated as 4–5/10 and reported that he had been pain free for 24 hours. He was treated a second time with 40 / 10 protocol and also treated for myofascial trigger points in the neck and shoulder muscles (see Chapter 7). He was told to reschedule for the following week.

He canceled the next appointment. He returned to the clinic 4 weeks later and said he didn't need treatment but only came to say thank you. He canceled his appointment because he had no pain and he spent the next month withdrawing himself from all of his medications. His pain level was a 2/10 and "I can live – have a life – at a 2/10."

Case #2

The patient was a 49-year-old woman referred by her management physician because he heard that there was a new treatment available. Her fibromyalgia started with an auto accident 18 years previously. She was on two different pain medications, sleep medication, muscle relaxants and medications for asthma and IBS. She rated her pain on the initial visit

as a 7–8/10 with the characteristic pain diagram. She complained of headaches, burning mid-scapular pain, hand, arm, leg, foot, neck and back pain, and jaw pain. She had developed acne, asthma, allergies and irritable bowel syndrome since her fibromyalgia diagnosis.

Her physical examination showed hyperactive patellar reflexes with adductor crossing, sensory hyperesthesia at C3, C4, C5 bilaterally and at C6 on the right. She had 14 out of 18 tender points tender to less than 2 pounds per square inch pressure as measured by algometer.

She was treated with 40 / 10 for the first time on December 8, 2000. Her pain went from a 7/10 to a 0/10. She had 20 in-office treatments between 12/8 and 3/15. She was treated with the cervical trauma fibro protocol and protocols for myofascial trigger points, facet joint pain, disc degeneration, TMJ, irritable bowel syndrome, adrenal support and asthma during her in-office visits. She had a small two channel microcurrent unit (manufactured by Rehabilicare, Minneapolis, MN) that provided 40Hz on one channel and 1Hz on the second channel to use daily at home as needed for pain management. She had 20-minute regional massages and a gentle form of chiropractic adjusting at each visit.

She was referred for physical therapy for spinal stabilization and strengthening, kept her appointments and was compliant with home exercises. She was referred for an epidural steroid injection at C5–C6 on the right and two sets of facet injections in the neck and one facet injection in the low back.

She was prescribed supplements for irritable bowel (digestive enzymes, friendly bacteria and soluble fiber) and adrenal support. She had a wonderful attitude and a supportive family and she declared that while she had fibromyalgia she was not planning on being a fibromyalgia patient forever.

On December 8 she had 14 of 18 tender points tender to less than 2 pounds per square inch pressure. On January 12 she had 11 of 18 tender points tender to four pounds per square inch pressure. On February 8 she had 7 of 18 tender points and no longer met the diagnostic criteria for fibromyalgia. She recovered in 2 months.

Her cervical range of motion improved by 40% and was pain free. Pain medication was reduced by 95% and taken only occasionally. Muscle relaxants were taken occasionally and reduced overall by 95%. She was sleeping well without medication. Her acne resolved when she was given an oil based form of vitamin A on the assumption that she did not convert beta carotene into the active form of vitamin A in her gut. Her digestion improved and the IBS resolved. She and her family were able to retire to their dream home in the Rocky Mountains.

During a follow-up phone call 7 years later she said that she had remained pain free for 6 years until she

developed ulcerative colitis after being given antibiotics for an infection. She said her fibromyalgia had returned after surgery but she knew she could get rid of it again by using her home unit. A second follow up some months later revealed that she had done just that.

Bibliography

Adler, G., et al., 1999. Reduced Hypothalamic-Pituitary and Sympathoadrenal Responses to Hypoglycemia in Women with Fibromyalgia Syndrome. American Journal of Medicine May.

Baker, Sidney, M.D., 1997. Detoxification and healing: The key to optimal health. Keats Publishing, New Canan, CT.

Bennett, G.J., 1994. Melzak, Wall, (Eds.), *Neuropathic Pain*: Textbook of Pain. 3rd edition Churchill-Livingstone, London, pp. 201–224.

Bennett, R.M., 1999. Emerging concepts in the neurobiology of chronic pain: evidence of abnormal sensory processing in Fibromyalgia. Mayo Clinic Proceedings 74, 385–398.

Bennett, R.M., et al., 1997. Hypothalamic – pituitary- insulin like growth factor-I axis dysfunction in patients with Fibromyalgia. J. of Rheumatology 24, 1384–1389.

Bendtsen, L., 1998. Evidence of qualitatively altered nociception in patients with fibromyalgia. Arthritis and Rheumatism 41, 1966–1971.

Bogduk, N., 1988. The innervation of the cervical intervertebral discs. SPINE 13, 2–8.

Bohlman, H., 1979. Acute fractures and dislocations of the cervical spine. Journal of Bone and Joint Surgery 61A, 1119–1142.

Busklla, D., Neuman, L., Valsberg, G., Alkalay, D., Wolfe, F., 1997. Increased rates of fibromyalgia following cervical spine injury: a controlled study of 161 cases of traumatic injury. Arthritis and Rheumatism 40, 446–452.

Cavanaugh, J.M., Ozaktay, A.C., Yamashita, T., Avramov, A., Getchell, T.V., King, A.I., 1997. Mechanisms of low back pain. Clinical Orthopedics 335, 166–180.

Chen, C., Cavanaugh, J.M., Ozaktay, A.C., Kallakuri, S., King, A.I., 1997.

Effects of phospholipase A_2 on lumbar nerve root structure and function. SPINE 22, 1057–1064.

Cloward, R.B., 1959. Cervical discography: Mechanisms of neck, shoulder and arm pain. Annals of Surgery 150, 1052–1064.

Crofford, L., 1998. Neuroendocrine abnormalities in Fibromyalgia and related disorders, the American Journal of the Medical Sciences. June 315 (6).

Crofford, L.J., Engleberg, N.C., Demitrack, M.A., 1996. Neurohormonal perturbations in Fibromyalgia. Bailliere's Clin Rheumatol 10, 365–378.

Crofford, L.J., Demitrack, M.A., 1996. Evidence that abnormalities of central neurohormonal systems are key to understanding Fibromyalgia and chronic fatigue syndrome. Rheumatology Disease Clinics of North America 22, 267–284.

Dessein, et al, 1999. Hyposecretion of adrenal androgens and the relation of serum adrenal steroids, serotonin and IgF1 to clinical features in women with Fibromyalgia. Pain 83, 313–319.

Galland, Leo, M.D., 1997. Four Pillars of Healing. Random House, New York, NY.

Guyton, A.C., 1986. Textbook of Medical Physiology. Seventh Edition, WB Saunders Co.

Henley, Jesse Lynn, M.D., Tired of being tired, 2001. Berkley Publishing group. Penguin Putnam, Inc.

Jeffries, William McK., M.D., 1996. Safe uses of Cortisol, 2nd edition Charles Thomas Publisher, Ltd, Springfield, Illinois.

Juhl, J., 1998. Fibromyalgia and the serotonin Pathway. Alternative Medicine Review 3 (5).

Kandel, E., Schwartz, J., 1985. Principles of Neural Science. 2nd edition Elsevier Science Publishing Co., Inc., New York, pp. 331–336.

Lombard, M.C., Larabi, Y., 1983. Electrophysiological study of cervical dorsal horn cells in partially deafferented rats. Advances in Pain research and Therapy. Raven Press, New York, pp. 147–154.

Maes, M., et al., 1998. Increased 24-hour urinary cortisol excretion in patients with PTSD and major depression, but not in patients with fibromyalgia. Acta Psychiatr Scand 98, 328–335.

Marshall, L.L., Trethewie, E.R., Curtain, C.C., 1997. Chemical radiculitis. A clinical, physiological and immunological study. Clinical Orthopedics 129, 61–67.

McCarron, R.F., Wimpee, M.W., Hudkins, P.G., Laros, G.S., 1987. The inflammatory effect of nucleus pulposus: A possible element in the pathogenesis of low back pain. SPINE 12, 760–764.

McMakin, C., 1998. Microcurrent Treatment of Myofascial Pain in the Head, Neck and Face. Topics in Clinical Chiropractic 5 (1), 29–35.

McMakin, C., 2004. Microcurrent therapy: a novel treatment method for chronic low back myofascial pain. Journal of Bodywork and Movement Therapies 8, 143–153.

McMakin, C., Gregory, W., Phillips, T., 2005. Cytokine changes with microcurrent treatment of Fibromyalgia associate with cervical spine trauma. Journal of Bodywork and Movement Therapies 9, 169–176.

Mendel, T., Wink, C.S., 1989. Neural elements in cervical intervertebral discs. Anatomic Record 223, 78A.

Moldofsky, H., Scaribrik, P., England, R., 1975. Musculoskeletal Symptoms and non-REM Sleep Disturbance in Patients with 'Fibrositis' Syndrome and Healthy Subjects. Psychosomatic Medicine. 37, 341–351.

Mountz, J.M., et al., 1995. Fibromyalgia in women: abnormalities of regional cerebral blood flow in the thalamus and the caudate nucleus are associated with low pain thresholds levels. Arthritis Rheum 38, 926–938.

Neeck, G., Riedel, W., 1999. Hormonal Perturbations in Fibromyalgia Syndrome. Annals New York Academy of Sciences.

Netter, F., 1991. Atlas of Human Anatomy. Ciba-Geigy plate 159.

Olmarker, K., Rydevik, B., Nordberg, C., 1993. Autologous nucleus pulposus induces neurophysiologic and histologic changes in porcine cauda equina nerve roots. SPINE 18, 1425–1432.

Olmarker, K., Blomquist, J., Stromberg, J., Nannmark, U., Thomsen, P., Rydevik, B., 1995. Inflammatogenic properties of nucleus pulposus. SPINE 20, 665–669.

Ozaktay, A.C., Cavanaugh, J.M., Blagoev, D.C., 1995. Phospholipase A_2 – induced electrophysiologic and histologic changes in rabbit dorsal lumbar spine tissues. SPINE 20, 2659–2668.

Ozaktay, A.C., Kallakuri, S., Cavanaugh, J.M., 1998. Phospholipase A_2 sensitivity of the dorsal root and dorsal root ganglion. SPINE 23 (12), 1297–1306.

Russel, I.J., Vipraio, G.A., Morgan, W.W., Bowden, C.L., 1986. Is There a Metabolic Basis for the Fibrositis Syndrome. The American Medical Journal. 81, 50–54.

Sapolsky, Robert, 1994. Why zebras don't get ulcers. WH Freeman and Company, New York.

Taylor, J.R., Twomey, L.T., 1993. Acute injuries to cervical joints. An autopsy study of neck pain. SPINE 18 (9), 1115–1122.

Teitelbaum, Jacob, MD, 2001. From Fatigued to Fantastic. Penguin Putnam, Inc New York, NY.

Treating shingles and oral and genital herpes

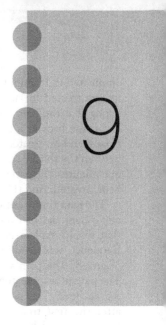

Shingles

Shingles is an infection of a dermatomal or cranial nerve by the herpes zoster virus. The herpes virus establishes a latent infection in the nerve that lasts for the life of the host and may become active at times of stress or immune system compromise (Steiner 2007). The pain usually begins during the viral prodrome and can last up to 3 weeks before red raised lesions and blisters break out along the course of the nerve. Herpes simplex virus 1 (HSV1) is part of the same family of viruses and causes "cold sores" or lesions around the mouth. Herpes simplex virus (HSV2) lies dormant in the genitals and causes recurrent outbreaks of lesions in the genital or anal area. All are related to the varicella or chickenpox virus and the Epstein–Barr virus is included in this class of viruses (Liu 2006).

Herpes zoster, or shingles, is caused by the varicella zoster virus (VZV) and may be found in individuals of any age. It is more common in immunocompromised HIV-AIDS patients and bone marrow transplant recipients and in the elderly who have an 8–10-fold increase of incidence compared to those under age 60, presumably due to reduction of T-cell mediated immunity seen with aging. Diabetes mellitus, surgery, spinal anesthesia, malignancies, and conditions associated with immune suppression such as steroid therapy, and immune-suppressive agents serve as predisposing factors and triggers for the appearance of VZV or shingles (Steiner 2007).

One frequency has been found to treat shingles and both oral and genital herpes. The frequencies, 230 Hz on channel A and 430 Hz on channel B, were discovered among Dr. Van Gelder's papers with the general description of being useful for viruses. When a patient came in with oral herpes in 1997 requesting treatment the frequency was used to determine if it would reduce the pain or change the normal course of the infection. The patient's pain was gone within 20 minutes although the treatment continued for an hour. The pain never returned and the blisters were gone the next day. The following week another patient presented with oral herpes and had the same response but it took two treatments in two days to achieve a permanent result. In subsequent years numerous patients with genital herpes and oral herpes have both responded in exactly the same fashion. Neither frequency by itself creates this effect; both frequencies must be used as a combination delivered simultaneously.

The following month a patient presented with symptoms of nerve pain but no mechanism of injury that would create nerve pain. He stated that he woke up in pain and had no idea what he had done to cause it. When the protocols for inflammation in the nerve did not reduce the patient's nerve pain, the frequency that had reduced the oral herpes virus was used on the chance that the frequency might be useful for the herpes virus in general and that the real cause of the pain might be shingles. The nerve pain started dropping immediately, was eliminated in 15 minutes, and the patient was treated for 60 minutes because he was sleeping and seemed too peaceful to be disturbed. He called the next day saying that the pain stayed down for about 8 hours and gradually returned but at a lesser level. He requested another treatment. He had the same response. The pain was

DOI: 10.1016/B978-0-443-06976-5.00009-5

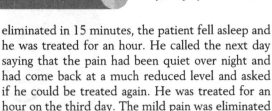

eliminated in 15 minutes, the patient fell asleep and he was treated for an hour. He called the next day saying that the pain had been quiet over night and had come back at a much reduced level and asked if he could be treated again. He was treated for an hour on the third day. The mild pain was eliminated in 5 minutes; the patient fell asleep for an hour while being treated. And this time the pain did not return.

The next time a patient came in with dermatomal nerve pain and had no history of injury or activity that would explain nerve pain the shingles/herpes frequency was used and the exact same response occurred. The pain was eliminated in 15 minutes. The patient was treated for an hour because he slept for an hour. The pain relief lasted about 6 hours after the first treatment, overnight at the second treatment, and became permanent after the third treatment. The pain returned at a much reduced level each time it was treated. One hour of treatment three days in a row prevented the blisters from breaking out and aborted the attack of what was presumed to be shingles in the prodrome.

If the vesicles of shingles have already appeared as either a rash or as blisters along the course of the nerve root the same frequency, 230 / 430, and treatment protocol are effective but the effect is not as dramatic. The pain is eliminated within 30 minutes and 3 hours of treatment within 3 days dries up the blisters, reduces the pain when it reoccurs and shortens the course from approximately 4 weeks to 3–5 days. The protocol has been modified by some practitioners to treat with 230 / 430 for 2 hours on one day only and the results have been similar. Pain is eliminated; blisters dry up and rash disappears in 3–5 days. No cases of post-herpetic neuralgia have been reported following treatment with FSM for shingles. Some practitioners have used this frequency to treat the aching and fatigue caused by recurrent episodes of Epstein–Barr virus.

This frequency combination is and has been so effective that it has been used to make a tentative diagnosis. The frequencies for reducing inflammation in the nerve (40 / 396) that are effective in dermatomal nerve pain will not reduce nerve pain caused by the herpes virus and may actually increase herpes generated pain. If this frequency, 230 / 430, takes away dermatomal nerve pain, or burning pain at the mouth or genitals then it is almost certain that the pain is being caused by one of the family of herpes viruses. There are hundreds of case reports describing positive effects from FSM practitioners around the US, the UK and Australia. The patients are always blinded to the frequency being used. No other frequency combination has been found that creates this effect. No patients with symptoms related to this virus have been found who do not respond to it. Controlled trials have been designed but none have been funded or carried out.

The immediate pain reduction and lasting pain relief suggest that something is happening to interfere with either viral structure or replication. The mechanism for this effect is unknown. Several mechanisms have been proposed but none have been tested. The herpes family of DNA viruses has a double stranded DNA molecule located within an icosapentahedral capsid surrounded by an amorphous protein material which is in turn encapsulated by an envelope that consists of polyamines, lipids and glycoproteins. The glycoproteins give the virus its distinctive properties and provide the antigens to which the host immune system can respond (Steiner 2007).

It is possible that some part of the viral capsid, the crystalline structure of the viral polymerases or the glycoprotein envelope, resonates at the frequencies created by 230Hz and 430Hz in an interferential field and is disrupted by the resonance. The frequencies found in the interferential field created by 230Hz and 430Hz would include coherent frequencies of 230Hz, 430Hz, 660Hz, and 200Hz. Any or all of these frequencies may participate in the observed clinical effect. When the frequency combination encounters the viral structure it is possible that it resonates with either the capsid membrane or glycoproteins in such a way as to dismantle it or change its structure in such a way that it cannot maintain its relationship with the nerve. It is also possible that the frequency resonates with the nerve in such a way that it makes viral attachment impossible, releases the virus into the circulation and makes it available to be dismantled by the immune system. This mechanism seems less likely because of the speed of pain relief and the length of pain reduction but it is possible.

Post-herpetic neuralgia (PHN) is more difficult to treat and does not respond to the protocols for shingles. The virus is gone within weeks of the active infection and the neuralgia may be caused by viral damage to the nerve. The treatment for PHN is focused on inflammation, calcium influx into the nerve and scar tissue between the nerve and the surrounding fascia, and reduction of central amplification created by deafferentation of the peripheral nerve. Thoracic nerve roots have sympathetic involvement which complicates PHN symptoms and treatment. The protocols for neuropathic pain discussed in Chapter 3 may be useful in PHN but it can be challenging to treat.

Shingles diagnosis

Shingles should be suspected when the history includes moderate dermatomal pain in any nerve root or pain in the head and scalp with no mechanism of injury that would account for it. Patients may rationalize the cause of the pain as being from some unusual activity such as working in the garden or carrying and lifting suitcases or "turning the wrong way". However, the pain is generally more severe than would be reasonable for any injury that would have been caused by some trivial activity.

For example a recreational weight-lifter thought he had a severely painful shoulder injury from lifting 40-pound suitcases because he woke up in pain after flying to his vacation destination and carrying the suitcases in the airport. It is not reasonable for someone who can repeatedly lift 180 pounds over his head to have level 7/10 pain created by lifting a 40-pound suitcase twice in one day. In this example, a sensory examination with a pin wheel revealed nerve hyperesthesia in the C4 and C5 dermatomes located on the shoulder. A simple sensory examination for sharp performed with a pin, a pinwheel or a sharp object like a paper clip will show the nerve to be irritated, hypersensitive and painful. If the history does not include a mechanism of injury for the disc or a traction injury that seems reasonable, then a treatment trial of 15 minutes with 230 / 430 can be used to confirm the suspicion. The treatment has been found to be effective enough that it may be used for differential diagnosis. If 230 / 430, the frequency for shingles and herpes virus, takes the pain away then the pain is caused by shingles until proven otherwise. The frequency is not useful for any other condition.

The majority of shingles cases in the elderly occur in thoracic nerve roots although any dorsal root ganglion may be involved (Bradley 2000). Thoracic nerve pain may present as abdominal pain or chest pain and may be mistaken for pain of visceral origin. A sensory examination for skin hyperesthesia, the first sign of nerve irritability, is a simple way to determine neural involvement and may avoid expensive and invasive diagnostic testing aimed at discovering a visceral cause for the pain.

Patients who have a history of oral or genital herpes are usually aware of the sensations experienced in the prodrome. These are usually described as burning or itching and there will be some local redness and swelling in the skin over the impending vesicle. If the diagnosis is uncertain, it may be prudent to wait for the lesion to erupt and culture it to determine if it is bacterial or viral or a 30-minute treatment trial with 230 / 430 can be done. After 10 years experience using this frequency in hundreds of clinical settings in several countries, it has been said that if the lesion is caused by the herpes virus treatment with 230 / 430 will change the pain and the course. If the frequency doesn't relieve the pain then a culture or reassessment is required to determine the source of the lesion.

Physical examination

Perform a sensory examination with a pin, pinwheel or a sharp object such as a paper clip. The sensory exam will show hyperesthesia in one or more dermatomes. Shingles should be considered and ruled out by doing a simple sensory examination any time there is moderate pain on the limbs, trunk, abdomen or head.

> ### Hydration
>
> - The patient must be hydrated to benefit from microcurrent treatment.
> - Hydrated means 1 to 2 quarts of water consumed in the 2 to 4 hours preceding treatment.
> - Athletes and patients with more muscle mass seem to need more water than the average patient.
> - The elderly tend to be chronically dehydrated and may need to hydrate for several days prior to treatment in addition to the water consumed on the day of treatment.
> - *DO NOT* accept the statement, "I drink lots of water".
> - *ASK* "How much water, and in what form, did you drink today before you came in?".
> - Coffee, caffeinated tea, carbonated cola beverages do not count as water.
> - Water may be flavored with juice or decaffeinated tea.

Treating shingles

A/B pair for shingles and herpes

230 / 430

The frequency for shingles is an A/B pair. The channel A frequency is not a condition and the B frequency is not a tissue. The frequency pattern created by 230Hz on A and 430Hz on B has the desired clinical effect.

Application

- **Current level:** 100–300µamps. Use lower current levels for very small or debilitated patients. Use higher current levels for larger or very muscular patients. In general higher current levels reduce pain more quickly. Do not use more than 500µamps as animal studies suggest that current levels above 500µamps reduce ATP formation while current levels below 500µamps increase ATP.
- **± Alternating or Biphasic Current:** Current is used in alternating mode for treatment of shingles and herpes. "Alternating DC current" is actually DC (direct) current that alternates its polarity from positive to negative during the machine duty cycle.

Waveslope

- Use a moderate to gentle waveslope.
- The waveslope refers to the rate of increase of current in the wave as it rises in alternating mode from zero up to the treatment current level every 2.5 seconds on the Precision Microcurrent. Other microcurrent instruments may have slightly different duty cycles and the waveform may change more or less frequently. A sharp waveslope has a very steep leading edge on the waveform, indicating a very sharp increase in current. A gentle waveslope has a very gradual leading edge on the waveform, indicating a gradual increase in current.
- Use a moderate to sharp waveslope for chronic pain. Use a gentle waveslope for acute pain or new injuries. A sharp waveslope is irritating in new injuries. Different microcurrent devices may provide different wave shapes and waveslopes but the reader may find them to be equivalent.

Technique

This is unattended treatment. There is no manual technique involved. Position the patient; position the contacts as described, set the frequency and turn on the unit; stay for a few minutes to ensure that the current is conducting and as soon as the patient relaxes and the pain begins to fall the practitioner may leave the room. Someone should check on the patient occasionally during the 1–2-hour treatment time. The patient may fall asleep and should be positioned comfortably and safely for this predictable response.

Lead placement for shingles

- Place the positive leads from channel A and channel B at the spine or in a warm wet contact that wraps the spine where the involved nerve roots exits.
- Place negative leads from channel A and channel B at the end of the involved nerve root.
- FSM typically uses graphite gloves to conduct the current. The graphite gloves need to be kept moist so they conduct the current comfortably. The contact for nerve treatment needs to wrap around the outflow of the nerve root as it exits from the spine. The graphite gloves, bare leads or alligator clips on leads can be placed in small warm wet towels or fabric sleeves.
- The positive leads in wet fabric contacts can cover a larger area and allow a broad contact around the neck or along the spine at the exiting nerve root.
- The negative leads wrap around the end of the dermatome being treated.

NOTE: The treatment is more effective if the negative lead is placed precisely at the end of the affected nerve root so it provides optimal current density. For example if the virus affects the C4 and C5 nerve root the positive contacts should wrap the spine and the negative contacts should wrap the upper arm just above the elbow.

- For the C2 nerve root place the positive leads in a wet contact around the neck and place the negative leads in a wet contact at the top of the head along a line between the ears.
- For the ophthalmic branch of Cranial V place one glove in a wet contact around the neck and the other glove in a wet contact placed from a line just behind the ears across the top of the head to the eye. Care should be taken not to let the contact touch the eye itself but it can be placed over the closed eyelid.
- For a patient who develops a headache or has shingles pain in multiple dermatomes there is reason to suspect spinal cord involvement. Place the red leads in a wet contact around the neck and the black leads in a wet contact around the feet or at the waist.

PRECAUTION: Herpes simplex encephalitis (HSE) is a very serious form of herpes infection with serious consequences and sequellae. HSE is a medical emergency and the prognosis is dependent on early initiation of treatment. If HSE is suspected due to headache, the presence of fever, personality changes, confusion, disorientation, seizures or focal neurological signs such as hemiparesis, oral antiviral therapy and medically appropriate supportive measures should be instituted without delay.

FSM may be of benefit in these cases as an adjunct but its use must not delay appropriate conventional therapy in this serious condition. If medical treatment or diagnostic measures are not available for some unavoidable reason then FSM may be used as sole temporary treatment if and only if no other treatment is available and only until such time as appropriate treatment becomes available.

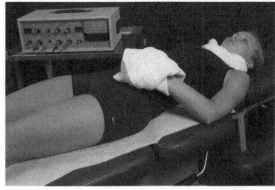

Figure 9.2 • Place the positive leads graphite glove wrapped in a warm wet fabric contact that is wrapped around the neck. Place the negative leads graphite glove in a warm wet fabric contact (hand towel) that is wrapped at the end of the involved nerve root, in this case the C6, C7 and C8 nerve roots.

See the placement as shown in the photographs (Figs 9.1 to 9.9).

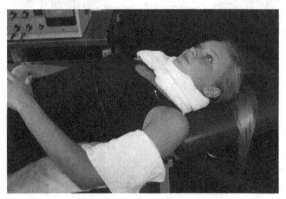

Figure 9.1 • Place the positive leads graphite glove wrapped in a warm wet fabric contact that is wrapped around the neck. Place the negative leads graphite glove in a warm wet fabric contact (hand towel) that is wrapped at the end of the involved nerve root, in this case the C4 and C5 dermatomes.

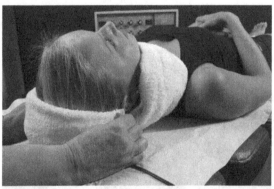

Figure 9.3 • Place the positive leads graphite glove wrapped in a warm wet fabric contact that is wrapped around the neck. Place the negative leads graphite glove wrapped in a warm wet fabric contact (face cloth) at the end of the C2 dermatome. The wet face cloth must make contact with the skin. This usually involves parting the hair and watching the machine to ensure that current is flowing. The contact may be propped, wrapped or clipped in place but occasionally it needs to be held by someone for the length of the treatment to make sure that it maintains conductivity.

Treatment time

Treat for 60 minutes on the first treatment and for each of the two subsequent treatments. Some practitioners use a single 2-hour treatment. Shorter treatments are not effective.

• **Prodrome:** If diagnosis is made early and treatment begins in the shingles prodrome, pain reduction begins within 10–20 minutes. Pain will return at a lower level about 6–12 hours after the first treatment. One hour of treatment on three consecutive days should abort the attack and the blisters should not appear.

• **Active infection:** If the patient is past the prodrome and the blisters or rash are already

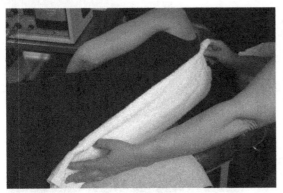

Figure 9.4 • Place the positive leads graphite glove wrapped in a warm wet fabric contact (hand towel) that is placed lengthwise under the patient's thoracic spine. Alligator clips may also be attached to the fabric contact as shown in Chapter 11. The treatment will last for 1–2 hours and the patient is more likely to be comfortable lying supine but may be treated in any comfortable position. Some patients have been treated while sitting in a recliner chair.

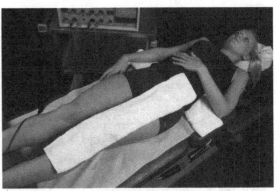

Figure 9.6 • Place the positive leads graphite glove or two leads attached with alligator clips to a warm wet fabric contact placed under the patient's low back making sure that it contacts the spine at T12 through L4. Place the negative leads graphite glove in a warm wet fabric contact (hand towel) that is laid lengthwise from L1 on the abdomen to L3 at the knee.

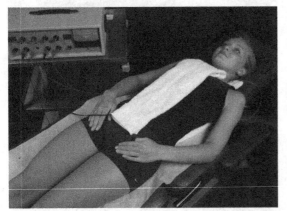

Figure 9.5 • Place the negative leads graphite glove wrapped in a warm wet fabric contact (hand towel) that is placed lengthwise down the trunk from collar bone to pubic bone. This allows treatment of several nerve roots simultaneously. The patient may be treated prone, supine or seated as long as the contact maintains good conductivity with the skin.

present, treatment should reduce or eliminate the pain in approximately 20 minutes but it may take as long as 60 minutes. Treat the patient for 60 minutes a day for 3 days or for as many days as necessary for the pain relief to become permanent. In general the blisters will scab over and the typical 6-week shingles course will be shortened to 3–5 days.

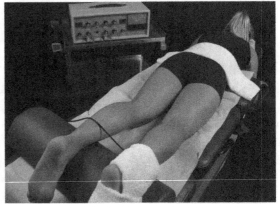

Figure 9.7 • Place the positive leads graphite glove or two leads attached with alligator clips to a warm wet fabric contact placed under the patient's low back making sure that it contacts the spine at L3 through S2. Place the negative leads graphite glove in a warm wet fabric contact (hand towel) that is wrapped around the distal leg and foot to provide current flow to all of the involved dermatomes. This patient is shown being treated prone but may be more comfortable positioned supine since they will be in this position for as much as 2 hours. If the patient has facet syndrome they most certainly cannot lay prone and must be positioned supine with the knees up and back flat. Disc patients may prefer lying prone. Patients are often treated in a recliner chair so they can be positioned comfortably and safely while they sleep for the 2-hour treatment.

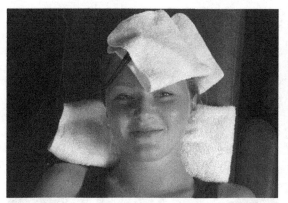

Figure 9.8 • Place the positive leads graphite glove in a warm wet contact that is under the patient's neck at the suboccipitals and mastoid process. Place the negative leads glove wrapped in a warm wet contact along the path of the ophthalmic branch of Cranial V, from a line just behind the ears across the top of the head to the eye. Care should be taken not to let the contact touch the eye itself but it can be placed over the closed eyelid.

Maintaining skin contact and conductivity in patients who have short hair is easy. Maintaining skin contact and conductivity in patients with longer hair takes more effort. The contacts need to be very wet instead of being well wrung out; the hair needs to be parted so the fabric is in direct contact with the scalp and the hair may even need to be wet to ensure adequate conductivity. Check conductivity indicators to ensure that current is flowing before leaving the patient unattended. The set up can be a bit messy and wet but the outcome is well worth the inconvenience.

Shingles case report

The patient was an 85-year-old male whose scalp rash had been diagnosed as actinic keratosis by his dermatologist one week previous to his visit to the chiropractor's office. The medication for the actinic keratosis was not helping his scalp pain and seemed in fact to be making it worse. The patient presented requesting FSM treatment for his scalp pain. Based on the diagnosis of actinic keratosis, the FSM treatment was directed at reducing inflammation in the skin and scalp with one contact on the back of the neck and one contact in a wet cloth on the top of the head covering the rash and the frequency was set at 40Hz on channel A and 116Hz on channel B. After 5 minutes the treatment to "reduce inflammation" caused the patient to complain that the cloth conducting the current on the scalp was too rough and irritating to the skin and seemed to be worsening

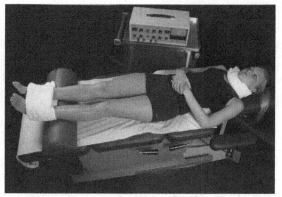

Figure 9.9 • This rare shingles distribution has only been seen once in the author's practice but this contact placement was effective in reducing pain and eliminating the blisters after three treatments in a 3-day period. Place the positive leads graphite glove or electrodes in alligator clips in a warm wet fabric contact (hand towel) that is wrapped around the neck. Place the negative leads graphite glove or electrode in alligator clips in a warm wet fabric contact (hand towel) wrapped around the patient's feet.

the pain. In general, the body uses inflammation to fight infection and a treatment whose purpose is to reduce inflammation will only make the pain worse if there is infection present.

Based on the report of increasing pain, the practitioner reassessed the location of the rash, considered the patient's age and general frail health, dismissed the dermatologist's diagnosis and changed the diagnosis to shingles in the ophthalmic branch of the fifth cranial nerve (V). The frequency was changed to 230Hz on channel A and 430Hz on channel B but no change was made to the position of the contacts or the current level. The pain stopped worsening, began to diminish within 10 minutes and after 30 minutes the patient was pain free. Treatment was continued for 90 minutes on the first day. The patient returned for one 60-minute treatment on each of the next two days but he was pain free after the first treatment. On the second day he reported that his eye "felt funny" although there was no change in vision. The scalp contact was moved forward until it covered the closed eyelid and the patient reported that the funny feeling was gone within 20 minutes. The eye symptoms did not return and the contacts were moved back from the eyelid to cover the scalp only for the third treatment. By the third day, the rash assumed the appearance of scabs sprinkled over the distribution of the ophthalmic branch of V and the scabs resolved with no further pain within 5 days.

Oral and genital herpes

Treatment protocol for oral and genital herpes

A/B pair for herpes

230 / 430
The frequency for the herpes virus is an A/B pair. The channel A frequency is not a condition and the B frequency is not a tissue. The frequency pattern created by 230Hz on A and 430Hz on B has the desired clinical effect. It appears to be effective against this entire class of viruses.

Application
- Current levels, biphasic polarity and waveslope are the same as for shingles.

Lead placement:
- **Oral herpes:** Place one graphite glove or electrode contact in a wet washcloth or small piece of fabric over the mouth. The fabric should be thoroughly wet but wrung out so it is not dripping. Place the other contact under the upper thoracic spine or behind the neck.
- **Genital herpes:** Place one graphite glove or electrode contact in a warm wet cloth under the sacrum and low back. Place the other graphite glove or electrode contact in a warm wet washcloth or small piece of fabric and place it over the vulva or genitals draping it from the pubic bone as far posterior as necessary. Include the anus if the lesions extend that far or if the history suggests that area may be infected. The fabric should be thoroughly wet but wrung out so it is not dripping.

Precaution: Treatment with this frequency has so far been universally effective at alleviating pain and skin lesions in both shingles and herpes; however, no controlled trials have been performed at this time and there is no information about its effect on viral shedding. Common sense and appropriate risk assessment should be applied to each individual case and the practitioner should decide whether to prescribe accepted oral antiviral medications in at-risk patients and use FSM treatment as an adjunct for pain management and to shorten the course of the infection on a case by case basis. FSM may be helpful in treating patients with renal problems who are not good candidates for antiviral therapy.

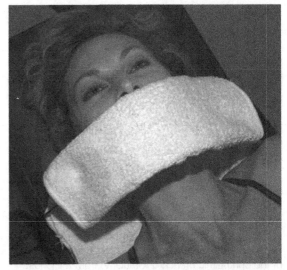

Figure 9.10 • Oral herpes: Place the positive leads graphite glove or electrode alligator clip contact in a wet wash cloth or small piece of fabric under the upper thoracic spine or behind the neck. Place the negative leads contact over the mouth. The fabric should be thoroughly wet but wrung out so it is not dripping.

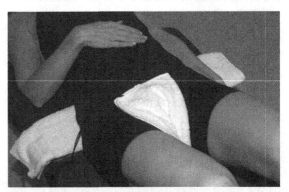

Figure 9.11 • Place the positive leads graphite glove or electrode alligator clip contact in a warm wet cloth under the sacrum and low back. Place the negative leads graphite glove or electrode alligator clip contact in a warm wet washcloth or small piece of fabric and place it over the vulva or genitals, draping it from the pubic bone as far posterior as necessary. Include the anus if the lesions extend that far or if the history suggests that area may be infected. The fabric should be thoroughly wet but wrung out so it is not dripping.

Oral herpes case report

The patient was a 27-year-old woman who presented with a severe outbreak of oral herpes. There were lesions visible encircling her mouth and covering most of the mucosal surfaces inside her mouth. She had pain with swallowing suggesting that there were lesions in her throat. She had a slight fever of 101 degrees Fahrenheit. She had a history of oral herpes but had never before had an attack this severe.

She was treated with microcurrent set at 230Hz on channel A and 430Hz on channel B. The graphite gloves were placed in a warm wet washcloth that was placed over her mouth as she lay supine. The other graphite glove was placed under her neck. The current level was set at 100µamps and the waveslope was set at moderate (5/10). The pain began to decline within 10 minutes and the patient fell asleep. She had the time and the treatment room she occupied was not needed and so she was allowed to sleep until she awoke 3 hours later.

At the end of the 3-hour treatment half of the blisters in her mouth had resolved, her throat was no longer sore, her temperature was normal and she was pain free. The rest of the lesions resolved with no further treatment by the next day. There has never been another case treated for this length of time but this isolated case is intriguing. It may be that 3 hours initial treatment may be sufficient to resolve shingles as well instead of 3 hours spread over three consecutive days.

Post-herpetic neuralgia

Post-herpetic neuralgia (PHN) is the most common neurological complication of herpes zoster. PHN is defined as pain in the distribution of the rash which persists beyond 4–6 weeks following shingles infection. The risk for PHN increases with age and almost half of patients over age 60 will develop PHN following the acute infection. The pain involves the affected nerve root; the constant pain is described as severe, burning, and stabbing and can be so disturbing as to lead to severe depression. PHN is said to be the leading cause of suicide in patients over the age of 65. The mechanisms behind PHN are not clear and there is speculation that it may be due to persistent viral infection in the dorsal root ganglia (DRG), structural damage to the DRG or the nerve following viral infection, or central mechanisms including long-term enhancement in synaptic excitability in the brain and the spinal cord or changes in the control mechanisms that allow both spinal cord and central sensitization.

Treating PHN requires a different strategy and is much more difficult than treating the acute phase of shingles but has been accomplished successfully often enough that treatment should be attempted. The treatment would be similar to that for chronic nerve pain with adhesions and central sensitization and is found in Chapter 3. The information required for a comprehensive treatment of this topic is beyond the scope of this book.

Bibliography

Bradley, W.G., Darhoff, R.B., Fenichel, G.M., Marsden, C.D., 2000. Neurology in clinical practice, third ed. Butterworth Heinemann, Boston.

Liu, S., Knafels, J.D., Chang, J.S., et al., 2006. Crystal structure of the herpes simplex virus 1 DNA polymerase. J. Biol. Chem. 281, 18193–18200.

Steiner, I., Kennedy, P.G., Pachner, A.R., 2007. The neurotropic herpes viruses: herpes simplex and varicella-zoster. Lancet Neurol. 6, 1015–1028.

Treating concussion, central pain and emotions

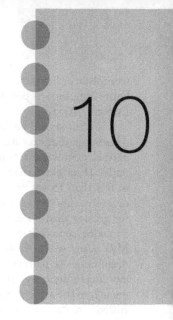

The term concussion as used in this chapter refers to two quite different concepts of "concussion". The first is the concept of a medically diagnosed concussion also called a traumatic brain injury (TBI) or closed head injury and is defined as an alteration in mental status, with or without loss of consciousness, accompanied by a brief period of amnesia after a blow to the head. The second, more subtle, concept means any shock or trauma to the system that has a direct or indirect impact on the medulla or brain stem.

A traumatic brain injury (TBI) is associated with loss of consciousness, post-traumatic amnesia in which the patient cannot remember the events leading up to the trauma for periods up to several days and focal neurological signs (de Kruijk 2002). A mild traumatic brain injury (mTBI), the most common form of concussion, is usually defined as one in which loss of consciousness (LOC) is less than 30 minutes and the Glasgow Coma Scale (GCS) score is more than 13 at the time of injury. A GCS score of 3 signifies deep coma and a GCS score of 15 signifies a fully alert and oriented patient spontaneously conversing and following commands. In an mTBI, the patient may have incomplete memory of the traumatic event and post-traumatic amnesia (PTA) of less than 24 hours and may have been dazed and confused at the scene without loss of consciousness. An example would be the driver of the target vehicle in a rear end accident who does not remember the sound of the impact or who does not remember anything between the time she saw the impact vehicle approaching and the time several minutes later when the police officer arrived at the car window (McCrea 2002, McAllister 2002, Ropper 2007, Ryan 2003).

Both TBI and mTBI are associated with post-concussive symptoms of cognitive, emotional and behavioral disturbances that can persist for months or years after the injury. These symptoms include headache, difficulties with attention, concentration and memory and the sequencing and processing of information, problems with mood including irritability, aggression and emotional lability, sleep disturbance, fatigue, dizziness and perhaps photophobia, hyperacussis or nausea although these tend to be more problematic immediately after the injury.

Incidence of traumatic brain injuries

There are 1.5 million traumatic brain injuries affecting 128 people per 100,000 in the United States every year and even though 85% are considered mild they result in significant disability and unemployment due to the cognitive, psychological and social dysfunction they cause (Ropper 2007). Sports and bicycle accidents account for the majority of cases among 5–14-year-olds and falls and motor vehicle accidents are the most common cause of concussion in adults. Post-concussive syndrome or post-concussive symptoms (PCS) refer to a constellation of signs and symptoms that may be reported after a TBI of any severity. Post-concussive symptoms affect up to 50% of mTBI patients at one month and 15–25% at one year. Some post-concussive patients never return to their pre-morbid function (Alves 1993, Middelboe 1992). Litigation and compensation factors involved in injuries sustained in the

DOI: 10.1016/B978-0-443-06976-5.00010-1

workplace or in auto accidents are thought to affect both symptom reporting and rates of recovery (Mooney 2005).

CT scans should be done to evaluate the need for neurosurgical intervention, even in the presence of a normal neurological examination, if the patient is under 16 or older than 65 years of age, has a GCS of less than 15 within 2 hours after the injury, two or more episodes of vomiting, retrograde amnesia for greater than 30 minutes prior to the trauma or is taking anticoagulants (Ropper 2007). CT and MRI scans while easily available and adequate to diagnose gross pathology such as hematoma, frank swelling or depressed skull fracture are not sensitive enough to show the subtle reductions in cortical perfusion, frontal and temporal hypometabolism and diffuse axonal injuries that have been demonstrated on PET or SPECT in mTBI patients with persistent PCS. Several studies have demonstrated abnormal frontal and temporal lobe activity with PET and SPECT scans in TBI/PCS patients whose CT and MRI scans were normal (Gross 1996, Ruff 1994, Humayun 1989, McCrea 2008).

Pathologies associated with TBI

Multifocal axonal injuries, increased permeability of the axonal membrane due to inflammation and activation of the glial system, disruption of axonal neurofilaments leading to disruption of axoplasmic flow and secondary axonal deafferentation in the areas of the brain served by the damaged axons have been observed after mild brain trauma in both human and animal studies (Oppenheimer 1968, Blumbergs 1994). Human postmortem studies have shown loss of cortical cholinergic afferents that would account for dysfunction in hippocampal cholinergic neurons and the resulting symptoms of memory loss and difficulty with information processing (Dixon 1994, Saija 1988, Murdoch 1998, Dewar 1996). Even mild brain injury has been shown to produce evidence of diffuse axonal injuries (Povlishock 1989, 1992, 1995). Sleep disturbances common in TBI patients are thought to be produced by injury to the reticular activating system that regulates sleep–wake cycles.

Imbalance, disequilibrium, particular problems with task sequencing, vision dependent balance and panic attacks during sleep or in visually complex settings may reflect damage to the endolymphatic system, eighth nerve or the vestibular apparatus in the inner ear. Damage to the inner ear can greatly confound and complicate PCS symptoms because some of the symptoms overlap but the diagnosis and successful treatments are completely different.

There are no universally effective treatments for post-concussive symptoms (Bazarian 2005). Tincture of time produces some recovery of function. Cognitive behavioral counseling for patients and their families at the time of the injury helps patients deal with the deficits, creates realistic expectations and reduces anxiety about symptoms. Medications and various strategies are used to modify post-concussive symptoms.

Complaints of sleep disturbance seen in 30–70% of TBI patients are particularly difficult to manage because medications for sleep disturbance such as the benzodiazepines and other sedative hypnotics mimic or exacerbate the post-concussive complaints of fatigue and cognitive dysfunction. But the sleep deprivation itself may exacerbate the post-concussive symptoms of cognitive dysfunction, fatigue, irritability and anxiety. Non-pharmacologic interventions such as the teaching and reinforcement of sleep hygiene and relaxation training promote functional recovery. The use of low dose anti-convulsant medication at night may be the best choice for medical management since it can address multiple symptoms of sleep disturbance, headache and chronic neck pain.

Dysfunction in the cholinergic, catecholaminergic and dopaminergic neurotransmitters may all contribute to cognitive impairment. It is clear that disruption in cortical cholinergic function is a primary source of cognitive dysfunction but some patients respond best to cholinesterase inhibitors and others to psychostimulants that increase catecholamine levels. Both classes of medications are intended to improve attention and working memory although it is advisable to start with low doses and titrate up in small increments (McAllister 2002).

In spite of these strategies symptoms from TBI persist for years following even mild head trauma and create significant disability. In 1999 the National Institutes of Health declared mTBI and post-concussive sequelae to be a major public health problem (NIH 1999).

Van Gelder's concussion model

The second concept of concussion is particular to one physician, a Dutch osteopath and naturopath from Australia who trained in England in the 1930s and came to practice in Vancouver, British Columbia in 1946 (Van Gelder 1985, 1989). Harry Van Gelder was mentioned in Chapter 1 of this text and it is he who bought the practice that came with the 1920s machine that came with the list of frequencies that allowed him to treat a multitude of physical conditions and complaints successfully using electromagnetic resonance along with other therapies. Although somewhat eccentric, Harry Van Gelder was beloved and acknowledged by those he treated as being superbly effective and skilled as a diagnostician and healer. He developed a more subtle concept of "concussion" to mean any shock or trauma to the system that had an impact on the medulla or brain stem. Van Gelder's skill, reputation and clinical outcomes lead to the consideration of this more subtle condition as a treatment focus.

Functions of the medulla

The medulla is located at the base of the brain and carries the ascending and descending tracts that connect the brain with the spinal cord. The medulla also gives rise to cranial nerve X, the vagus nerve. The vagus influences every vegetative function including, but not limited to, respiration and bronchodilation, heart rate and blood pressure and digestion through its regulation of the esophagus, stomach, small intestine, gall bladder, and the secretions of the pancreas and stomach. It contributes to immune system regulation by regulating secretions in the thymus. It supplies the motor parasympathetic functions of all of the viscera except the adrenal glands.

In Van Gelder's model of injury and illness, trauma to the medulla made it function inefficiently and created dysfunction in all of the vegetative systems including the immune system, the cardiovascular system and the digestive system. The trauma to the medulla also created dysfunction in the pituitary and the endocrine organs it regulates by changing regulatory impulses in the fibers that connect the medulla to the pituitary.

The trauma to the medulla could be physical and caused by a fall, a blow to the head or any sort of physical injury that stretched or stressed the neck and brainstem. The trauma could be from emotional shock producing a flood of impulses from the viscera pouring into the medulla via the vagus. The medulla effectively becomes overloaded by overwhelming input rather like a circuit breaker that switches off during a power surge causing the system to function less effectively. The trauma could be from "chill" or any sort of event such as infection, exhaustion or toxic exposure that shocks the viscera creating a flood of impulses from the viscera through the vagus to the medulla causing it to "switch" into something like a "safe mode". The vagus and the medulla simply function less effectively than they did prior to the trauma. The analogy between a computer or power system and the medulla moving into a less effective but "safe mode" is an apt one. The "safe mode" preserves the most important critical functions and allows for repair and recovery at some later time.

In Van Gelder's model, trauma leads to "paralysis" which leads to "allergy reaction" and reduction in secretions and vitality. "Paralysis" does not refer to a true medical paralysis or complete loss of function. Once again the analogy to the loss of function when a computer "locks up" and loses the ability to move to the next step is most apt. Computers move smoothly from one step to the next because of a continual flow of "do this – then do that" lines of instruction. The computer "locks up" because it has lost the line of code that tells it what to do next and becomes "paralyzed". The frequency to remove "paralysis" is Van Gelder's conceptual equivalent of the computer command "control–alt–delete" that reboots the computer system.

In Van Gelder's system, as well as in our medical understanding of physiology, the body's first response to any dysfunction is to release histamine as a way of starting the inflammatory cascade. The third problem, after "trauma" and "paralysis" that assails the medulla as it moves into "safe mode" is a histamine release or allergy reaction making the medulla less efficient by reducing both secretions and vitality and initiating inflammation as a means of repair and recovery. The loss of efficiency in the immune, digestive and endocrine systems caused by the malfunction in the medulla and vagus leads to a variety of allergy reactions and health issues while the system slowly initiates the repair process.

Treating the "constitutional factors"

Van Gelder became a physician at a time when the concept was developed that genetic factors could be turned off or turned on by life events or exposures predisposing the person to various illnesses. These genetic factors were called "constitutional factors" and probably correspond to what modern genetics

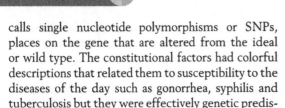

calls single nucleotide polymorphisms or SNPs, places on the gene that are altered from the ideal or wild type. The constitutional factors had colorful descriptions that related them to susceptibility to the diseases of the day such as gonorrhea, syphilis and tuberculosis but they were effectively genetic predispositions to various ailments.

The practicing clinician will be familiar with the relationship between susceptibility to illness and patient family histories even if the concept of constitutional factors is not familiar. If every one of 100 people in a room is exposed to a certain bacterium only a certain percentage will contract the disease while some will fight it off successfully and a few seem not to even notice the exposure. Why is that? Van Gelder would say that the patients who fell ill had the genetic "constitution" that made them susceptible to the bacterium. Modern physicians trained in immunology and genetics would say that the immune systems of the patients who fell ill were less effective in fighting the bacterium because the minute receptors on the lymphocytes were less vigorous in defense. One interpretation of the event is more poetic and the other is more scientifically informed but different susceptibilities to illness are a known fact no matter how one chooses to interpret the causation.

The same patterns become apparent when interpreting patient family histories of illness. Physicians take a family history because it gives clues about what the individual's risk is of contracting certain diseases. One patient will have a family history in which every adult over the age of 40 has diabetes as well as some primary relatives who have asthma and a few with multilevel disc disease and one with sarcoidosis. No one in the family suffers from alcoholism or psoriasis. The genes or SNPs would almost surely be related to inflammation and insulin regulation and the constitutional factor is related to the susceptibility to tuberculosis. Another patient will have a family history replete with stroke, heart disease, degenerative but not rheumatoid arthritis and hypertension but no one has diabetes, psoriasis or psychosis. Another will have psoriasis, eczema, irritable bowel as a personal diagnosis and in the family history but no family history of heart disease or diabetes. Another patient will have a family history replete with alcoholism and psychosis or other mental illnesses but no incidence of diabetes or heart attack. These patterns in family medical history are familiar to every practicing physician whether one chooses to interpret them in the light of modern genetics

or in the light of turn of the century medical practice. Van Gelder's device had one specific frequency that seemed to neutralize all of the constitutional factors.

Using Van Gelder's model

Van Gelder's model of restoring the patient to full function involved clearing "concussion" from the medulla, restoring secretions to the pituitary, turning off constitutional factors and the final step was to restore "vitality" to the system and "balance the energy centers." This model is clearly not part of mainstream medical training or practice and it would be simpler not to teach it as part of an FSM pain treatment program taught to traditionally trained physicians.

A 6-week trial was done in which the "concussion protocol" was not performed on any of the week's 90 patients in order to assess whether it was actually essential to the outcomes achieved. The patients but not the practitioners were blinded to the change in treatment protocol. Within a few weeks it became clear that outcomes, while not quantified, had declined and treatment results were less favorable even when every other therapy and protocol were applied as before. By the end of the 6-week trial the "concussion protocol" was again used on a regular basis and outcomes returned to their normal positive level in the week's 90 patients. Subsequent shorter trials with both the patients and the practitioner blinded produced the same pattern of effect on outcomes.

Van Gelder's reputation as a master physician and healer was the original reason for considering using and teaching his more subtle concussion model. The model continues to be used and taught because it produces results that cannot be achieved if it is not used. It is left to the reader to decide from personal experience whether treatment of this more subtle interpretation of concussion contributes to positive outcomes in pain management.

Concussion protocol treatment outcomes

Treatment for this mild form of "concussion" described by Van Gelder was among the first FSM protocols used in practice. Patients reported improvements in sleep, mood and general wellbeing that were both subtle and profound sometimes years after a mild head injury and even when they could recall no head trauma. Encouraged by these results, FSM was used in patients with post-concussive symptoms from brain trauma, including TBI, mTBI and stroke. One to four treatments produced consistent profound improvements in sleep, mood, cognitive function, information processing, emotional stability and fatigue in hundreds of case reports from over 1000 practitioners after 12 years of use. Only the headache has proven to be somewhat resistant to treatment. In seriously injured patients more than four treatments may be necessary and the improvements may never last for more than a few days if neural tissue has been lost. Significant objective and subjective improvements have been observed in multiple case reports from numerous clinical centers in the US and abroad.

Concussion protocol increases serotonin

The data acquired through micro-immunochromatography demonstrated that the concussion protocol produced a significant but probably temporary increase in serotonin levels. Serotonin decreased during the treatment that reduced pain in fibromyalgia patients (see Chapter 8). When the pain reached 0/10 VAS or had stopped decreasing the protocol was changed and for the next 30 minutes the patient was treated with the "concussion protocol". The patient was blinded to the change in treatment. Serotonin levels dropped during the pain reducing portion of the treatment in every patient treated and rose with use of the concussion protocol from an average of 175.75ng/ml ($\pm$ 40.20) to 244.34ng/ml ($\pm$ 76.05) in each of 16 different patients whose samples were collected during the 2-month test period. The normal range for serotonin is 100–300ng/ml.

The average increase in serotonin in the 30 minutes from the zero VAS time point to the end of the concussion protocol was 68.59 $\pm$ 54.79 for a 39% increase. One patient's serotonin level more than doubled increasing from 155.2 to 337.6ng/ml. The Wilcoxon Signed Ranks Test result was Z = -3.52 p<0.001.

These anecdotal reports give some basis to pursue an organized controlled trial including neuroimaging such as PET and SPECT scans to provide some objective evidence to validate the observed clinical improvement.

Diagnosing concussion

If the patient presents acutely after head trauma, the practitioner should perform whatever neurological examination is within their training and scope of practice. If the patient has not been evaluated in an emergency department, has focal neurological signs, is under 16 years of age or older than 65 years of age, had a GCS of less than 15 within 2 hours after the injury, had two or more episodes of vomiting after the injury, retrograde amnesia for greater than 30 minutes prior to the trauma or is taking anticoagulants, the practitioner should order a CT scan to rule out intracranial lesions or hemorrhage.

The acute signs of concussion may include headache, nausea, photophobia, sleepiness, irritability and mental confusion including problems with word finding, memory and orientation. The acute concussion protocol is described below and would be used in this patient if the CT scan were negative or if the injury was not severe enough to require a CT scan.

Unless the practitioner reading this text is a neurologist it is unlikely that the patient's presenting complaint will be post-concussive symptoms. The PCS symptoms may be incidentally mentioned in passing or not mentioned at all in a patient that is some months or even years post head injury.

The systems engineer referred for treatment of chronic neck and shoulder pain provided a rambling, tangential and disorganized history of the auto accident that occurred 2 years previously but did not complain of having post-concussive symptoms. When asked she admitted that she was having trouble organizing projects at work, was fatigued and had trouble sleeping but attributed these problems to pain. A typical systems engineer without post-concussive symptoms provides an organized, sequential and detailed history often presented in writing. The brain MRI ordered after this patient's visit showed a small focal lesion said to be unrelated to the trauma although no basis for this determination was provided.

Treatment with FSM and nutritional supplements helped reduce the symptoms. The diagnosis was based on observation and questioning when the quality of the history did not match the patient's job description and presumed premorbid level of function. The basic concussion protocol included in this chapter was used on this patient in addition to more advanced protocols for chronic concussion in other areas of the brain and her symptoms were significantly improved.

There were frequencies for five general sections of the brain on the list of frequencies acquired from Van Gelder – the forebrain, midbrain, hindbrain, medulla, pineal and pituitary. The midbrain is the site of the thalamus. Concussion and post-concussive symptoms can affect any or all brain areas and questions should be asked that query the functions of each part of the brain so it can be determined which areas are most in need of treatment. Treating these areas of the brain requires a level of understanding of neurology and an appreciation of the profound effects that can be produced by FSM on nervous system tissue that are not generally available to students reading a basic level FSM text in pain management. There are protocols for treatment of acute brain injuries and chronic brain conditions taught in the FSM Core and Advanced seminars and the student who has an interest in treating these conditions would find these courses useful.

- **History:** Directed questioning may reveal symptoms the patient does not associate with the injury. Be aware that the patient may not be an accurate historian or may simply lack the self awareness to assess their own performance and cognitive function. When there is any doubt the patient's family should be consulted.
- **Memory and decision making problems:** Are you having any problems with being forgetful? Are you having any unusual problems with memory for numbers, names, facts or words? Is decision making any more of a problem for you now than it was before the accident?
- **Task sequencing:** Is it difficult for you to accomplish projects that require multiple steps? Are you having problems performing errands in sequence, getting a meal on the table, or planning multistep projects?
- **Sleep disturbance:** Are you having any problems with getting to sleep or staying asleep?
- **Fatigue:** Are you more fatigued than you were before the injury? Do you fatigue more easily than you did before the injury?
- **Mood:** Are you more anxious, irritable, or depressed than you used to be? Do your moods shift more easily than they used to? Do you find yourself yelling or losing your temper more often than is normal for you?
- **Balance and co-ordination:** Do you have any new problems with balance? Can you walk around your home when you get up at night in the dark

or do you need a light on? Do you fall or bump into things more often than usual?
- **Hormones:** Are you having any menstrual cycle irregularities (progesterone and estrogen balance)? Are you having any prostate symptoms (testosterone and estrogen balance)? When did you start having problems with acne (testosterone excess)? Have you had any weight gain since the trauma (insulin and blood sugar regulation)? Has your libido changed from what is normal for you (testosterone)? Do you awaken with hot flashes or have episodes of sweating since the accident (cortisol, estrogen)? Are you more fatigued than seems normal? Do you have difficulty performing or recovering from exercise? Are you depressed for no apparent reason (growth hormone)?
- **Imaging:** Unless the patient has severe symptoms or meets the criteria that require a CT scan acutely it is not necessary to order routine diagnostic imaging. MRI, PET and SPECT scanning are more revealing in chronic mTBI and the practitioner is encouraged to find a neurologist specializing in brain injuries as a referral resource.

Treating concussion – the concussion protocols

Hydration

- The patient must be hydrated to benefit from microcurrent treatment.
- Hydrated means 1 to 2 quarts of water consumed in the 2 to 4 hours preceding treatment.
- Athletes and patients with more muscle mass seem to need more water than the average patient.
- The elderly tend to be chronically dehydrated and may need to hydrate for several days prior to treatment in addition to the water consumed on the day of treatment.
- *DO NOT* accept the statement, "I drink lots of water".
- *ASK* "How much water, and in what form, did you drink today before you came in?".
- Coffee, caffeinated tea, carbonated cola beverages do not count as water.
- Water may be flavored with juice or decaffeinated tea.

Frequencies

Channel A/condition frequencies

The frequencies, listed in the usual order of use, are thought to remove or neutralize the condition for which they are listed except for 81, 49 / which are thought to increase secretions and vitality respectively

- Emotional component   970 /
- Remove trauma   94 /
- Restore function   321 /
- Remove Histamine   9 /
- Inflammation   40 /
- Chronic Inflammation   284 /
- Support secretions   81 /
- Vitality   49 /
- Stop bleeding   18 / 62
- Fibrosis   51 /
- Sclerosis   3 /
- Calcium influx   91 /
- Remove opiates   19, 43, 46

A / B Pairs

6.8 / 38
- Remove or reset constitutional factors.
- 6.8 / 38 is an A/B pair in which channel A is not a condition and channel B is not a tissue. The desired effect is created by the two frequencies delivered simultaneously in an interferential field. This frequency combination appears to neutralize all of the genetic factors described by Van Gelder and the physicians of the early 1900s and generally makes people feel more grounded and steadier.

35 / 102
- Balance the energy centers.
- / 102 was the frequency on Van Gelder's list for the pineal gland which secretes melatonin and regulates sleep wake diurnal cycles. Melatonin is a powerful antioxidant and has some anti-tumorgenic activity in preventing breast cancer and other cancers. In Van Gelder's understanding, this frequency also resonated with the energy center at the top of the head known as the "crown center" when combined with 35 / on channel A. If the practitioner's belief system does not include the concept of energy centers, then the frequency

can be used with the intention to simply address the physical structures. This frequency combination usually makes patients feel lighter and more relaxed. The affect of the frequency combination and the outcomes achieved do not appear to be affected by the practitioner's belief system.

Channel / B tissue frequencies

There is some debate in the FSM community as to what anatomical brain structures are included in each area. The divisions are probably imprecise and some-what arbitrary. Response to treatment helps to disclose what functions reside in which brain part in any particular patient.

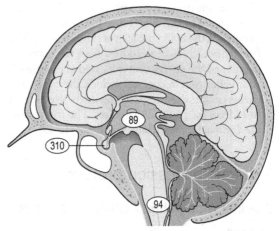

Figure 10.1 • The frequencies for portions of the brain treated with the concussion protocol or treated to remove central pain are shown in the diagram above. / 94 is the frequency for the medulla. / 310 is the frequency for the anterior pituitary. / 89 is the frequency for the midbrain and is used for pain syndromes involving the thalamus.

Medulla: ___ / 94
- The medulla, brain stem, or myelencephalon includes the medulla oblongata and the medullary pyramids. The medulla contains the motor and sensory pathways to the body and the face and the vital centers regulating the cardiac, respiratory and vasomotor systems.

Midbrain: ___ / 89
- The "midbrain" is part of the mesencephalon and includes the tectum, the pretectum, the inferior and superior colliculi, the cerebral peduncle, the midbrain dorsal and ventral tegmental areas,

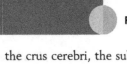

the crus cerebri, the substantia nigra, and the cerebral aqueduct and may also include third ventricle, thalamus, hypothalamus, subthalamus, subcortical system, the amygdala (limbic system), hippocampus (limbic system). For the purposes of this chapter it has been found to successfully treat central pain and is assumed to address the thalamus and periventricular, responsible for central pain.

Anterior pituitary: ___ / 310
- The anterior pituitary regulates the hormonal body processes, sexual maturation, sexual function, physical maturation, growth height and form through its secretions of gonadal regulatory hormones.

Solar plexus: ___ /200
- The solar plexus is an archaic term for the celiac nerve plexus of the vagus nerve just below the sternum in the epigastric area of the abdomen. This frequency is thought to address both the nerve plexus and the energy center located in this area. If your belief system does not include the concept of energy centers then the protocols can be used simply to address the physical structures. The frequencies used and outcomes achieved will not change.

General concussion protocol

Channel A condition / Channel B tissue

94 / 200 – Nervous tension
- Literally translated this frequency removes "trauma" from the solar plexus but Van Gelder used it to reduce nervous tension. It is observed to have a calming effect and to begin increasing serotonin levels.
- Treatment time: Use this frequency for at least 1–2 minutes depending on clinic time demands and the patient's condition. If the patient is very tense and time allows this frequency may be used for up to 5 or 10 minutes.

970 / 200 – Emotional tension
- Literally translated this frequency combination balances the emotional component or removes emotional stress from the "solar plexus" and Van Gelder described it as reducing emotional tension. It is observed to have a calming effect and begins increasing serotonin levels.
- Treatment time: Use this frequency for at least 1–2 minutes depending on clinic time demands and

the patient's condition. If the patient is very tense and time allows this frequency may be used for up to 5 or 10 minutes.

94 / 94
- Remove concussion from the medulla.
- If the memory of some recent trauma is replayed in slow motion in the mind's eye it will become apparent that there are two parts to any trauma. The first is the pain of the physical injury. The second is the "fact" of the trauma and the surprise or shock to the system that it represents. It is the "fact" of trauma and the shock to the system that is thought to be removed by using 94 /.
- Treatment time: In general all of the frequencies in the "concussion protocol" are used for 2 minutes each but if time allows and the patient's condition requires it 94 / 94 has been used for as long as 10 minutes. If time allows, the indicators such as tissue softening or warmth discussed in Chapter 2 can be used to determine when it is time to change the frequency. If the practitioner and the patient are not sensitive to tissue softening or a feeling of warmth or induced euphoria, the practitioner can use the frequencies in a standardized protocol for 2 minutes each with good effect. The automated FSM units run each of the frequencies for 2 minutes.

321 / 94
- "Reboot" or remove paralysis from the medulla.
- Treatment time: Use for 1–2 minutes each or for as long as there is a positive response if time allows it.

9 / 94
- Remove allergy reaction or histamine from the medulla.
- Treatment time: Use for 1–2 minutes each or for as long as there is a positive response if time allows it.

49 / 94
- Restore vitality from the medulla.
- Treatment time: Use for 1–2 minutes each or for as long as there is a positive response if time allows it.

94 / 310
- Remove concussion from the anterior pituitary.
- Treatment time: In general all of the frequencies in the "concussion protocol" are used for 2 minutes each but if time allows and the indicators such as tissue softening or warmth demonstrate that patient's condition requires it, 94 / 310 has been used for as long as 10 minutes.

321 / 310

- Reboot or remove paralysis from the anterior pituitary.
- Treatment time: Use for 1–2 minutes each or for as long as there is a positive response if time allows it.

9 / 310

- Remove allergy reaction or histamine from the pituitary.
- Treatment time: Use for 1–2 minutes each or for as long as there is a positive response if time allows it.

81 / 310

- Restore or increase secretions in the pituitary.
- Treatment time: Use for 1–2 minutes each or for as long as there is a positive response if time allows it.

49 / 310

- Support or restore vitality in the pituitary.
- Treatment time: Use for 1–2 minutes each or for as long as there is a positive response if time allows it.

6.8 / 38

- Remove or reset constitutional factors arising from trauma, chill, exhaustion, toxic exposure or emotional shock. This frequency combination is an A/B pair always used together for treating "constitutional factors". It appears to neutralize all of the genetic factors described by Van Gelder and the physicians of the early 1900s and generally makes people feel more grounded and steadier.

49 / 37

- Restore vitality in females.

49 / 39

- Restore vitality in males.

49 / 00

- Restore vitality in general.
- This version is used in any automated FSM unit. There has never been an adverse or paradoxical reaction when a gender specific vitality frequency was used on an opposite gender.

35 / 102

- Balance the energy centers.
- /102 was the frequency on Van Gelder's list for the pineal gland which secretes melatonin and regulates sleep wake diurnal cycles. Melatonin is a powerful antioxidant and has some anti-tumorgenic activity in preventing breast cancer

and other cancers. In Van Gelder's understanding, this frequency also resonated with the energy center at the top of the head known as the "crown center" when combined with 35 / on channel A. If the practitioner's belief system does not include the concept of energy centers, then the frequency can be used with the intention to simply address the physical structures. The affect of the frequency combination and the outcomes achieved do not appear to be affected by the practitioner's belief system.

 Box 10.1

Summary for standard concussion protocol

- 94, 970 / 200
- 94, 321, 9, 49 / 94
- 94, 321, 9, 81, 49 / 310
- 6.8 / 38
- 49 / 37 for females
- 49 / 39 for males
- 35 / 102
- Alternating current ±

When to use the general concussion protocol

The general concussion protocol as described by Van Gelder for "restoring health" is used on virtually every patient regardless of the presenting complaint for which they are being treated. For patients whose primary complaint is head injury the concussion protocol is used on the first visit and on every subsequent visit until maximum improvement has been achieved.

The general concussion protocol should be used on the second treatment visit for most chronic pain patients unless a head injury was involved in the mechanism that created the presenting complaint. Pain produces "concussion" in Van Gelder's concept of medulla overload via visceral input so treating the concussion without reducing the pain is self defeating. Treat to reduce the pain first if possible then treat with the concussion protocol. Patients may return and ask for repeat treatment with the concussion protocol and this is not a problem. It has been used daily with no ill effects observed. The practitioner is advised to self treat at least once a week and any time there is unusual stress.

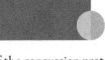

If the concussion protocol is to be used on infants, treat the mother and have her hold the child with skin contact. It has been used in autistic children and adolescents, a wide range of pain and general medicine patients and in the elderly and there has been no report of adverse effects occurring with use of the general concussion protocol on any patient except as noted below.

Precaution side effect – induced euphoria

The concussion protocol often produces a profound euphoric affect that is more pronounced the first few times it is used. Some patients become very relaxed and many will fall asleep. This temporary phenomenon will wear off as the other frequencies are used at the end of the treatment protocol. The patient will remain relaxed and should come to full function within an hour or so after treatment. Most patients are in full possession of their faculties by the time they are ready to leave the clinic and most report sleeping better on the night of the treatment.

Precaution: The practitioner should take care to ensure that the patient is safe to drive before allowing them to leave the clinic. In extreme cases patients have been warned against making important financial decisions until the effect has worn off.

Precaution side effect – dizziness

A very small percentage of patients who have vestibular injuries respond to the frequency 94 / 94 by becoming dizzy. No patient should be left unattended during the first treatment until the response to 94 / 94 has been assessed. This may be simply a very strong euphoric effect that has been interpreted as being vertiginous but it is not pleasant and may be concerning to the patient. The effect stops as soon as the frequency is changed away from 94 / 94 to some other channel A frequency. Use the remaining portion of the concussion protocol and avoid using 94 / 94. 94 / and other brain frequencies may be used with no ill effect. Only 94 / 94 has been observed to produce this temporary effect. In extreme cases if the side effect persists the patient may need one dose of an over-the-counter motion sickness pill to reverse it. This side effect has only been observed in a very small percentage of patients who have vestibular injuries. Not all patients with vestibular injuries will respond to 94 / 94 by becoming dizzy. If it occurs the patient should be evaluated at a vestibular testing center or by a vestibular specialist.

Treatment application

- **Current level:** Average current level 100μamps. Use lower current levels around 40–60μamps for children or very small or debilitated patients. Use higher current levels closer to 200–300μamps for larger or very muscular patients. Do not use more than 500μamps as animal studies suggest that current levels above 500μamps reduce ATP formation while current levels below 500μamps increase ATP.
- **± Polarization:** Current is used in alternating mode. Alternating DC current is actually pulsed DC (direct) current that alternates its polarity from positive to negative.
- **Waveslope:** Use a moderate to waveslope for the general concussion protocol and chronic brain issues. Use a gentle waveslope in acute brain injuries. The waveslope refers to the rate of increase of current flow on the leading edge of the square wave. A sharp waveslope has a very steep current up ramp on the leading edge of the ramped square wave and a gentle waveslope has a gradual current up ramp on the leading edge.
- **Patient position for all concussion applications:** The patient can be placed in any comfortable position in which the body is well supported. Patients can become very relaxed during this protocol and may fall asleep so the head and trunk should be well supported.
- **Lead placement for all concussion applications:** The nervous system is an information processing system and is designed to respond to input in the form of patterns that include frequencies and even thought or emotion (Pert 1997, Lipton 2005). Consequently the frequencies for any brain structure seem to have an effect no matter where in the body they are applied. The leads can be applied any place that is convenient as long as the current and frequencies from the two channels cross in an interferential pattern.
- **Graphite gloves at the neck or abdomen:** The two positive electrodes may be placed in the jacks cemented to the back of one graphite glove and the two negative electrodes may be placed in the jacks cemented to the back of the second graphite glove. Graphite is a good current conductor and the glove itself may have an additional positive effect for reasons not completely understood. The gloves should be sprayed or moistened with water

to improve conductivity or placed in small wet fabric contacts such as a wash cloth and placed on the skin of the abdomen and back, or on the front and back of the cervical spine.

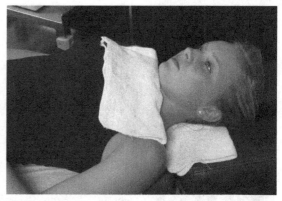

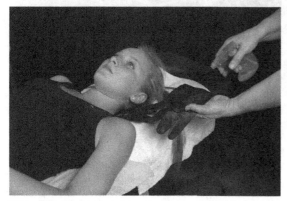

Figure 10.4 • Place the two positive leads from channel A and channel B in a warm wet fabric contact (face cloth) using either a graphite glove or two alligator clips attached to the contact. Place the two negative leads from channel A and channel B in a warm wet fabric contact (face cloth) using either a graphite glove or two alligator clips attached to the contact. Position the contacts to ensure that they do not touch each other, which would direct current to the contacts instead of the patient and do not touch the patient's ears which would send current through the brain.

Figure 10.2 • The graphite gloves must be moistened with water in order to conduct current comfortably. Dry graphite gloves create a strong prickling or stinging skin sensation and are quite uncomfortable. Ordinary tap water contains enough minerals to make it an effective conducting medium. Make sure the gloves are wet and place them flat on the skin with good contact. The skin will produce minute amounts of moisture from the galvanic skin response during treatment that will maintain comfortable conductivity for the average treatment.

It is not necessary to run the current or the frequencies through the brain in order to affect the brain tissues. **DO NOT run current through the brain.**
• **Adhesive Electrode Pads:** Place adhesive electrode pads anywhere on the patient's body such that the current from channel A and the current from channel B crosses in three dimensions. For example if the positive lead from channel A is placed on the back of the right shoulder then the negative lead from A can be placed on the lower left abdomen. Then the positive lead from channel B would be placed on the back of the left shoulder and the negative lead from channel B would be placed on the lower right abdomen.

Treating central pain

When to treat central pain

The normal function of the thalamus in the midbrain is pain suppression. The rapid reduction of the sharp pain that follows abrupt contact between the shin and the edge of the coffee table is produced when the midbrain suppresses the ascending pain signals from the anterior tibia. Injuries to this part of the brain can change it from a pain suppressor into a pain generator.

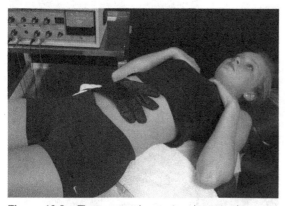

Figure 10.3 • The concussion protocol uses only alternating current so habit is the only consideration that directs placement of positive and negative leads. One moistened glove with the two positive leads from channel A and channel B should be placed on the low back. And the other moistened glove with the two negative leads from channel A and channel B should be placed on the abdomen. The photograph shows a towel under the low back but the graphite glove could be used without being wrapped in the fabric contact.

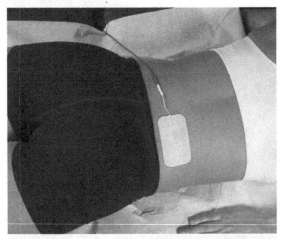

Figure 10.5 • The gel electrode pads can be used if they are more convenient. The pads need to be placed so the current and frequencies from the two channels make an "X" and cross through the patient in an interferential pattern. Place the gel electrode pads attached to the positive lead from channel A on the right side of the low back.

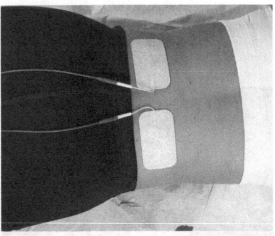

Figure 10.7 • Place the gel electrode pad attached to the positive lead from channel B on the left side of the low back. The gel electrode pads attached to the positive leads from channel A and channel B should be side by side at the low back as shown.

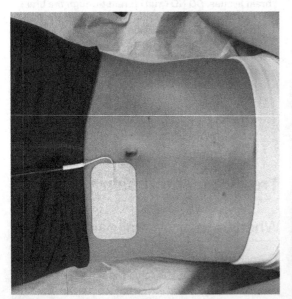

Figure 10.6 • Place the gel electrode pads attached to the negative lead from channel A on the left side of the abdomen.

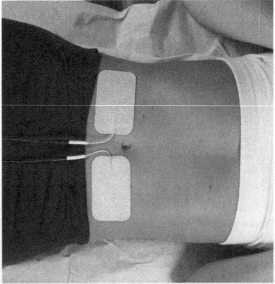

Figure 10.8 • Place the gel electrode pads attached to the negative lead from channel B on the right side of the abdomen. The gel electrode pads attached to the negative leads from channel A and channel B should be side by side on the abdomen as shown.

Central pain arises from deafferentation injuries that affect the thalamus and pain processing centers in the brain. The full body pain is described as intolerable, aching, burning, stabbing, deep, boring, sharp, dull and emotionally bothersome to a degree not seen in any other type of pain. Central pain can occur after any brain trauma such as surgery, a stroke or head injury that affects the pain processing centers in the brain. If the stroke or brain injury was on the right side of the brain the patient will have pain on the left side of the head and body. If it is in the central portion of the thalamus it will be bilaterally symmetrical and will include the head and face (see Fig. 10.9). Central pain is unresponsive to opiates and to most medications and refractory to virtually every treatment.

Central pain can also develop after spinal cord injuries that create deafferentation in the pain pathways in the spine. If the pathways are just chemically deafferented then the protocol described in Chapter 8 appears to reduce inflammation in the cord and effectively "re-afferent" the pain pathways. But if the spinal column has been traumatized and the pain pathways are physically disrupted then treating the cord will not be effective and the brain must be treated. This kind of pain is seen in paraplegics, quadriplegics and patients with cord traction injuries.

The protocol to reduce central pain involves "reducing inflammation" in the "midbrain" – 40 / 89. This protocol has been used to resolve central pain successfully in numerous patients in different facilities around the US. The results have been consistent and there have been no negative effects and no side effects beyond the induced euphoria already described. If the damage is due to a stroke and there has been loss of brain tissue structure as well as function the pain relief has been temporary, perhaps only 12–24 hours. If the protocol reduces pain the first time it will reduce the pain every time it is used. The pain relief does not diminish with repeated use as it does with TENS devices. The pain reduction seems to be more lasting with repeated use but will always be temporary if the physical structure is severely damaged. The protocol is presented here in the hopes that expanded use will bring relief to patients with central pain and encourage study of the phenomenon.

Central pain case report

The patient was a 42-year-old male referred for FSM therapy from Kaiser Premanente pain clinic and accompanied to the appointment by a care giver.

He had an aneurysm burst at the age of 28 and developed right-sided central pain at the age of 35. When he presented for treatment, his pain was rated as a 7/10 on a 0–10 visual analog scale while he was taking 100mg of oral morphine daily with the option to increase the dose to 150mg as needed. His pain diagram covered the right side of his body from the top of his head to the bottom of his right foot and there was a brace on his right lower leg. The right-sided headache was his primary complaint. His lower extremity reflexes demonstrated clonus. His MRI showed extensive tissue scarring in the left peri-ventricular area of the brain.

His was the first case of central pain ever seen at the clinic and he was told that, while treatment would be offered, it was considered very unlikely that treatment would be successful. His caregiver suggested that we follow the request of the referring physician in the name of compliance and the patient consented to treatment. The contacts were set up from neck to feet (Fig. 10.9) because the nervous system is polarized positive from neck to feet according to Becker (1985). The frequencies were chosen on the basis of what had been found to be effective in fibromyalgia (40 / 10) but the tissue was changed to the midbrain known to be the site of central pain. After 20 minutes of treatment, the patient was asked about his headache. He replied in a quizzical tone that "It appears to be gone." In another 20 minutes he was pain free.

The pain returned within 24 hours but at a reduced level and when he returned for treatment the next day it was back to a 6–7/10. Treatment eliminated the pain again and this time it remained reduced for 48 hours. But it always returned. When the first automated unit became available it contained the protocol found to be effective for him and the patient could eliminate or manage his pain by using the protocol for central pain on the unit three times a week. He remained on a very low dose of morphine primarily to prevent having to deal with the detoxification process. These results have been reproduced on a number of patients with central pain resulting from surgeries, head trauma or strokes. So far, there has been no one with central pain who did not experience pain relief.

Treatment protocol for central pain

19, 43, 46 / 89, 45

• Remove opiates from the midbrain and nervous system. Patients with central pain may be on opiate medication. For some reason the presence

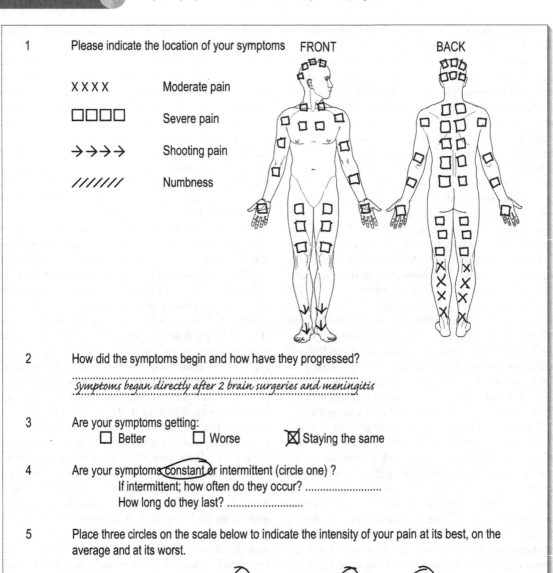

1   Please indicate the location of your symptoms   FRONT   BACK

X X X X   Moderate pain

☐☐☐☐   Severe pain

→ → → →   Shooting pain

/ / / / / / /   Numbness

2   How did the symptoms begin and how have they progressed?

symptoms began directly after 2 brain surgeries and meningitis

3   Are your symptoms getting:
     ☐ Better   ☐ Worse   ☒ Staying the same

4   Are your symptoms (constant) or intermittent (circle one) ?
          If intermittent; how often do they occur? ....
          How long do they last? ....

5   Place three circles on the scale below to indicate the intensity of your pain at its best, on the average and at its worst.

     0   1   2   3   ④   5   6   ⑦   8   ⑨   10
     No pain...Worst pain imaginable

Figure 10.9 • This is the pain diagram of someone with central pain onset on the day after she had a second brain surgery to remove the second part of a pituitary tumor. It is similar to the pain diagram seen with fibromyalgia from spine trauma (CTF) except that it includes the face and head. This feature helps distinguish central pain from CTF. Central pain includes the head; fibromyalgia from spine trauma does not. Using 40 / 89 on this patient with current polarized positive from neck to feet reduced her pain from 7–8/10 to a 0/10 in 45 minutes.

of opiates slows the effectiveness of the FSM protocol. Experience shows that using these frequencies for 2–3 minutes each speeds up the pain reduction. If the patient is not on opiate medication there is no need to use this frequency combination.

• Treatment time: Use each frequency combination for 2–3 minutes each. A higher dose of opiate medication generally requires a longer use of the frequency to remove it. If the patient's pain increases while these frequencies are being used the desired effect has been achieved and the frequencies should be changed immediately to 40 / 89.

Reduce pain

40 / 89

- Reduce inflammation / in the midbrain.
- Polarized Positive Current + applied from neck to feet is optimal.
- Treatment time: Use this frequency until the pain is reduced from its likely incoming 7–8/10 VAS level until it stops declining. This process may require up to 60 minutes. In every case treated to date the pain has been reduced to a 0–2/10 within 60 minutes. This protocol reduces central neuropathic pain and central pain amplification only. It will not reduce local orthopedic pain. For example if the patient has both a broken foot and central pain, 40 / 89 will reduce the central pain but the foot pain may still be at a 5–6/10 level, although the elevated endorphins seen with this protocol usually reduce the orthopedic pain to some extent as well.

CAUTION: If the patient has full body pain that is NOT from central sources and the midbrain is performing its normal function of pain suppression, using frequencies to reduce the activity of the mid brain reduces central suppression and causes the pain to increase temporarily.

This protocol is only effective for true central pain. Do not use it for other types of pain. If use of 40 / 89 increases pain it is best to rethink the diagnosis. Use 81 / 89 to reverse the effect of increased pain.

Precaution side effect – induced euphoria

The central pain protocol produces a profound euphoric affect that is more pronounced the first few times it is used. Some patients become very relaxed and many will fall asleep. This temporary phenomenon should wear off as the other frequencies are used at the end of the treatment protocol. The patient will remain relaxed and should come to full function within an hour or so after treatment. Most patients are in full possession of their faculties by the time they are ready to leave the clinic and most report sleeping better on the night of the treatment.

Precaution: The practitioner should take care to ensure that the patient is safe to drive. In extreme cases patients have been warned against making important financial decisions until the effect has worn off.

Treat the midbrain

970, 94, 321, 9, 40, 284, 51, 3, 91, 81, 49 / 89

- Remove the emotional component, trauma, paralysis, allergy reaction, inflammation, chronic inflammation, fibrosis, sclerosis, and calcium influx and restore secretions and vitality / in the midbrain.
- Once the pain has been reduced, treat the midbrain to "remove the pathologies" that made it a pain generator. This appears to make the pain reduction more lasting but there is no guarantee that pain relief will be permanent. The adage that "FSM cannot put tissue back that is not there" applies to brain tissue as well as other tissues. The frequency 40 / 89 appears to be able to restore function in some way that alleviates the pain for variable periods of time. Using the frequencies above may improve tissue function so that pain relief may be longer lasting. There have been no negative effects observed from their use but common sense and prudent professional judgment should be exercised by the treating physician if side effects are observed.
- **Treatment times:** All of the frequencies used to treat the midbrain once the pain is eliminated are used for 1–2 minutes each on the automated FSM microcurrent units but if time allows and the patient's condition requires it any of the condition frequencies, except for 81/ can be used for several minutes. Experience shows that 81 / may actually increase secretions in the midbrain as demonstrated by changes in patient behavior and function. This frequency should be used with respect and for no more than 1–2 minutes.
- The indicators such as warmth and softening can be used to determine when it is time to change the frequency. If the practitioner and the patient cannot feel the tissue softening or warmth, the practitioner can use the frequencies in a standardized protocol for 2 minutes each with good effect. Practitioners using manual microcurrent devices can change frequencies every 2 minutes and can customize the protocol depending on the patient's symptoms and response.

Box 10.2

Summary for central pain

USE ONLY FOR CENTRAL PAIN
Remove opiates if necessary
- 43, 46 / 89, 45

Reduce pain
- 40 / 89

Treat the midbrain pathologies
- 970, 94, 321, 9, 40, 284, 51, 3, 91, 81, 49 / 89

Treatment application

Stenosis precaution

If there is dense scar tissue or bony stenosis of the nerve root or spinal cord or if a disc fragment is compressing a nerve root or the spinal cord, the patient's pain may increase when polarized positive current is applied. If the patient is positioned comfortably, it is the only time the pain will increase during treatment with polarized positive current. Pain may increase in the dermatome or at the spine or both. Assess patient position to determine whether it is contributing to the pain increase.

Stop treating immediately if pain goes up during treatment. Move the patient to a seated position if possible. Move the contacts to the abdomen, reduce current levels and change the current from polarized positive to alternating. Use 40/10 to reduce the increase in pain. If this is going to reduce the reaction it will do so in 5–10 minutes. If the pain continues to increase, stop treating with current. The pain should go back down in a few hours although it may take up to 24 hours to reduce to baseline. Return to 40/89, change the current to alternating and place the contacts on the abdomen and spine.

This reaction is diagnostic. The physical examination findings caused by brain injuries will confound the examination finding suggestive of cord stenosis. But the patient is always entitled to more than one complaint. This reaction suggests the need for imaging to confirm the presence of spinal cord compression or stenosis.

Patient position for treating central pain

The patient can be placed in any comfortable position in which the body is well supported. The patient will become very relaxed during this protocol and may fall asleep so the head and trunk should be well supported.

Lead placement for treating central pain

The nervous system is an information processing system and is designed to respond to input in the form of patterns that include frequencies and even thought or emotion. It is not necessary to run current through the brain in order to affect the brain.

Graphite gloves wrapped in a warm wet towel at neck and feet

The two positive electrodes should be placed in the jacks cemented to the back of one graphite glove or into two red alligator clips and the two negative electrodes should be placed in the jacks cemented to the back of the second graphite glove or into two black alligator clips. Graphite is a good current conductor and the glove may have an additional positive effect for reasons not completely understood. The graphite glove with the positive leads can be wrapped in a warm wet towel that is wrapped around the neck. The graphite glove with the negative leads can be placed in a warm wet towel that is wrapped around the feet. This set up appears to have the most rapid positive effect.

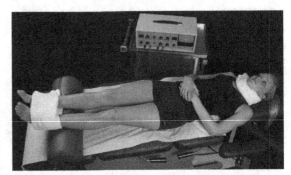

Figure 10.10 • Central pain seems to respond best when the contacts are placed at the neck and feet using polarized positive current. Place the two positive leads from channel A and channel B in a warm wet fabric contact (hand towel) using either a graphite glove or two alligator clips attached to the contact. Wrap the positive leads contact around the patient's neck.

Place the two negative leads from channel A and channel B in a warm wet fabric contact (hand towel) using either a graphite glove or two alligator clips attached to the contact. Wrap the negative leads contact around the patient's feet. The fabric should be wet but wrung out thoroughly. Cover the patient with a blanket to keep them warm as the contacts cool during the treatment.

Graphite gloves at the abdomen and spine

If the patient has spinal cord stenosis or for some other reason does not tolerate polarized positive current flow from neck to feet the gloves should be sprayed or moistened with water or placed in small wet fabric contacts such as a hand towel and placed directly on the skin of the abdomen and back. The protocol is slightly less effective when applied this way. The pain is not reduced to the same degree and is reduced more slowly with this application but it is still more effective than any other treatment available for central pain.

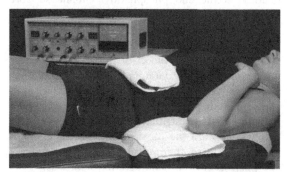

Figure 10.11 • If the patient has spinal stenosis or for some other reason does not tolerate current polarized positive from neck to feet the central pain protocol may be applied with the contacts at the back and abdomen.

Place the two positive leads from channel A and channel B in a warm wet fabric contact (face cloth) using either a graphite glove or two alligator clips attached to the contact. Place the positive leads contact behind the patient's low back. Place the two negative leads from channel A and channel B in a warm wet fabric contact (face cloth) using either a graphite glove or two alligator clips attached to the contact. Place the negative leads contact on the patient's abdomen. The fabric should be wet but wrung out thoroughly. Cover the patient with a blanket to keep them warm as the contacts cool during the treatment.

Graphite gloves may be moistened and used directly on the skin as shown above but if the gloves become dry the current will sting or prickle and be uncomfortable. The wet fabric ensures that the contacts stay moist. The current flow should be sub-sensory as long as the gloves are moist.

Electrode pads

Place adhesive electrode pads on the patient's body such that the current from channel A and the current from channel B cross in three dimensions. For central pain if the positive lead from channel A is placed on the right side of the spine at the neck then the negative lead from A can be placed on the left foot.

The positive lead from channel B would be placed on the left side of the spine at the neck and the negative lead from channel B would be placed on the right foot.

- Channel A – left neck – right foot
- Channel B – right neck – left foot

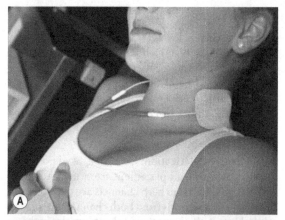

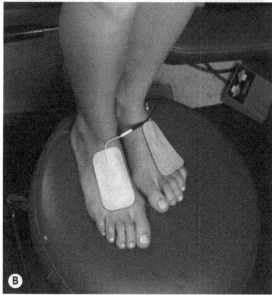

Figure 10.12 • The gel electrode pads may be used if they are more convenient. The pads need to be placed so the current and frequencies from the two channels make an "X" and cross through the patient in an interferential pattern. Place the gel electrode pads attached to the positive lead from channel A on the left side of the neck. Place the gel electrode pad attached to the negative lead from channel A on the right foot. Place the positive lead from channel B on the right side of the neck and the negative lead from channel B on the left foot.

Channel A – Left neck – Right foot
Channel B – Right neck – Left foot

It is not necessary to run the current or the frequencies through the brain in order to affect the brain tissues. DO NOT run current through the brain.

Current level

- Average current level 100µamps. Use lower current levels around 40–60µamps for children or very small or debilitated patients. Use higher current levels closer to 200–300µamps for larger or very muscular patients. Do not use more than 500µamps as animal studies suggest that current levels above 500µamps reduce ATP formation while current levels below 500µamps increase ATP.
- **+ Positive Polarization:** Current is used polarized positive with lead placement from neck to feet. Positive leads from both channels are placed at the neck; negative leads from both channels are placed at the feet. If the patient tolerates polarized positive current it appears to reduce pain more quickly than using alternating current at the abdomen and spine. If the patient has spinal stenosis there will be an increase in mid-scapular pain (see warning box) and the patient must be treated with alternating current applied at the abdomen and low back.
- **± Alternating DC Current:** Alternating current mode is pulsed DC (direct) current that alternates its polarity from positive to negative. Alternating current is used when the contacts are placed at the abdomen and spine and when cord stenosis prevents use of polarized current.

Waveslope

Use a moderate to waveslope for treating central pain. Use a gentle waveslope in acute brain injuries that create central pain. The waveslope refers to the rate of increase of current flow on the leading edge of the square wave. A sharp waveslope has a very steep current up ramp on the leading edge of the ramped square wave and a gentle waveslope has a gradual current up ramp on the leading edge.

Adjunctive therapies

Brain injuries and central pain involve inflammation and activation of glial cells as well as reduced axonal transport. Treatment with FSM is thought to change the membrane protein configuration and reduce inflammation. Maintaining the changes achieved by FSM treatment is best achieved when the nutritional environment supports the desired state.

Nutritional support

Omega 3 essential fatty acids EPA/DHA reduce inflammation and DHA is an important component of neural membrane tissue. These lipids are found in lipid-rich animal sources such as salmon and halibut. Tuna must be consumed with care due to its tendency to be contaminated with mercury. Phosphatidyl serine and phosphatidyl choline support membrane stability. Fish oil supplements should be certified free of mercury by the manufacturer.

Lipoic acid is an important anti-oxidant that is thought to cross the blood–brain barrier. Glutathione, co-enzyme Q10, vitamin C, vitamin E and other anti-oxidants should be taken in a balanced diet or in supplement form. Professional grade supplements manufactured by nutritional companies who market to physicians are the most reliable source of these nutrients due to their quality control procedures and pharmaceutical manufacturing standards.

Behavioral support

When recovering from a brain injury or central pain the patient should be coached to think of it as they would recovery from any other physical injury. Rest, sleep and good sleep hygiene are important. Regular bedtimes in a quiet room free from electronic stimulation such as televisions and computers should be observed. If diurnal rhythms have been lost and the patient finds that they become more awake at night and take hours to become alert in the morning there are two possible strategies. The first is to sleep when sleepy as long as the patient is able to sleep for 8–9 hours a day in at least 90-minute segments. The second is to attempt to restore normal diurnal rhythm using melatonin taken one hour before desired bed time to quiet the adrenals at night and help achieve deeper sleep. Take herbs, licorice, B6, B5 and vitamin C in the morning to help increase adrenal stimulation.

Seek professional help from a neuropsychologist who specializes in brain injuries. If such advice is not available some common sense approaches can be suggested by any compassionate practitioner. Advise the patient to seek mental stimulation as tolerated such as puzzles, word games, reading or listening to certain classical composers, or books on tape.

If the exercise is too frustrating or fatiguing choose a less demanding task until the brain recovers more function. Television, especially commercial television with its quick, visually and emotionally stimulating content and style, should be avoided. Avoid emotional strain and the occasions of conflict as much as possible especially if emotional lability is part of the symptom profile.

Gentle exercise such as walking or swimming provides increased circulation without jarring the brain as would happen with running or more vigorous forms of exercise. Avoid the occasions of re-injury such as bicycle riding, basketball or other contact sports, horseback riding or riding motorcycles. Once the brain and balance have recovered completely the patient may choose to resume such stimulating exposures but avoiding them during the recovery period is wise. Modifying such choices may be challenging for patients if the judgment centers in the brain that regulate such choices are impaired.

Emotional balance

When to treat for emotional states

The frequencies to balance or neutralize strong emotions came from Van Gelder along with the frequencies for concussion, emotional tension and nervous tension. The channel A frequency is 970Hz and the channel B frequency is the frequency for the organ associated with that emotion in Chinese medicine.

The frequencies do not remove the emotions but rather seem to reduce the intensity with which they are felt and the impact that they have on the nervous system and pain syndromes. Response to these frequencies has been consistent over the 11 years in which they have been used. Patients are never told what frequency is being used and are blinded to the intended effect. The practitioner treating the patient can observe the response and feel the characteristic tissue softening that occurs when the frequency is "correct".

Emotional frequency case report

A fairly stoic, long-term clinic patient presented with a recurrence of his chronic low back pain. He rated his pain as 5–6/10; worse with any movement. Unlike his previous treatments, at this treatment the protocols for nerve, muscle, disc and facet involvement produced no softening of tissue and no reduction of pain after 15 minutes. This was such an unusual response for him that when he confirmed that he was well hydrated, the frequencies for emotions were used out of desperation without informing the patient that they were being used. The characteristic muscle softening and pain reduction happened within a few minutes especially with the frequencies for fear, grief, and resentment. He commented that his back pain was going down and asked what had finally been effective. The response to the emotional frequencies prompted a reply with a question, "Before I tell you what frequency was used can I ask how things are going at home?" His response, "You mean besides the fact that my marriage is in the toilet? Why do you ask?" "I asked because the frequencies for emotions were the only ones that reduced your back pain and softened the muscles. You responded with muscle softening to grief, resentment and fear and not at all to anger. Does that match what is going on?" He affirmed that the response matched his experience. His back pain resolved and his marriage survived the rough patch.

Treat with emotional frequencies when treatment for physical pain sources does not produce the expected effect. Every physical injury or condition creates an emotional effect so treating for emotional balance is a good strategy in almost any condition. Some patients are clearly more emotionally reactive than others and they benefit greatly from use of these protocols.

If the patient talks incessantly about their emotional reaction to a trauma, accident, event, medical or surgical procedure, the emotional balance protocol reduces the strength of their reaction. Athletes who are injured rarely talk about the emotional impact of the injury or their emotional state at the time of the injury. The frequencies seem to dissipate the emotional load and reduce the impact of the emotion on the physical tissue – without requiring that the emotion be disclosed or discussed.

The responses to these frequencies have been consistent. There is no way to blind the observer and there is no way to objectively evaluate something as subtle as the degree of fear or anger felt or expressed or its effect on the body so it is unlikely that these frequencies will ever be studied in a controlled trial. But the reader is encouraged to use them in combination with the concussion protocol and observe the effects.

Treatment times

Use these frequencies for 1–2 minutes each depending on clinic time demands and the patient's emotional state. If the patient has a very strong specific emotion and time allows, any particular frequency may be used for up to 5–10 minutes.

- 94 / 200 – Nervous tension
- 970 / 200 – Emotional tension
  - Always start with these two frequencies first
- 970 / 562 – Mental tension
  - 970 / Sympathetic nervous system
- 970 / 35 – Anger
  - 970 /Liver
- 970 / 38 – Resentment
  - 970 / Gallbladder
- 970 / 27 – Fear or Terror
  - 970 / Colon
- 970 / 23 – Fear, over concern, worry
  - 970 / Kidney
- 970 / 37 – Hurt feelings
  - 970 / Bladder
- 970 / 17 – Grief
  - 970 / Lung
- 970 / 33 – Restoring Joy
  - 970 / Heart

Application

- Use alternating or biphasic current ±.
- Use the same current levels, waveslope, and electrode placement as for whatever other protocol has been used. It is not necessary to change any parameter.
- The emotional frequencies are more effective when used in combination with the concussion protocol.

How to use the frequencies for emotions

Start with the basics 94, 970 / 200 for 1–2 minutes each and then think about how emotions combine themselves. Pure emotion is rare. Fear is usually behind anger. Anger and fear are usually behind resentment and hurt feelings. Mental tension makes it all worse. Grief is always a combination of responses. Anger combines with grief and says "Why couldn't you save my husband or child?" Resentment combines with grief and says, "How could you die and leave me with all this?" Worry combines with grief and says, "What if something happens to my other child?" or "Did I do something wrong?" The opposite of love and happiness is fear. Emotions are always a mix.

Emotions are mediated by brain and endocrine function. The midbrain and forebrain structures that modulate emotional response are sensitive to the neurotransmitters involved in stress. Reducing "mental tension" improves response to the other emotional frequencies. Additional protocols for emotional conditions are available in the FSM advanced training seminars.

Box 10.3

Summary of Emotion Frequencies

Nervous tension	94 / 200
Emotional tension	970 / 200
Mental tension	970 / 562
Anger	970 / 35
Resentment	970 / 38
Fear or Terror	970 / 27
Concern, worry	970 / 23
Hurt feelings	970 / 37
Grief	970 / 17
Restoring Joy	970 / 33

Case report

- Catherine Willner, MD. Neurologist – Durango Neurological Associates, Durango, Colorado

FSM concussion protocol

The concussion protocols are among the most useful standard protocols available to practitioners of FSM. Over the years in our clinical practice, the range of situations where use of the concussion protocol has been appropriate continues to expand. In retrospect, it has helped to consider the broader meanings associated with the term, "concussion." Though what follows is a brief discussion about the typical aspects of concussion, thinking about clinical situations where there is a sudden change in the ability to process information or simply to function on automatic pilot, because of some shock to the system, is a useful way to think about concussion. We learn about the environment from the earliest days of life on this planet, integrating complex sets of information and become able to process them to allow us to function without thinking about some very important information that we process subconsciously on a continual basis. The very core of experience in everyday life is dramatically impacted when these automatic processes no longer function according to our expectations.

Considerations in concussion

Sustaining a concussion clinically implies trauma to the head and its contents which includes the brain and the structures to which it connects (the olfactory organs, eyes, brainstem and spinal cord being the structures at significant risk for injury). It goes without saying (but sometimes it seems to be overlooked) that this includes potentially painful injury to skull, ranging from contusion all the way to fracture. In the case of the latter, the risk for pain is obvious but in the former, when the acute swelling in the scalp resolves, the reasons for persistent head pain or headache may seem less obvious. Localized trauma to the nerves to the scalp, which is also a very vascularized tissue, can lead to chronic pain in the region of the injury. As regards injury to the contents of the skull, the components of the brain most at risk depend on the type of impact, and discussion is beyond our scope. However, it is also important to keep in mind that, when a person sustains a concussion, there has likely also been other injury to the body, and all of the changes associated with such injury are going to be processed by a brain that has been traumatized.

Some of the typical sequelae will depend on the extent of trauma, with varying degrees of altered awareness extending from transient changes to extended periods of coma. The portions of the brain at obvious risk for injury in trauma are those which are adjacent to bony structures, especially the petrous portions of the temporal bones, but the brainstem is quite vulnerable because of typical types of motion that can strain the normal anatomical

relationships that support the brain, but allow the brainstem to descend to become the spinal cord. Any type of motion with sudden disruption of the pattern of that motion can result in traction on the brainstem. It is important to remember that almost any structure which communicates with the rest of the body by neural connection traverses the brainstem or areas adjacent to it in the neck (such as sympathetic traffic following the arteries to the brain).

Consequences of concussion

Clinical accompaniments of concussion include changes in cognitive functions of many different types including attention, processing, memory and especially multi-tasking. Vertiginous symptoms and problems with equilibrium, balance and co-ordination are frequent, as are headaches, which have a variety of characteristics. For more extensive review of the clinical symptoms, the reader is referred to references on the topic. It is relevant, however, to review the structures localized within the brainstem which include most of the cranial nerve nuclei (other than functions of olfaction and vision, in the sense of perception, however the oculomotor nuclei reside in the brainstem and dysfunction will lead to perceptual problems because of the possibility of altered or dysconjugate movement of the two eyes simultaneously).

Our perception of the environment and our ability to function in gravity or with movement is a combination of many different sensory inputs, including the primary sensory input from the vestibular organs. But these strong stimuli are also matched to input from binocular vision, binaural hearing, and our joint perception and perception of movement in gravity sent through sensory input from our limbs and trunk, as well as the head and neck. Acute dysfunction in the vestibular organs is usually obvious and manifests itself as vertigo or severe disequilibrium. But subtle dysfunction which can occur either as an acute trauma to the peripheral vestibular input resolves or as a "mismatch" in the co-ordination of the multiple other signals is typical of the pathology associated with concussion. And though not the only remaining other structures that can be altered by concussion, the balance between sympathetic and parasympathetic functions occurs for many functions at the level of the brainstem including the higher anatomical structures which innervate the pupils, the outflow for innervations of vascular responses, heart rate and rhythm alterations, and gustatory stimuli. Discussion of this complex group of functions is beyond our task, but it makes consideration of these complex interactions imperative when one addresses issues to be addressed in any patient who has sustained even a very mild concussive injury.

FSM concussion protocol

If one reviews the standard FSM concussion protocol, it becomes obvious the emphasis on possible pathological states or alterations which are targeted within the structures traditionally localized to the brainstem and some other deeper structures in the brain. Physical, even gentle, traction injury can lead to swelling, and fluid shifts, upregulation of inflammatory signaling, which is typically acute but can become chronic, as well as a change in the activation of the supportive cells, including possibly chronic inflammation (microglial activation) or astrocytic gliosis, depending on the extent of the trauma. Treating these parameters as conditions would then lead to use of those in the protocol.

We have used the FSM concussion protocol for patients who have sustained mild traumatic brain injuries with significant success. Ours is a small office and as such the discussion which follows is mostly anecdotal, however, we have, in several patients, tested some functions pre- and post-treatment and demonstrated improvement after using the full concussion protocol. Though many practitioners have reported problems with vestibular complaints in association with certain frequency patterns, we have not had that experience in this office such that it prevented treatment.

Case report
(Catherine Willner, MD, Durango, Neurological Associates, Durango, Colorado)

Our initial experience with the full concussion protocol involved treating three college students who sustained mild concussive symptoms following head trauma. The first was injured during a hockey game when she struck the wallboards with her head. Though she was wearing a regulation helmet, the impact was strong enough that her helmet was damaged and she was additionally struck by another player such that both head strikes were on the right side. She was dazed for about 60 seconds but did not think that she lost consciousness. She noticed a headache developing over the next few hours, accompanied by disequilibrium and mild nausea. Her cervical muscles were strained and gradually tightened over the next several

hours. She has some mild recurrence of a previous cervical radicular pain in her left arm without any weakness or dysesthesias. This incident occurred during the week before her semester final examinations were scheduled and she had several papers and examinations that would be due or occur within 10 days. Her persistent headache and other symptoms persisted in severity to the point that she could not focus to study or complete the work on papers she had already started. She presented 3 days after the injury for clinical evaluation. On the abbreviated test of mental status, all of her answers were correct, though her processing was quite slow. She spontaneously recalled three of the four words she had been asked to remember and after missing the first, recalled it spontaneously just before she would have been given a hint to recall it. This was similar for naming objects she had been asked to remember.

There were no signs of increased intracranial pressure or nuchal rigidity. The only physical finding was stiffness in the cervical musculature and minor reflex changes on the right at C5–6, a known finding in this patient previously. Smell was completely intact and there were no frontal release signs. There was no nystagmus, and ocular movements and reflexes to assess for central vestibular dysfunction were normal. There was no weakness and cerebellar and sensory functions were intact. She had undergone a non-contrasted CT scan of the brain in the emergency room at the local hospital which was reviewed and was unremarkable including bone windows. After attention to adequate hydration, using water and a mineral supplement, we offered her frequency-specific microcurrent therapy (FSM), and using leads from back to sternal area, we ran the "full concussion protocol". She fell asleep during the treatment after about 5 minutes. When the treatment was completed, she awakened easily, reporting that her headache and cervical tightness were significantly improved. Her headache prior to treatment was described as a tight band with mild throbbing bilaterally. Those features were gone and she reported that the level of discomfort related to the headache had decreased from a 6/10 to 1–2/10. Though we could not exclude the impact of sleep in reducing her pain, she repeated the protocol twice more on consecutive days and during the next treatment reported similar reduction in pain without falling asleep. Additionally, after the first treatment, she awoke and demonstrated to the technician that she still remembered both the words and names of objects on the test she had taken earlier that morning. Her pronouncement of the eight words was quick and accurate. She also reported that her arm symptoms were nearly gone after the second treatment, though there was no focused treatment used for radicular or cervical symptoms.

This patient was so thrilled with her response that she sent a friend from school who had sustained a concussion when she fell from her mountain bike about 3 weeks earlier. This young woman had hit a small patch of ice on a trail and fell over the handle bars, hitting her head. She thought that she might have lost awareness for about 2–3 minutes at the scene. As she was alone, she could not be completely sure about the time. She sustained contusions but no other serious injuries. She had also been evaluated at the ER after the injury and was cleared, also having labs and a CT scan of the brain (without contrast). Her persistent symptoms included headache (global, intermittently severe, sharp and throbbing with nausea when it was more severe) and dizziness which was worse with movement but not characteristic of benign positional vertigo. The vertigo gradually started to improve and by the time she was referred to try frequency-specific microcurrent, her headache was rated as intermittently a 3/10. Her major problem was that she was also having trouble concentrating to study for her final examinations. She would lose focus and fall asleep or lose interest and find that she had to exercise to stay awake and the exercise, even only mild exertion, would reproduce her headache symptoms. She came well hydrated, and underwent two consecutive full concussion protocol sessions, reporting that after these treatments she felt nearly back to normal and was able to study easily and did well on her finals. Though only an anecdotal report, she was so pleased with the outcome that she recruited a third patient to try the treatment.

This young man was also a mountain biker and participated in semi-professional races on a regular basis. He had fallen during a training session and hit his head. Though his injury was not considered severe by his interpretation, he had persistent headaches, intermittently and found that he was having some trouble juggling expectations. On further questioning he characterized the issue as problems with multi-tasking. He would work construction regularly for income and typically could finish carpentry quite easily. He had observed that his skills seemed less on target and he would frequently have to ask his co-workers how to accomplish tasks he had previously done without effort. Though he was not a seasoned carpenter, this change in his performance was concerning to him. He did admit that he had been sleeping longer and feeling less rested after a night's sleep. Both the latter two patients passed an abbreviated test of mental status without any problems, though they were both slower than they thought that they should be in doing simple math problems and explaining proverbs. Recall was not impaired and attention was fine to simple tasks. Their examinations were neurologically normal as well. He noticed complete resolution of the headaches after the first treatment and only repeated the treatment about a week later at which time he reported that he had been to work during the week without problems in his skill sets.

None of these three patients had a history of migraine. The first woman had a history of cervical problems which would wax and wane but she did not have further symptoms of concussion after her three treatments and she also went on to pass all of her exams and complete her papers on time. She also returned to the office intermittently to focus on treatment of her cervical problems managing them easily with FSM treatments combined with physical therapy programs.

Because of the observation that this woman's cervical issues were improved only using the concussion protocol, our technician started to use a shorter version of the concussion protocol on any patient who presented with more than one obvious problem. As we introduced this approach about a year after she had been in the office, she started to record the number of treatments on other problems required to help patients and observed that most patients required fewer focused treatments when we started with some version of the concussion protocol. This was especially true with patients who had sustained any form of physical injury prior to the onset of more focused symptoms.

Collected case reports

We did accomplish a very small pilot study on 10 patients with symptoms of mild concussion, ranging in age from 19 to 44, all of whom were classified with mild closed head injury without focal findings. None had sustained any more than a minute of altered consciousness. We performed tests of mental (math problems, verbal similarities) and physical agility (puzzle and peg placement) and accuracy pre- and post-treatments and demonstrated, on average a 35% improvement in performance following a second treatment done within 3 days. This is obviously not a well controlled experiment but we did test three other head injury patients and retest them without treatment in 3 days and they had less than 5% improvement on the scores used. Even though this data is very limited, it is our greatest hope that trials could be applied in larger settings. Given the frequency of head injury in the military especially during active duty in combat, it would be wonderful to be able to assess this treatment in that setting. Treatment done in traditional settings for head injury is usually supportive rehabilitation, when done best, it is tied to psychometric retraining. Combining such approaches with use of FSM would be a wonderful opportunity for further assessment and if our observations hold true in a larger population, this would be a significant addition to the treatments available at this time in the typical clinical setting.

Bibliography

Alves, W., Macciocchi, S., Barth, J.T., 1993. Postconcussive symptoms after uncomplicated mild head injury. J. Head Trauma Rehabil. 8, 48–59.

Bazarian, J.J., McClung, J., Shah, M.N., Cheng, Y.T., Flesher, W., Kraus, J., 2005. Mild traumatic brain injury in the United States, 1998–2000. Brain Inj. 19, 85–91.

Becker, R.O., Seldon, G., 1985. The body electric: electromagnetism and the foundation of life. Quill, William Morrow, New York.

Blumbergs, P.C., Scott, G., Manavis, J., et al., 1994. Staining of amyloid precursor protein to study axonal damage in mild head injury. Lancet 344 (8929), 1055–1056.

De Kruijk, J.R., Leffers, P., Menheere, P.P., Meerhoff, S., Rutten, J., Twijnstra, A., 2002. Prediction of post-traumatic complaints after mild traumatic brain injury: early symptoms and biochemical markers. J. Neurol. Neurosurg. Psychiatry 73, 727–732.

Dewar, D., Graham, D.I., 1996. Depletion of choline acetyltransferase but preservation of M1 and M2 muscarinic receptor binding sites in the temporal cortex following head injury: a preliminary postmortem study. J. Neurotrauma. 13, 181–187.

Dixon, C.E., Bao, J., Bergmann, J.S., Johnson, K.M., et al., 1994. Traumatic brain injury reduces hippocampal high affinity (3H) choline uptake but not extracellular choline levels in rats. Neurosci. Lett. 180, 127–130.

Gross, H., Kling, A., Henry, G., et al., 1996. Local cerebral glucose metabolism in patients with long-term behavioral and cognitive deficits following mild traumatic brain injury. J. Neuropsychiatry Clin. Neurosci. 8, 324–334.

Humayun, M.S., Presty, S.K., Lafrance, N.D., et al., 1989. Local cerebral glucose abnormalities in mild closed head injured patients with cognitive impairments. Nucl. Med. Commun. 10 (5), 335–344.

Lipton, B., 2005. Biology of belief, mountain of love. Elite Books, Santa Rosa California.

McAllister, T.W., Arciniegas, D., 2002. Evaluation and treatment of postconcussive symptoms. NeuroRehabilitation 17, 265–283.

McCrea, M.A., Kelly, J.P., Randolph, C., Cisler, R., Berger, L., 2002. Immediate neurocognitive effects of concussion. Neurosurgery 50, 1032–1040.

McCrea, M.A., 2008. Mild traumatic brain injury and postconcussion syndrome: the new evidence base for diagnosis and treatment. American Academy of Clinical Neuropsychology/Oxford University Press, New York.

Middelboe, T., Andersen, H.S., Birket-Smith, M., et al., 1992. Minor head injury: impact on health after 1 year. A prospective follow-up study. Acta Neurol. Scand. 85, 5–9.

Mooney, G., Speed, J., Sheppard, S., 2005. Factors related to recovery after mild traumatic brain injury. Brain Inj. 19, 975–987.

Murdoch, I., Perry, E.K., Court, J.A., et al., 1998. Cortical cholinergic dysfunction after human head injury. J. Neurotrauma 15, 295–305.

National Institutes of Health, 1999. NIH consensus development panel on rehabilitation of persons with traumatic brain injury. J. Am. Med. Assoc. 282, 974–983.

Oppenheimer, D.R., 1968. Microscopic lesions in the brain following head injury. J. Neurol. Neurosurg. Psychiatry 31 (4), 299–306.

Pert, C., 1997. Molecules of emotion. Touchstone Publications, Simon and Schuster, Inc., New York.

Povlishock, J.T., Coburn, T.H., 1989. Morphopathological change associated with mild head injury. In: Levin, Eisenberg, Benton, (Eds.), Mild head injury. Oxford University Press, New York, pp. 37–53.

Povlishock, J.T., Erb, D.E., Astrug, J., 1992. Axonal response to traumatic brain injury: reactive axonal change, deafferentation and neuroplasticity. J. Neurotrauma. 9, 189–200.

Povlishock, J.T., Christman, C.W., 1995. The pathobiology of traumatically induced axonal injury in animals and humans: a review of current thoughts. J. Neurotrauma. 12 (4), 555–564.

Ropper, A.H., Gorson, K.C., 2007. Concussion. N. Engl. J. Med. 356, 166–172.

Ruff, R.M., Crouch, J.A., Tröster, A.I., et al., 1994. Selected cases of poor outcome following a minor brain trauma: comparing neuropsychological and positron emission tomography assessment. Brain Inj. 8, 297–308.

Ryan, L.M., Warden, D.L., 2003. Post concussion syndrome. Int. Rev. Psychiatry 15, 310–316.

Saija, A., Robinson, S.E., Lyeth, B.G., et al., 1988. The effects of scopolamine and traumatic brain injury on central cholinergic neurons. J. Neurotrauma. 5, 161–170.

Van Gelder, H., 1985. Inner peace through the process of knowing: essays in metapsychology. Robert Martin Outsound Publishing, Merry Land West, New South Wales, Australia.

Van Gelder, H., 1989. The process of healing: a field theory approach. Robert Martin Outsound Publishing, Merry Land West, New South Wales, Australia.

Frequency-specific microcurrent in clinical practice

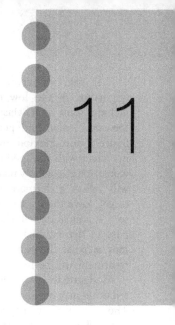

The history chapter describes how FSM was developed, the mechanisms chapter described how we think it has its effects, the treatment chapters describe how to use FSM to treat specific conditions and this chapter will describe how to integrate it into clinical thought and practice.

The pain management applications of FSM are easy to document and use but the implications and experience of using frequency patterns to change physical conditions in biological tissue are profound. The softening, warmth and relaxation response that occurs when the frequency is correct can be perceived to varying degrees by most practitioners. The ability to perceive the frequency response follows a bell-shaped curve in any given class of students at an FSM seminar. On one end of the curve are practitioners who are so sensitive that they become light-headed, euphoric, warm and wobbly. On the other end of the curve are those students who perceive nothing at all when different frequencies are used during the practicum sessions. And the bulk of the class has an experience that is someplace in between the two extremes.

The resonance response affects an arena of perception that most people do not normally attend to even though almost everyone probably has the capacity. It is as if we are born with auditory apparatus but live in a silent world until someone points out the sounds that can be heard. The same is true with the resonance response. We live in an environment filled with electromagnetic signals but most of them are not coherent and most are not noticed until the phenomenon is isolated and presented in an educational setting.

Using frequency-specific microcurrent in clinical practice creates a profound change in outcomes and expectations and ultimately requires a change in practice mechanics and patient flow to produce optimal results.

The diagnosis matters

Changes in patient history and physical examination

The change begins with the patient history and physical examination. In some medical settings the history may be simple and even perfunctory because the treatment options for a particular patient will be identical no matter how the patient arrived at his symptoms. FSM treatments are very specific and so the diagnosis must be equally specific. For example if the patient presents with "leg pain" and pain medication, such as non-steroidal anti-inflammatory medications or opiates are the only available treatment option then the mechanism of injury and the exact nature of the pain generators are not material. Pain medication is the only treatment option and correcting the source of the pain, while desirable, is not a consideration. But if the patient presents to an FSM practitioner with "leg pain" the diagnosis is the primary consideration because the treatment must be specific to the condition if it is to be successful.

What tissue is it? What is wrong with it?

The FSM practitioner asks, "What tissue is causing the pain? And what pathology in this tissue is making it a pain generator?"

DOI: 10.1016/B978-0-443-06976-5.00011-3

"Leg pain" may come from dermatomal nerves originating in the low back and the history will include some mechanism of injury that includes forward flexion and perhaps rotation that would injure a disc. Flexion, including driving and sitting in a chair with slumped posture, will make the pain worse; extension may make the pain better. The pain will follow a dermatomal nerve pattern and will travel down the leg to the big toe or heel. The sensory examination will show hyperesthesia or numbness in dermatomal nerves. A "straight leg raise" may increase the pain in the leg or foot. The FSM treatment will be for the nerve and the disc.

Moderate to severe "leg pain" in a nerve root distribution may begin after some insignificant activity. The sensory exam may show nerve hypersensitivity but reflexes are normal, flexion doesn't increase the pain and the mechanism of injury (slight) does not match the severity of the pain (moderate to severe). The FSM treatment will be for shingles in the L2, L3, L4 or L5 dermatome.

"Leg pain" may also come from low back facet joints. The posterior joints create "leg pain" that usually goes down the back or front of the thigh to the knee and follows a scleratomal or joint referral pattern. The pain will be worse with sitting and with low back extension and may be better while lying supine with the knees up and the back flat. The pain will increase during the physical examination when the facet joints are compressed as the patient lies prone. The FSM treatment must address the facet joints and the psoas and lumbar paraspinal muscles if it is to be successful.

"Leg pain" may come solely from myofascial trigger points in the lumbar spine, gluteals or the leg muscles. It may have started after some overuse injury, from chronic postural strain, or trauma or a fall. The history may include some metabolic cause of myofascial trigger points such as hypothyroidism, significant emotional stressors or after use of lipid-lowering drugs. Statins have a considerable risk of causing muscle pain even after the patient has been taking them for some months and may be overlooked as a cause of pain because of the time lapse between initial medication use and the onset of symptoms. The whole class of lipid-lowering medication carries this risk which is minimized with the prescription because of the perceived benefit. The history points the way to this diagnosis and the FSM treatment must address the cause of trigger points in muscles in order to successfully resolve the pain.

"Leg pain" may also be due to referred pain from the sacroiliac, hip or knee joints. The history and physical examination will be specific and positive for dysfunction in those joints. FSM treatment and supportive therapies will be effective if specific to the local joint pathology.

The myofascial protocol calls for treating the nerve, then the muscle and then the spinal discs, facets and finally the peripheral joints. This protocol provides the context for treating all of the causations of "leg pain" mentioned above except shingles. The practitioner experienced in physical medicine who enjoys differential diagnosis may produce relief more quickly but anyone following the protocol will be able to provide a positive outcome in most patients treated.

This change in detail in the history, physical examination and diagnosis is achieved over time and assisted by the patient's response to treatment. Experience has shown that when the treatment is not effective either the patient is dehydrated or the diagnosis is incorrect. This positive response to treatment becomes apparent within a single 30-minute treatment session and the rapid feedback shortens the learning curve once the practitioner learns to trust the response.

Equipment

Applying frequency-specific microcurrent to a patient requires a two-channel microcurrent instrument that produces a ramped square wave, pulsed, direct current output that can be set to deliver between 20 and 600µamps. This is current in millionths of an amp and cannot be provided by a TENS unit even though most microcurrent devices are approved in the USA and other countries in the category of TENS. The machine must be able to run the current in either alternating or polarized positive mode. New injuries require a gentle waveslope and very chronic conditions require a sharp waveslope, so a variable waveslope is ideal. The two channels must be independent and capable of providing a different three-digit specific frequency accurately on each channel.

All of the research and experience in frequency-specific microcurrent has been performed with an analog two-channel microcurrent unit, the Precision Micro, manufactured by Precision Microcurrent, Inc. (Newberg, Oregon) and sold by Precision Distributing, Inc. (Vancouver, Washington). But there are numerous units available, digital or analog, which supply the same electronic parameters which should be capable of reproducing the results described in this text.

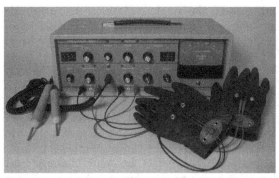

Figure 11.1 • The Precision Micro (Precision Microcurrent Inc., Newberg, OR, USA) shown here with leads attached to graphite gloves and cotton tipped probes attached to the front panel din plug, is an analog two-channel microcurrent device that produces frequencies accurate to three digits using a variable ramped square wave pulse train on each channel. The current varies between 10 and 600μamps and the frequencies and current can be set independently on each channel. The battery operated device delivers pulsed alternating or polarized positive or polarized negative DC current. Company standards require that the frequencies be accurate to 0.5 Hz. FSM research has been done using this unit but any microcurrent device may be used that provides the same current, polarization, wave shape and frequency parameters.

The reader is advised to evaluate units based on the required electronic parameters, availability, service policies and price.

Units such as the Precision Micro require someone to change the frequencies manually and are perfect for attended therapy in clinics specializing in physical medicine, pain management or physical therapy. But individualized hands-on treatment is not ideal for a busy practice setting in which similar conditions are treated in numerous patients and unattended treatments are preferred. The only units programmed with the frequency protocols described in this text are supplied by Precision Distributing. The HomeCare, AutoCarePlus, CustomCare and SportsCare are preprogrammed with some of the protocols described in this text but are not easily modified for treatments that must be customized during the session. The AutoCarePlus and Sports-Care can hold on one frequency combination, skip a frequency, or go back to the last frequency used. These units are only sold to practitioners who have taken the FSM course because they include protocols for visceral and neurological conditions not covered in this text.

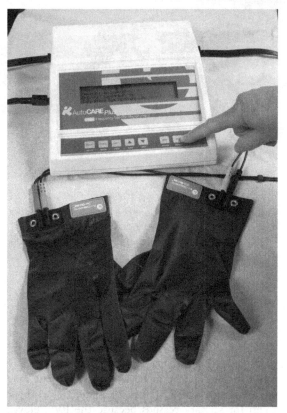

Figure 11.2 • The AutoCarePlus runs 83 frequency protocols by sequencing automatically through a list of programmed frequencies for each protocol. It has a manual mode that allows the unit to hold on a frequency combination, skip forward to the next frequency combination, and go back to the last frequency combination in the sequence or to customize but not store a frequency choice. This unit is regulated as a TENS device and cannot make any claims beyond that which could be made for a TENS device. The screen shows only initials that indicate the frequency sequences being delivered. This unit is only sold to practitioners who have completed the FSM Core seminar.

Precision Distributing has made available a small automated unit preprogrammed with only the protocols described in this text. The FSM PainCare will run these protocols for the average times described in the text and will have a manual mode that allows for some customization. It can be purchased by any practitioner whose practice scope or license includes the ability to purchase, use or prescribe electrical stimulation devices.

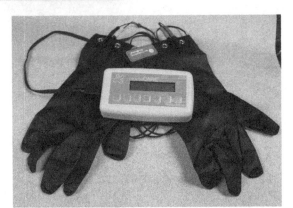

Figure 11.3 • The HomeCare is a pocket-sized unit that runs 22 protocols described in the text box. It is intended for patient home use and has no manual mode.

Conduction choices

There are a variety of conductive gloves for various electrical stimulation uses available through different providers. Silver-yarn knit gloves are stretchy and fit a wide range of hand sizes comfortably. They are difficult to clean in between patients but may be used with a PVC (vinyl, non-latex) glove over them for sanitary reasons because the PVC gloves conduct current when they are wet or stretched. The silver on the nylon mesh oxidizes when exposed to chlorine bleach or iodine cleansers and becomes non-conductive. The silver-yarn knit gloves are generally more expensive than the graphite gloves and can be found on the internet from various providers.

Graphite conductive gloves are sold by Precision Distributing. The graphite gloves cannot be left in the sun or exposed to chlorine bleach, iodine-based cleansers or UV light. They need to be kept free of oil in order to maintain conductivity and must be washed only with hot water and grain or ethyl alcohol such as vodka. They are considered a temporary electrode and are not warranted by the manufacturer because they are somewhat fragile and subject to damage by misuse. With good care they usually last one to two years but exposure to oil or bar soap can make them irreversibly non-conductive in minutes.

The graphite gloves have certain advantages that may make the extra care worthwhile. They are flexible and easy to wear and use for manual therapy, and appear to create what is probably a magnetic field associated with the circular electron path around the glove that has a subtle but distinct effect. For some reason, which possibly exists only in the author's

imagination, the graphite gloves seem to provide an additional effect not found with adhesive electrode pads. It is left to the reader to decide based on personal experience. The graphite gloves must be wet with plain tap water to conduct current comfortably. The cart holding the machine should be equipped with a small water dish or spray bottle for moistening the gloves. If the gloves become dry the current will prickle and sting so it is best to moisten them before the patient has this unpleasant experience. The contact becomes "skittery" just before it begins to sting but it is best to moisten the gloves each time a frequency is changed.

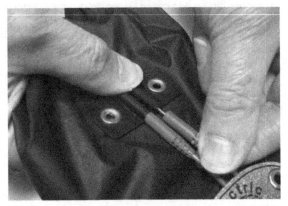

Figure 11.4 • Care must be taken to stabilize the jacks when inserting the leads.

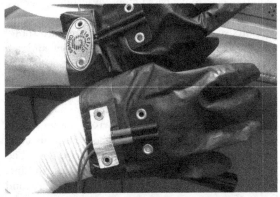

Figure 11.5 • Latex or nitrile gloves are worn under the graphite glove to insulate the practitioner from the current flow. Two positive leads, one from channel A and one from channel B, are connected to the pin jacks cemented onto the cuff of one graphite conductive glove. Two negative leads, one from channel A and one from channel B, are connected to the pin jacks on the back of the other glove. The frequencies and current from both channels "cross" in the area between the gloves forming the required interferential field.

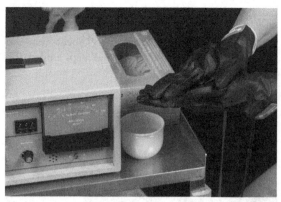

Figure 11.6 • The treatment room cart is set up with the machine, the latex or nitrile insulating gloves, a small dish of water that can be changed after each patient and a small spray bottle filled with water set up on the top shelf. Dip the fingers of the graphite glove in the water and then rub the hands together to distribute the water evenly over the glove surface.

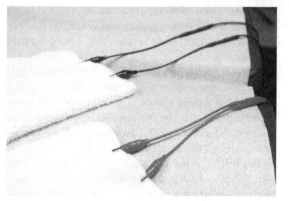

Figure 11.7 • The two positive leads from channel A and channel B are connected to two red alligator clips which are then attached to a moistened fabric contact such as a hand towel or face cloth to create a long flexible electrode. The two negative leads from channel A and channel B are connected to the two black alligator clips which are then attached to another moistened fabric or graphite contact to form a long flexible electrode. The two contacts should be positioned so the current and frequencies cross in the body area being treated and so that they do not touch each other.

The practitioner can also use "alligator clips" to attach the leads to a conductive fabric such as small hand towels, wash cloths, or even single-use paper towels wet with warm water. The graphite gloves can be wrapped inside a piece of wet fabric allowing the same option. When attached to the machine by alligator clips, the wet fabric becomes a long flexible conductive surface or electrode and can wrap around the neck or low back, lay along the length of the spine, wrap around a knee, ankle, elbow or wrist, hand or foot. Any sort of long flexible fabric or graphite electrode will be useful for treating regional pain or dermatomal nerve pain.

Alligator clips can be purchased inexpensively at any commercial electronic supply store. A high quality clip with minimal resistance is recommended to reduce current loss into the conductor. The machines are constant current generators and will increase the voltage as needed to overcome resistance and ensure that the current flowing to the patient is equivalent to what the device has been set to deliver. If the resistance in the conductive medium is too high the machine may reach its maximum voltage output before the desired current can be achieved. If this happens, and the resistance is too high, the machine will show less than 100% conductance on the current flow indicators. The practitioner can decrease the current until 100% of the current set can be conducted or change the conducting medium and re-hydrate the patient to improve conductivity.

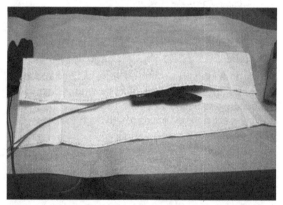

Figure 11.8 • The hand towel or any similar convenient fabric contact is first thoroughly wet with warm water, then wrung to eliminate excess moisture and folded lengthwise into thirds with the graphite glove in the middle. This arrangement converts the entire towel into one long electrode.

Adhesive electrode pads can be used to conduct the current and are available in a wide range of sizes and shapes. Sanitary considerations require that each patient have their own set of gel adhesive electrodes and that these electrodes be labeled and stored in the patient chart or in some central place in the clinic.

Graphite electrodes adhered and moistened with conductive gel for each application are a little messier but less expensive to use because they can be used on indefinite numbers of patients. Some patients are sensitive to adhesives and the chemicals in the gels and this consideration may limit usefulness of this method for those patients. The adhesive pads must be arranged so that the current and frequencies from the two channels cross and intersect in three dimensions through the area being treated.

Regardless of the medium used to apply the current the practitioner needs to keep in mind the need to create an interferential field in the area to be treated where the current and frequencies from the two channels cross. The positive leads from both channels need to be positioned so that the current flows through the area being treated in three dimensions to the negative leads from both channels. The photographs provide illustration of the principle.

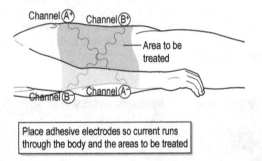

Place adhesive electrodes so current runs through the body and the areas to be treated

Figure 11.9 • When using the adhesive electrode pads the leads from the two channels must be arranged so that the current and frequencies from the two channels cross and intersect in three dimensions through the area being treated.

Setting up the treatment room

The ideal treatment room arrangement provides a variable height table that allows the practitioner to work with optimal body biomechanics during the treatment and allows the patient to be positioned comfortably no matter what their pain complaint may be. If patients are going to be treated with unattended current and protocols from automated units they may be treated while lying on tables or seated in reclining chairs as long as their position is supported and comfortable.

The equipment should be placed on the top shelf of a sturdy metal or plastic cart or trolley that has room for the machine plus a water spray bottle or small plastic dish for the water needed to keep the

graphite gloves moist, and a box of the latex or nitrile gloves required to isolate the current from the practitioner. The frequency summary sheet may be laminated so it is waterproof and kept under the machine for easy access.

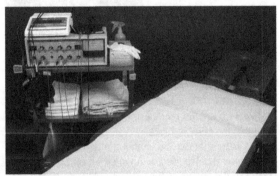

Figure 11.10 • The treatment table in this photograph (Hill Tables) has adjustable supports and cushioning for prone or supine patient positioning and is adjustable in height for practitioner comfort. Any table can be used that suits the practitioner's preference and allows for proper practitioner body mechanics during treatment. The cart is shown with two machines, the Precision Micro manual unit and an AutoCarePlus automated unit, the insulating gloves, the water spray bottle on the top shelf and gowns and spare dry towels on the second shelf. The practitioner sits on an adjustable height rolling stool for easy mobility and comfort.

If a flexible wet contact is going to be used for conducting current then the treatment room or some space nearby should be set up to make them available and convenient. A supply of dry hand towels or rolls or stacks of dry paper towels can be kept on the cart or on a shelf in the treatment room or nearby supply area as long as there is a warm water faucet and basin nearby in which to moisten them. Some practitioners keep a supply of hand towels wet and warm for the day's patients in an electric warmer like a "crock-pot". Adjust the water temperature so there is no risk of scalding to either patients or employees. Using a microwave to warm a wet towel produces isolated hot spots which can burn a patient and is not recommended.

The bottom shelf or shelves of the cart can be used to store patient gowns, a supply of towels, a small soft blanket to use as a drape and bolsters or pillows used for patient positioning and comfort. The options for equipment and room set-up are virtually unlimited and depend on practitioner training and preference and the types of patients being treated. The details are left to the reader to explore and experience.

If the wet contacts are not disposable then some accommodation must be made for laundry management. Some clinics have a washer and dryer on site and find it most economical to do the laundry daily in-house. If a laundry service is used the added cost can be balanced against the convenience of having clean towels supplied once or twice a week. If disposable paper contacts are used then some consideration should be given to how to recycle the paper.

Patient hydration

In order for FSM to be effective the patient must be hydrated. For most patients this means drinking 1 to 2 quarts of water in the 3 to 4 hours prior to treatment. The boxed alert below appears in every treatment chapter and some version of it should be posted on the wall in the waiting room of every FSM practitioner. Hydrated patients require that the clinic have easy access to toilet facilities.

Hydration

- The patient must be hydrated to benefit from microcurrent treatment.
- Hydrated means 1 to 2 quarts of water consumed in the 2 to 4 hours preceding treatment.
- Athletes and patients with more muscle mass seem to need more water than the average patient.
- The elderly tend to be chronically dehydrated and may need to hydrate for several days prior to treatment in addition to the water consumed on the day of treatment.
- *DO NOT* accept the statement, "I drink lots of water".
- *ASK* "How much water, and in what form, did you drink today before you came in?".
- Coffee, caffeinated tea, carbonated cola beverages do not count as water.
- Water may be flavored with juice or decaffeinated tea.

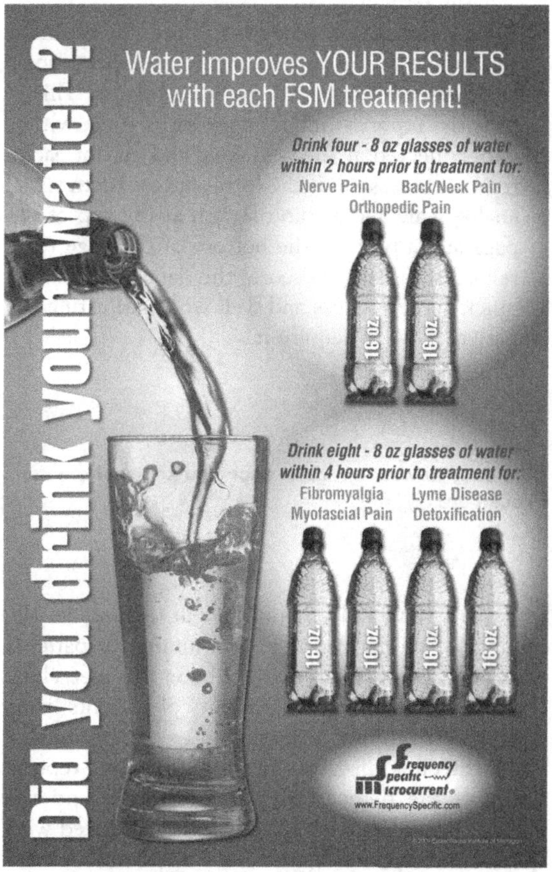

Figure 11.11 • Hydration is so important to successful treatment that one creative practitioner, Vanessa Cayle, PT created this hydration poster and placed it on the waiting room and treatment room walls (© Vanessa Cayle, reproduced with kind permission).

Patient flow

For some practitioners the 20–60-minute treatment time required for FSM therapy is compatible with appointment time slots already in use and, for some, scheduling will need to be adjusted to accommodate the longer appointments. If the practitioner cannot afford to spend 20–30 minutes of individual time with a patient, a clinical assistant can be trained to administer FSM treatment for the various conditions covered in this text. If a clinical assistant performs the treatment in one treatment room, the clinician is free to start a patient interview or close a patient appointment in additional rooms in 5–10-minute slots.

Once a patient has been assessed, the automated units allow unattended treatment for conditions that don't require manual therapy. The patient can be treated with unattended protocol for 30 minutes and then seen for manual therapy in the last 15 minutes by either the practitioner or a skilled assistant. If the space is available and the patient demand justifies it, the practitioner can expand the number of rooms and the number of clinical assistants almost indefinitely. Eight rooms and six clinical assistants seem to be the maximum workable in larger pain management or physical medicine practices and four rooms and two or three assistants is more easily managed.

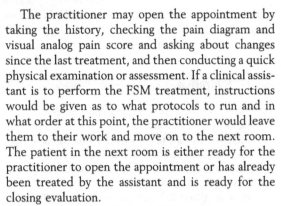

The practitioner may open the appointment by taking the history, checking the pain diagram and visual analog pain score and asking about changes since the last treatment, and then conducting a quick physical examination or assessment. If a clinical assistant is to perform the FSM treatment, instructions would be given as to what protocols to run and in what order at this point, the practitioner would leave them to their work and move on to the next room. The patient in the next room is either ready for the practitioner to open the appointment or has already been treated by the assistant and is ready for the closing evaluation.

The patient should give a pain score report at the beginning and at the end of every treatment. It only takes a minute and it is invaluable for patient management and data collection to demonstrate efficacy of treatment for research, or for the patient or for a third party, such as an insurance company, that is paying for treatment. The patient should fill out a questionnaire that documents function instead of pain at regular intervals. If the pain remains the same but function improves that is a positive response to treatment and should be documented.

If the patient reports at the beginning of an appointment that the treatment isn't helping, a quick check of the post-treatment pain scores will show that the patient has been pain free at the end of the last four treatments and has returned with the pain score reduced from the previous incoming pain score at each of the last three treatments. So the pain returns at some point between treatments but to a lesser degree than was present before. The data helps to reassure the patient and helps the clinician to ask questions to discover the source of the patient's frustration.

In a different instance, the pain score data may make it clear that the patient is no longer making progress. The patient comes in at a 5/10 VAS and leaves at a 2/10 VAS with an identical pain diagram at each of the last six once-a-week appointments.

The data gives a starting point for the conversation about:

1. **Treatment frequency:** How soon does the pain return and would twice a week treatments instead of once a week treatments for a few weeks help make the response more lasting? What do time and finances allow?

2. **Treatment goals**: What does the patient want from treatment and is the pattern acceptable? After 12 years in chronic pain the patient may be

thrilled with 4 days of a level 3–4/10 pain between treatments. Or perhaps the patient envisions a pain free life and is frustrated with the pattern of improvement and return. Treatment goals should be a collaborative decision making process. The patient is allowed to vote. Some fibromyalgia patients cannot envision a pain free life and devise a treatment schedule that leaves them in just enough pain so that they have what they need to navigate their emotional and social landscape.

3. **Treatment program:** Can the patient do the prescribed exercises or home treatments consistently or does the prescribed home program need to be modified? Are they prone to overdo prescribed home programs or do they tend to forget and do half of what is prescribed? The only way to find out is to have a judgment free conversation and then modify the prescription to suit the patient.

4. **Treatment expectations:** Is the present situation acceptable to the patient and what expectations do they have for treatment at this point? This progress report is much more easily done with data collected at the beginning and end of each treatment session. If the forms have a 10cm visual analog scale and a pain diagram at the top of the page and a place at the bottom of the page to record a verbal pain score, the data collection is quick and effortless and well worth adjusting the patient flow to acquire it.

It's easy to walk on water once you know where the rocks are

Patient flow and scheduling will depend on the number of rooms available, the number of patients who need to be treated in an hour to meet clinic revenue needs and the complexity of patients being treated. This in turn will depend on the number of hours the clinician wants to work, the clinic reputation and the demographics of the clinic and the clientele. Patients with fibromyalgia associated with spine trauma occupy a treatment room and an automated unit for 60–90 minutes but only require supervision for 10–20 minutes of that time or perhaps manual therapy for specific regional complaints for up to 20 minutes. If treatment rooms are very

Date_____

Patient Name _____

Please rate your current pain level below

0_____10

No pain   Worst pain

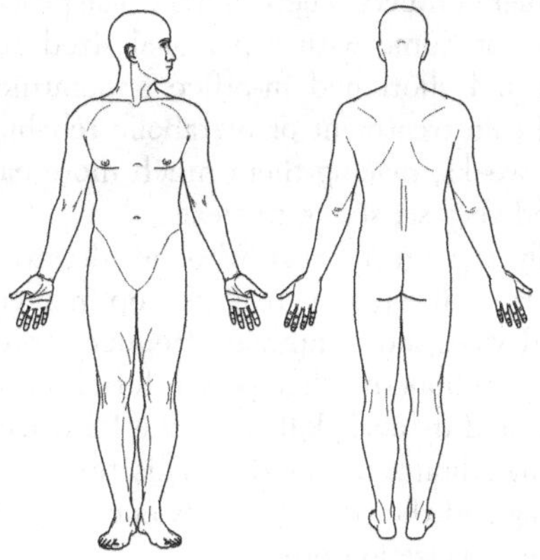

Practitioner progress notes   Please mark affected areas

_____
_____
_____
_____
_____
_____
_____
_____
_____
_____
_____
_____
_____
_____
_____
_____
_____
_____
_____
_____
_____
_____
_____
_____
_____
_____

Practitioner signature

_____

Figure 11.12 • This chart note sheet is an example of a simple form that can be used to document pain scores and a pain diagram at the beginning of each treatment. The pain diagram can help distinguish between different pain generators by providing pattern recognition for the practitioner before the history begins. This sample has blank lines for notes but any convenient format can be used depending on the practitioner's profession. If electronic chart notes are being used the patient should be given a sheet with a 10cm line and a body diagram to fill out at each visit.

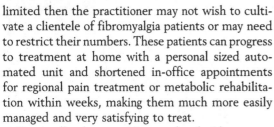

limited then the practitioner may not wish to cultivate a clientele of fibromyalgia patients or may need to restrict their numbers. These patients can progress to treatment at home with a personal sized automated unit and shortened in-office appointments for regional pain treatment or metabolic rehabilitation within weeks, making them much more easily managed and very satisfying to treat.

Eventually the practitioner who decides to use FSM will personalize it and create the optimal combination of devices and equipment, frequency protocol references, adjunctive therapies, referral sources, patient flow and manual skills to make FSM useful and satisfying adjunct to practice. This text is only the beginning and the practitioner is encouraged to enjoy the personalization process.

Billing and charting

Every practitioner in every health care profession is required to keep chart notes that document the treatment delivered to patients. The chart notes provide a record of services performed during the therapeutic encounter that supports billing for the treatment provided. If the practitioner has a cash practice or works in an environment that does not include insurance billing, be grateful and skip to the next paragraph. To provide support for billing, the chart needs to document the complexity of the condition and the time spent with the patient. If the condition is complex and requires a longer visit, it is reimbursed at a higher rate but the complexity has to be reflected in the number or severity of diagnosis or documentation of the topics discussed and the amount of time spent in patient contact. Each profession is reimbursed at a different rate for the cognitive evaluation portion of the treatment. The chart needs to document what modalities were used and for how long. FSM treatments are billed as "attended electrical stimulation" in 15-minute time units for insurance reimbursement as if it were a TENS device because the device is classified as a TENS device by governmental regulatory agencies such as the FDA in the US or the TGA in Australia. It can be combined with manual therapy, trigger point therapy or proprioceptive neuro facilitation (PNF) and each of those modalities is billed as a separate service. Detailed advice on billing and coding is beyond the scope of this text and the practitioner should consult a professional in this area for more complete information.

Even if the practitioner does not bill insurance the chart notes serve as something akin to a laboratory notebook for the clinician's reference. If the clinician wants to know how the patient responded, the record of the treatment and the response should be in the chart notes in as much detail as possible so that a positive response can be reproduced and a negative response can be avoided.

For an FSM practitioner this means documenting the patient's condition, the frequency protocols used and the response. It may be a fine point, but for complete accuracy, the practitioner should simply list the frequencies used and not interpret the frequency action. When 13 / 396, 142 are used to "remove scar tissue between the nerve and fascia", it may decrease pain with motion and increase range of motion but there is no way to say with complete certainty that the frequency combination is actually dissolving scar tissue between the nerve and fascia. It acts as if it is dissolving scar tissue but there is no way to prove that claim. It is far more accurate to report 20 degrees of flexion with pain before treatment, use of 13 / 396, 142 and then 40 degrees of pain free flexion after treatment with that frequency combination.

In modern practice the chart note is also a medical-legal document in the event of any unfortunate treatment outcome that might lead to a malpractice lawsuit. Risk management advice dispensed by malpractice insurance companies suggests that every patient encounter be recorded with the thought in mind that the practitioner may end up in court or before a review board. In addition to being good advice in general, this recommendation is another reason to avoid making claims in the chart notes about the effect of a given frequency. If 40 / 116, 480, 783, 157 are used on a red and swollen joint, it is easier to defend and more accurate to report that those frequencies reduced redness and swelling and increased range of motion by a certain amount than to say that the frequency reduced inflammation in the immune system, joint capsule, periosteum and cartilage. If asked in a legal setting what the frequency was used for the practitioner is not in the position of making an unsupportable claim. "The treatment reduced redness and swelling" is an observation by a trained and licensed professional. "The treatment reduced inflammation" is an entirely different statement which cannot be supported.

If the patient has any side effects from treatment such as a detox reaction, it is important to make note of the reaction along with the instructions given to prevent it or manage it. Any conversation or interaction regarding positive or negative effects of treatment should be recorded in as much detail as space and time allow.

Marketing

In general, the use of FSM to treat pain patients increases patient volume and clinic revenue even though it increases overheads by requiring the purchase of machines and consumables like adhesive electrode pads and towels. Detailed marketing advice is beyond the scope of this text because marketing is constrained by the individual practitioner's finances, personality and preferences and, in some cases, by statute and licensing board regulations.

Experience suggests that the ideal marketing tool is a satisfied pain free patient who tells everyone, including their friends, family, referring physician and fellow pain patients, about their positive outcome. Sending out preprinted thank you notes to referring physicians and a preprinted welcome card to new patients and having an incentive program for patients who refer new patients are simple inexpensive touches that can improve patient relations and increase patient flow.

The learning curve

Every new skill acquired has a certain learning curve. The practitioner usually starts at a place of **"unconscious competence"**, completely comfortable with a familiar skill set that produces desired outcomes and unaware of any effort required to use it. When any new skill is learned this equilibrium is upset.

The practitioner moves to a period of **"conscious incompetence"** in which he is not very skilled at the new technique and is aware of the lack of proficiency but is also enthusiastic enough about the rewards and the promise of improvement to keep practicing. This is the most uncomfortable part of learning any new skill and with luck, persistence, practice, good learning tools and rapid feedback it is brief. This portion of the FSM learning curve lasts about 3 months depending on how many patients are treated per day. The average practitioner needs to treat approximately 10–20 patients with similar complaints such as shoulder or low back pain or nerve pain to move through to the next phase.

The summary sheet that comes with this text provides the frequencies and summary protocols at a glance. This eliminates the need to memorize the frequencies and helps shorten the time to competence. It can be copied and laminated for durability and easy access. Learning the frequencies and the protocols can proceed from practice and repetition and may be almost effortless for some practitioners and may be a struggle for others. Some motivated and enthusiastic practitioners will memorize the numbers and protocols very quickly because they can and because they enjoy the process. Both approaches have advantages and which is chosen depends solely on practitioner preference. The photographs in the text and in the summary boxes may shorten the time required to become comfortable with the mechanics of placing electrodes on the patient for treating different conditions in different parts of the body but it is still a matter of trial and error and takes time, repetition and may involve some problem solving. The learning curve and acceptable solutions will be different for every practitioner and every patient.

If the practitioner survives the "conscious incompetence" phase and has the personality, intellect and tools to make it to the next phase, the rewards of **"conscious competence"** make the transition worthwhile. "Conscious competence" produces better outcomes with less effort because the practitioner knows what to do to produce an effective treatment even though it takes some conscious thought. In the case of acquiring skill in using FSM, making the correct diagnosis becomes easier; patient set-up requires little if any thought, and choice of the appropriate or optimal treatment protocol becomes more easily apparent. This phase is more comfortable and may last for months or years depending on the practitioner and the conditions being treated.

The conscious competence phase may be prolonged because the patients being referred for treatment tend to become more challenging over time. Every difficult patient who has been successfully treated seems to know six people just like themselves who also need care. Eventually the case load that seemed difficult at first looks easy by comparison and the practitioner develops improved diagnostic and treatment skills by continually treating more and more complex cases. This growth in skill set requires conscious effort and prolongs the conscious competence phase.

The practitioner moves almost imperceptibly into the next and final phase returning to **"unconscious competence"** having fully integrated the new skill set and using it to produce successful outcomes

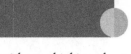

without thinking about the process. The average FSM practitioner requires perhaps a year or two to achieve this level of comfort.

Rapid feedback accelerates the learning curve

The rapid changes in tissue texture and pain provide immediate feedback during treatment and shorten the learning curve dramatically. If the practitioner has to wait hours, days or weeks to determine whether a specific application of the new skill has been successful, it takes longer to learn because the feedback that distinguishes between correct and incorrect choice of action is so delayed. The rapid feedback available with use of FSM shortens the learning curve once the practitioner learns to notice it and then learns to believe what can be felt. The occasional patient who experiences or reports positive response to treatment 24 hours after the treatment instead of noticing it immediately is the rare but disconcerting exception to this rule.

At first, when there are so many new things to notice and to attend to – doing a more detailed history and physical examination, operating the machine, positioning and setting up the patient for treatment, instructing an assistant, reading the frequency list, integrating the examination findings with the patient's palpation, deciding and then wondering about the diagnosis, to mention a few – the clinician has little time or attention to devote to noticing the tissue response. But, as some of these issues become routine there is more time and attention available to notice the response to treatment. There will be times when the response is so immediate and profound as to grab the attention but it may not be obvious in every case at first.

The profound change in state that occurs when the proper frequencies are used has been described as "disorienting" because it is unlike anything experienced with any other form of treatment in common use. One practitioner described his difficulty at the end of the first day of class with the statement, "Everything I thought I knew about muscles, or even matter, and how it works has just changed. It is disorienting." It is almost impossible to describe the change in words because it is such a palpatory phenomenon and is akin to describing the sunrise to a blind person. The tissue simply rapidly profoundly changes state when it responds to the correct frequency.

Muscle tissue that is hard, tough, scarred, firm, rigid, "gnarly" or stiff begins to soften and within minutes feels "smooshy", like pudding in a plastic sack. The areas of tissue that have not responded to that frequency or set of frequencies stands out amidst the smooshy tissue and can then be addressed with additional frequency choices. The residual firm tissue will respond and assume the pudding-like consistency when the appropriate frequency combination is applied and so on until the area being treated is comfortable and uniformly soft. It has to be experienced to be believed. Skeptics are forgiven in advance because there really is no reason to believe that this phenomenon is possible until it is experienced.

For the author there was one learning curve for noticing this softening as a palpatory change and a separate learning curve for believing that it had happened. There is a third and final learning curve in which this response is taken for granted and its presence or absence is used to determine the choice of treatment. Patience is recommended during this part of the FSM learning process as each phase may require weeks or months of experience. Thousands of patient treatments were required before the author fully appreciated this phenomenon.

Managing patients

FSM is one of few treatment modalities with a problem caused by the speed of positive outcomes. When a patient with chronic nerve pain or fibromyalgia from spine trauma has been in pain for more than 10 years and becomes virtually pain free in 90 minutes it is almost disorienting. There is an emotionally challenging dissonance between the pain the brain expects and the comfort the patient is currently experiencing.

In a very real sense, the patients literally do not know who they are if they are not in pain. Pain has limited and defined every aspect of life and function for years and now it is gone. Imagine and attempt to appreciate the challenge that presents itself to the patient. They have to change or reduce medication levels, rediscover their boundaries, learn what they can and cannot do now on almost a daily basis through rehabilitation until the recovery process is complete. They have to dare to be willing to hope that the pain relief and physical recovery will persist. They have to dare to hope again when the inevitable temporary setback occurs. They have to be willing to believe that recovery is possible. They have to be patient when recovery stalls and it becomes apparent that it will never be complete. The recovery process takes time but occurs faster with FSM than with almost any other treatment modality and the practitioner needs to learn how to support the patients emotionally and physiologically during this process. The learning curve is different for every practitioner and his or her patients in this situation. There is no way to give specific guidance on exactly what to do or how to do it during the recovery phase and it is only possible to advise the practitioner to prepare for its inevitable appearance.

When a regional pain patient with neck or shoulder pain, for example, achieves increased range of motion and reduction of pain in two to three treatments the challenge is less profound but still present. The compensations created by the body in response to the dysfunctional tissue are no longer necessary or appropriate. The patient will notice the compensations once the original problem is gone and may think that they are a new problem and become concerned.

Experience will make these "compensation events" predictable and the wise practitioner will learn to warn patients about this phenomenon before it happens. "We just increased the range of motion in your neck by 50% in 30 minutes and there is going to be some reaction someplace in your body to this change. I cannot tell you what the reaction will be or where it will be because it is different for everyone but I can guarantee that something somewhere will be different. It may be as simple as the fact that your upper back and shoulders will feel tighter in the areas we didn't treat. The neck moves farther and more easily and the shoulders and upper back are being asked to move in ways not possible for years so they will feel tighter. This is not a new problem; it is a response to an improvement and is very good news. Or, the response may be something as strange as low back pain or leg cramps. Whatever it is we will be able to treat it when it comes up."

Patients may experience an increase in thirst during treatment or shortly after treatment. Increasing current flow and ATP energy production requires water molecules to form a contiguous semiconductor layer all throughout the body in the fascia. It could be that the brain senses this need and increases the desire for water. Whatever the cause, it is not uncommon for patients to report increased thirst during and after treatment and they should be encouraged most strongly to increase water intake.

Managing expectations and limitations

The last area of patient management is peculiar to the rapid responses seen with FSM treatment – management of expectations on the part of both the patient and the practitioner. Once the patient has experienced the effects of increased range of motion and decreased pain, stabilized ligaments, or elimination of nerve pain, improved cognitive function and emotional stability it is hard to imagine that anything is impossible.

It is difficult to describe the excitement and pleasure that accompany each successful treatment. Using FSM is fun and even veterans of 18 years in practice find renewed joy, delight and stimulation in producing the rapid results in routine patients. The joy becomes addictive and each success creates the expectation that the next success will be as easily achieved.

Eventually the practitioner will encounter a new patient, or a new condition in a patient successfully treated for some other condition in which the desired relief simply cannot be achieved. When this occurs during the early years of experience with FSM it is not as surprising as when it happens after several years of experience creating changes formerly thought to be impossible. After a few years using FSM the formerly impossible result becomes the expected outcome. The challenge is not the unsuccessful treatments; the challenge lies in the unrealistic expectations. No treatment is ever 100% successful.

Be realistic, expect a miracle
  But be patient, the impossible takes slightly longer than the difficult

A phone call from a practitioner who was treating a patient with moderate Parkinson's disease brought this situation into stark relief. The practitioner described treating a patient with the characteristically rigid posture, difficulty walking, loss of fluid motion and tremor seen with moderate Parkinson's disease. She described her success in reversing these symptoms in a single 60-minute treatment allowing the patient to walk normally and move fluidly without tremor or rigidity. She asked in frustration what she was doing "wrong" because the improvements would only last 3 days. She lost sight of the fact that the improvements themselves, however temporary, were miraculous and it was the expectation of a permanent resolution that was unrealistic. She was not ever able to produce a permanent resolution in this patient but by managing her expectations she and the patient were both content with once a week treatments that restored function temporarily and improved his quality of life.

The frequencies cannot put tissue back that is not there. They can restore function, especially in neural tissue, reduce inflammation, dissolve scar tissue and restore secretions by providing a frequency pattern that apparently changes cellular function. But frequencies cannot put tissue back that is not there. There are some degrees of scarring that so damage the tissue it cannot be restored to its former state. The interactions between damaged and compensating tissues are so complex and so restricted that FSM seems to have little lasting impact on them. These failures are frustrating and humbling and often leave the practitioner wondering if there isn't some treatment protocol that could be devised if enough was known.

There are some emotional predispositions and psychological responses to early childhood trauma or pain that are so severe that nothing FSM can do will restore emotional peace and normal central pain processing. The dedicated curious practitioner can acquire additional skills, knowledge, tools or referral options in nutritional support, evaluation and biochemical manipulation of neurotransmitter levels, hypnosis, and different types of therapies helpful in modulating emotional responses. Navigating this process requires more thought and inventiveness than knowing how to spell and dose the newest anti-depressant medication. FSM is likely to be necessary but not sufficient to achieve success in these complicated patients. And sometimes nothing seems to help. The persistent practitioner with a hopeful or desperate patient may eventually find a solution if they search long enough.

These less than optimal responses keep the clinician humble. No matter how successful FSM has been in treating similar cases the clinician is advised to avoid making promises or being or appearing overconfident. As the practitioner's level of experience increases so usually does the degree of difficulty of patients being referred for treatment.

Never make promises

It is much easier to "under promise and over perform" by exceeding expectations than it is to come back from the disappointment of unrealistic expectations that have not been met. When a patient presents with nerve pain, it is much more prudent to allow that FSM has pretty good success in treating nerve pain and that a trial of treatment would be worthwhile.

"It can't hurt and might help" is a favorite FSM phrase

And the final advice for the practitioner who will use FSM to treat more and more difficult patients is to "Participate fully in the process but don't get attached to the outcome." Eventually there will be patients who cannot be helped for whatever reason. Pain patients invite compassion in the dedicated physician or practitioner of every profession who treats them. Participating fully in the process of discovering the pain generators, treating them appropriately, providing emotional and nutritional support and physical reconditioning is challenging and stimulating, creating hope and the vision of the opportunity for healing for the practitioner and the patient.

Participate fully in the process but don't get attached to the outcome

Frustration and despair await those who become attached to the outcomes. And frustration makes it easy to misdirect the blame from the failed treatment to the patient. Pain patients are routinely told that the pain is "all in their head" by frustrated physicians who do not understand or appreciate the diagnosis or have the tools to treat the pain. There is no way for anyone to know enough to help every chronic pain patient who walks in the door. And eventually, every FSM practitioner will have patients who cannot be helped. There is no one to blame.

If there is no attachment to the outcome, there is no frustration and no need to blame anyone or anything for the failure. If the therapeutic process is its own reward and the ego does not need the patient to recover for its own satisfaction then, in the end, compassion remains. The outcome is simply an outcome and compassion can help the patient manage when the outcome is not a cure.

The practitioner and the patient form a team that works for recovery. Healing is not something that the practitioner does to the patient. It is a collaborative effort between the patient and the practitioner with FSM as a third collaborator.

FSM beyond this text

Some patient responses will require frequencies and ways of thinking that are not within the scope of this text. For example, a patient who was injured in a severe auto accident 24 years previously was treated for neck and shoulder pain. Her cervical range of motion increased from pre-treatment flexion of 30 degrees to post-treatment flexion of 60 degrees and the neck and shoulder pain resolved. And then during the night after treatment the patient experienced lower leg and foot muscle cramps. The patient had been warned to expect some unpredictable reaction as a result of the increased range of motion in the neck and so called to report the painful leg cramps the next day.

What could possibly connect the neck with the calves and feet? It might have been pure coincidence but the timing of the leg cramps and a cursory knowledge of neurology made that an unlikely and remote possibility. The potential solution and how to arrive at it are obvious to those with more advanced training and experience in FSM.

There are frequencies for the spinal cord in Chapter 8 and for the dura in the FSM advanced course. The spinal cord contains sensory and motor tracks that carry signals between the brain and the muscles in the legs and feet, the dura covers the cord and they travel together through the neck inside the spinal column. When the neck moves, the cord and the dura have to slide through the spinal canal during the movement like a cable moving inside a piece of moving flexible conduit. If the neck has not moved to more than 30 degrees of flexion in 24 years, then the dura and the cord have not moved in 24 years and could be expected to become adhered to the canal during that time. Increasing range of motion in the neck from 30 degrees to 60 degrees in a 40-minute treatment after 24 years of restricted movement by working on the muscles, discs, and facet joints (but not the dura or the cord) would reasonably be expected to cause problems in the untreated tissue. The increased movement would tug on the adhesions between the cord and the dura and the dura and the canal, create traction in neural pathways in the cord

and probably inflammation in tethered regions of the cord and dura. It would not be surprising if this inflammation led to leg cramps in this particular patient. At least this was the hypothesis formed when the patient called. There had to be a connection between the increased motion and the leg cramps and this seemed the most likely possibility.

The solution was to treat the cord and the dura to remove inflammation and adhesions while the patient flexed forward to move the cord and dura through a complete range of motion. Initially the patient could feel restrictions and pain in the spine and pain in the lower legs at 20 degrees of forward spinal flexion. Instructed to return to an upright position and then to try trunk flexion again after a few minutes with the frequencies running from neck to feet, her range increased by 10 degrees. After repeating this movement during 20 minutes of treatment to remove "inflammation and scar tissue" from the "cord and the dura" she gradually flexed further forward with each repetition until she was sitting with her chest on her thighs and her hands on the floor for the first time in 24 years. The pain and range of motion in her neck improved even more with this treatment and the leg cramps were never again a problem.

The ability to treat the condition helped to create the hypothesis and then test it. The response to treatment suggests that the dura and the cord became inflamed and adhered to each other because of the injuries to the disc created by the accident 24 years previously.

• "Inflammation leads to chronic inflammation leads to fibrosis, adhesions, hardening, and scarring." This progression of pathology is universal and the ability to disrupt it by dissolving adhesions and removing inflammation in minutes using frequencies presents treatment possibilities not available through any other means.

The treatment possibilities change the diagnostic possibilities. It would never occur to most (non-FSM) practitioners to connect increased range of motion in the neck with leg cramps unless there was a way to treat the spinal cord and dura to remove the hypothesized inflammation that was causing the cramps and dissolve the hypothesized adhesions that were limiting range of motion. It is entirely possible that the adhesions would have dissolved in time due to the effects of increased motion but it was educational and revealing to double range of motion in the trunk and reduce the tone in the calf muscles in 20 minutes. The time frame in which the changes were created eliminates the possibility that anything other than the frequency-specific intervention was responsible for the change.

These more advanced frequencies and concepts are available to those who wish to move beyond this introductory text to the full FSM Core seminar course and then progress to the advanced frequencies and physical medicine or visceral medicine advanced course material.

The frequency response creates profound changes in physical tissue and gives us a glimpse of the energetic reality behind matter and physical appearance. The power for healing and pain relief inherent in the frequency response should be used with compassion, skill, humility and wisdom.

The mission statement for frequency-specific microcurrent is

To reach every patient in pain who wants to be helped
    By training practitioners who can treat them
    And to teach, research, practice and write about
FSM in such a way that it thrives

Index

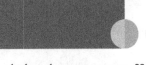

Printed in the United States
By Bookmasters